Atlas of Clinical Hematology

SECOND EDITION

Editor-in-Chief

James O. Armitage, MD

Professor, Internal Medicine
Section of Hematology and Oncology
Nebraska Medical Center
Omaha, Nebraska

With 13 Contributors

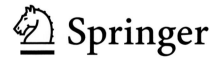

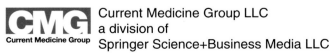

Current Medicine Group LLC
a division of
Springer Science+Business Media LLC

CURRENT MEDICINE GROUP LLC
a division of SPRINGER SCIENCE+BUSINESS MEDIA LLC
400 Market Street, Suite 700 • Philadelphia, PA 19106

Senior Developmental Editor . . . . Elizabeth Rexon
Editorial Assistant. . . . . Juleen Deaner
Cover Design . . . . Wieslawa Langenfeld
Design and Layout . . . . William Whitman
Illustrators. . . . . Wieslawa Langenfeld and Maureen Looney
Creative Director. . . . . Wendy Vetter
Assistant Production Manager . . . . Megan Charlton
Indexer . . . . Holly Lukens

Library of Congress Cataloging-in-Publication Data

Atlas of clinical hematology / editor, James O. Armitage ; with 13 contributors. -- 2nd ed.
    p. ; cm.
 Includes bibliographical references and index.
 ISBN 978-1-57340-276-7 (alk. paper)
 1. Blood--Diseases--Atlases. 2. Hematology--Atlases. I. Armitage, James O., 1946- II. Title.
 [DNLM: 1. Hematologic Diseases--diagnosis--Atlases. 2. Hematologic Diseases--therapy--Atlases. WH 17 A8812 2008]

RC636.A85 2008
616.1'500222--dc22

2007031999

ISBN 978-1-57340-276-7

For more information, please call 1 (800) 427-1796 or (215) 574-2266 or email us at inquiry@phl.cursci.com

www.currentmedicinegroup.com

10 9 8 7 6 5 4 3 2 1

Printed in China by Hong Kong Graphics & Printing Ltd.

This book was printed on acid-free paper

Hematologic malignancies are not rare diseases, with approximately 100,000 new cases each year in the United States. Although patients with these disorders can sometimes be cured, unfortunately most will eventually die of their disease. Thus, hematologic malignancies are quantitatively, and not just qualitatively, important.

Many of the important advances in the understanding and treatment of patients with cancer have come from the study of hematologic malignancies. In the 1940s, Hodgkin disease was found to be the first cancer to respond to chemotherapy using nitrogen mustard. In the late 1940s, childhood leukemia was first put into remission using antifolates. In the 1960s, Burkitt lymphoma was shown to be sometimes curable with chemotherapy, and childhood acute lymphoblastic leukemia was shown to be curable with combination chemotherapy. Shortly thereafter, Hodgkin disease, and subsequently large cell non-Hodgkin lymphoma, were found to be curable with combination chemotherapy. Bone marrow transplantation was developed for the treatment of hematologic malignancies and has cured many patients who would otherwise have died.

The study of hematologic malignancies has continued to lead the way in the development of new approaches to cancer therapy. Antibodies, with or without radiolabels, targeted at surface antigens on lymphoid and myeloid cells have provided important new treatment options. Studies using gene arrays have made it possible to identify previously unknown subtypes of lymphoma and provide new prognostic information. These same approaches offer the possibility of allowing a better choice of therapy for individual patients and, thus, a higher cure rate.

Our understanding of these disorders of lymphoid and myeloid cells continues to advance. The mechanism of blood coagulation and the factors that predispose to thrombosis and bleeding are increasingly well understood. A variety of new therapies have recently become available to treat patients with both hypercoagulable states and a predisposition to bleeding. Disorders of mature red cells and granulocytes remain common problems in the practice of medicine, and with the development of clinically available hematopoietic growth factors, management has improved.

Hematology is a particularly visual science. It has always been possible to look at blood cells and their progenitors in the bone marrow with comparative ease. Of all the areas of medicine, hematology is perhaps the one most amenable to presentation in an atlas such as this. The second edition of the *Atlas of Clinical Hematology* describes the exciting advances occurring in hematology and presents them in an attractive and useable way.

James O. Armitage, MD

CONTRIBUTORS

Karen L. Chang, MD
Medical Director
Department of Clinical Pathology
City of Hope National Medical Center
Duarte, California

Bruce D. Cheson, MD
Professor of Medicine
Head of Hematology
Georgetown University Hospital
Lombardi Comprehensive Cancer Center
Washington, District of Columbia

Bertrand Coiffier, MD, PHD
Professor and Head
Department of Hematology
Hospices Civils de Lyon
Pierre-Benite, France

Joseph M. Connors, MD
Clinical Professor, Medical Oncology
Department of Medicine
British Columbia Cancer Agency
University of British Columbia
Vancouver, British Columbia, Canada

Steven R. Deitcher, MD
President and Chief
 Executive Officer
Hana Biosciences
South San Francisco, California

James M. Foran, MD, FRCPC
Assistant Professor of Medicine
Director
Hematology/Oncology Fellowship Program
Chair
Hematologic Malignancy Working Group
Department of Medicine
University of Alabama at Birmingham
Division of Hematology/Oncology and
 Comprehensive Cancer Center
Birmingham, Alabama

Stephen J. Forman, MD
Chair
Hematology and Bone Marrow
 Transplantation Program
City of Hope National Medical Center
Duarte, California

Randy D. Gascoyne, MD, FRCPC
Clinical Professor of Pathology
Department of Pathology
British Columbia Cancer Agency
Vancouver, British Columbia, Canada

John D. Jackson, Jr., PhD
Associate Professor
Department of Pathology and Microbiology
University of Nebraska Medical Center
Omaha, Nebraska

Chin-Yang Li, MD
Professor
Department of Laboratory Medicine
 and Pathology
Mayo Clinic College of Medicine
Rochester, Minnesota

Sagar Lonial, MD
Associate Professor
Hematology and Oncology
Director of Translational Research
B-Cell Malignancy Program
Associate Director
Hematology/Oncology Fellowship Program
Winship Cancer Institute
Emory University School of Medicine
Atlanta, Georgia

John G. Sharp, PhD
Professor of Genetics, Cell Biology,
 and Anatomy
Professor of Radiology and
 Radiation Oncology
University of Nebraska Medical Center
Omaha, Nebraska

Ayalew Tefferi, MD
Professor of Medicine
Department of Internal Medicine
Mayo Clinic
Rochester, Minnesota

CONTENTS

Chapter 1

Non-Hodgkin Lymphoma 1

Bruce D. Cheson and Bertrand Coiffier

Diagnosis and Pretreatment Investigation 2
B-cell Lymphoma 7
T-cell Lymphoma 18
Prognostic Factors 22
Treatment 28
Treatment of Specific Clinical Situations 41
Site-specific Treatment Strategies 45
Treatment Strategies Based on the Initial Treatment Response 47
Follow-up 50
Conclusions 50

Chapter 2

Hodgkin Lymphoma 53

Joseph M. Connors and Randy D. Gascoyne

Pathology 53
Staging 58
Treatment 59
Late Effects, Complications, and Follow-up 61

Chapter 3

Plasma Cell Disorders 63

Sagar Lonial

Monoclonal Gammopathy of Undetermined Significance. 64
Multiple Myeloma 67
Variant Forms of Multiple Myeloma 77

Chapter 4

Myeloid Disorders 85

James M. Foran, Karen L. Chang, and Stephen J. Forman

Acute Myeloid Leukemia 86
Myelodysplastic Disorders 109
Myeloproliferative Disorders. 118
Myelodysplastic Syndromes/Myeloproliferative Disorders 136

Chapter 5

Disorders of Hemostasis and Thrombosis 141

Steven R. Deitcher

Normal Hemostasis 141
Clinical Presentation. 148
Platelet Disorders 150
Qualitative Platelet Disorders 156
Coagulation Disorders 157
Acquired Hemophilia 159
Von Willebrand Disease. 159
Anticoagulation-associated Bleeding 160
Thrombotic Disorders 161
Clinical Thrombosis 163
Warfarin-induced Skin Necrosis 167
Vascular Disorders 168

Chapter 6

Anemias 175

Ayalew Tefferi and Chin-Yang Li

Red Cell Changes 178
Microcytic Anemia: Iron Deficiency Anemia 180
Microcytic Anemia: Thalassemia 183
Microcytic Anemia: Not Associated with Either Iron Deficiency or Thalassemia 184
Normocytic Anemia 185
Macrocytic Anemia 195
B_{12} Deficiency 196

Chapter 7

Hematopoietic Stem Cells and Cytokines 201

John G. Sharp and John D. Jackson, Jr.

Index. 223

CHAPTER 1

Non-Hodgkin Lymphoma

Bruce D. Cheson and Bertrand Coiffier

Non-Hodgkin lymphomas are cancers of the immune system that originate from B or T lymphocytes and, rarely, from natural killer (NK) cells. They encompass an extremely heterogeneous group of diseases based on the histologic subtypes, genetic features, clinical presentations (nodal and/or extranodal), tumor behavior (localized vs disseminated), and the response to treatment. This heterogeneity has important prognostic and management implications: given the existence of so many variants and their multiple possible manifestations, it is often difficult to predict outcome in a given patient. However, in the past 10 years, the leading international lymphoma treatment centers have undertaken collaborative analyses that have helped to define the various disease entities [1,2], the generally recognized prognostic parameters [3–5], and standard therapeutic options [6–8]. As a result, it is often possible to select a treatment appropriate to a particular patient's risk profile. The aim of all lymphoma treatment is to prolong high quality survival or to achieve cure in these curable histologies.

The incidence of lymphoma has been increasing but the causes are unknown [9]. A small proportion are related to infectious pathogens and immune errors induced by the environment or age.

Diagnosis of the lymphoma requires an excisional biopsy to provide sufficient tissue for morphologic, immunophenotype, and genotype evaluation by an experienced hematopathologist because of the difficulty of the diagnosis in at least one fourth of the cases [10]. The classification of lymphomas has been simplified during the past few years and is based on genotypic abnormalities with their immunophenotypic and morphologic correspondences.

Outcome is related to lymphoma subtype, extension of the disease, and the patient's characteristics. Treatment decision is a complex act that includes the patient. It is based on the lymphoma subtype and on the presence or absence of prognostic parameters. In a few cases, standard treatments exist, but usually it is good clinical practice to include the patient in prospective studies designed to improve our knowledge on this disease and to improve the patient's outcome.

Infectious Agents Involved in the Development of Lymphomas

Pathogens	Lymphomas Associated with Virus	Putative Mechanisms Leading to Lymphoma
HIV	Diffuse large B-cell lymphoma [11], Burkitt's lymphoma, Castleman disease, Hodgkin lymphoma	Depression of immune functions with activation of *c-MYC*, inactivation of *p53*, and infection with EBV [12]
HTLV-1	ATL	Inactivation of tumor suppressor genes mediated by Tax [13]
EBV	Burkitt's lymphoma, T-NK-cell lymphoma (nasal type), post-transplant lymphomas	Chronic latent infection with encoding of two proteins that inhibit apoptosis (BHFR1 and LMP-1)
HHV-8	Kaposi's sarcoma, primary effusion lymphoma, Castleman disease	Coinfection with EBV, viral protein expression
HCV	Splenic marginal zone lymphoma, mixed cryoglobulinemia [14]	Unconvincing evidence [15]
SV40	Diffuse large B-cell lymphoma, follicular lymphoma [16]	Inactivation of *rb* and *p53* genes
Helicobacter pylori	Gastric MALT lymphoma [17]	Chronic antigen stimulation followed by secondary activation of NF-κB pathway [18]
Borrelia burgdorferi	Cutaneous MALT lymphoma [19]	
Chlamydia psittaci	Ocular adnexal lymphoma	
Campylobacter jejuni	Immunoproliferative small bowel disease	

Figure 1-1. Viruses and other pathogens involved in the development of lymphomas. The cause of lymphomas is supposed to be immune deregulation, but the specific immune defects are not fully understood as well as the influence of viruses, genes, chemicals, radiation, diet, and aging on the complex immune system. Viruses and other infectious agents play a critical role in the development of lymphomas. They operate by depressing immune functions (HIV), by inhibiting apoptosis-regulator genes (Epstein-Barr virus [EBV], human T-cell leukemia/lymphoma virus-1 [HTLV-1]), or by chronic inflammation (*Helicobacter pylori*). Some associations are well established, such as HTLV-1 and adult T-cell leukemia/lymphoma (ATL), EBV and T- and natural killer (NK) cell lymphoma; others are less demonstrated (hepatitis C virus [HCV], simian virus 40 [SV40]). Exposure to potential environmental toxins, *eg*, herbicides, chemicals such as hair dyes, and naturally occurring compounds such as wood preservatives, has also been implicated as a risk factor for lymphoma. MALT—mucosa-associated lymphoid tissue.

DIAGNOSIS AND PRETREATMENT INVESTIGATION

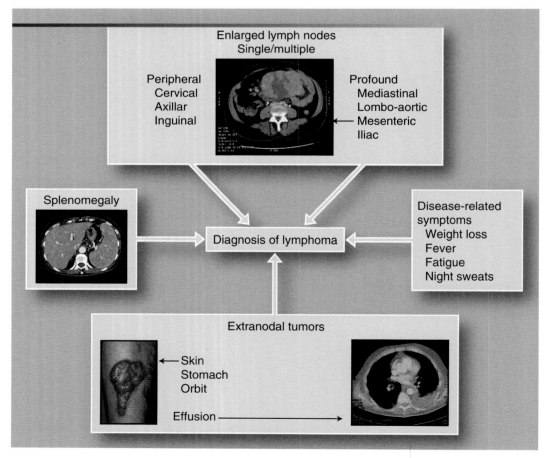

Figure 1-2. Clinical presentation. Lymphoma may be diagnosed as a result of organ involvement or disease-related symptoms.

Diagnostic Studies for Lymphoma

Setting	Type of Analysis	Expected Results
Standard	Morphology	Subtype
	Histology	
	Cytology	
	Immunohistochemistry, flow cytometry	B- or T/NK-cell lymphoma
Prospective studies	Cytogenetics	Chromosomal abnormalities
	PCR analysis	Gene rearrangement
	Genetic abnormalities	Oncogene expression
	Molecular profiling	Gene profile signature

Figure 1-3. Diagnostic studies for lymphoma. The diagnosis of lymphoma always requires a biopsy followed by pathologic analysis including cytology and immunology. CD20 or CD3 antigen–positive tissue indicates a B- or T-cell lymphoma, respectively. Further analysis of fresh or frozen material is often useful for diagnosis in difficult cases, which can account for up to 30% to 40% of the total. Such analyses may also reveal biologic or molecular markers of an adverse prognosis. In all difficult cases, and in patients participating in prospective studies, the diagnosis must be confirmed by one or more pathologists specializing in the diagnosis of lymphoproliferative disorders. NK—natural killer; PCR—polymerase chain reaction.

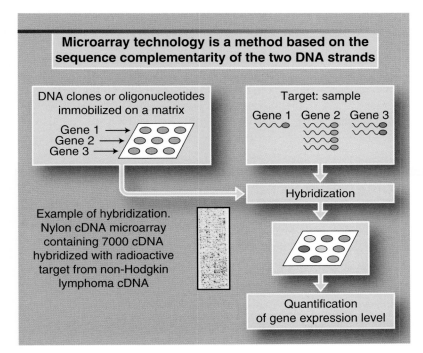

Figure 1-4. Microarray technology. This method is based on the sequence complementarity of the two DNA strands. DNA clones for genes of interest are obtained and amplified by polymerase chain reaction. Aliquots are printed on a matrix (nitrocellulose membrane, coated glass microscope slides, silicate glass) using a computer-controlled, high-speed robot. Total RNA from the sample is labeled by reverse transcription using radioactivity or fluorescence. Finally, signal intensities on scanned images are quantified by computer analysis.

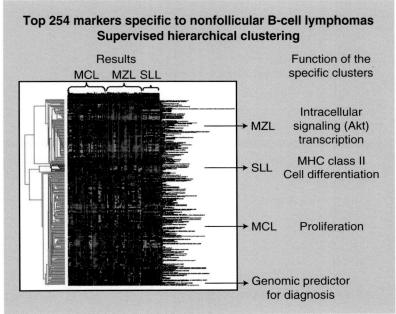

Figure 1-5. Markers specific to nonfollicular B-cell lymphomas. Some genes or groups of genes are preferentially expressed in certain lymphoma subtypes and not in others, allowing the confirmation of diagnosis in difficult cases. Some genes or groups of genes are preferentially expressed in poor-prognosis cases and not in good-prognosis cases, allowing the determination of outcome for some patients, the selection of the best treatment for the individual patient, but also the recognition of important genes for the appearance of resistance to treatment or histologic progression. MCL—mantle cell lymphoma; MHC—major histocompatibility complex; MZL—marginal zone lymphoma; SLL—small lymphocytic lymphoma.

Full Pretreatment Work-up for Lymphoma Patients

Clinical examination

    Detailed interrogation in search of symptoms of possible involvement (ECOG scale or Karnofsky index), fatigue

    Peripheral lymph nodes, spleen and liver, extranodal locations

    B symptoms (weight loss, fever, night sweats)

CT of neck, thorax, abdomen, pelvis

FDG-PET where indicated

Specialized investigations, *eg*, gastrointestinal endoscopy, brain CT scan are indicated if there is clinical evidence of possible involvement

Measurement of the different tumor masses

    To establish a prognosis (tumor > 10 cm)

    To have baseline status to evaluate the response

Bone marrow biopsy with imprints is required

Exploratory lumbar puncture recommended in aggressive lymphomas (see later)

    Because of the adverse prognostic implication of such a location

    Because of the specific treatment modalities required in case of such a location

Routine pretreatment laboratory screening

    Complete blood count with blood slide review

    Hepatic, renal, cardiac work-up

    Serum LDH level

    Serum β_2-microglobulin levels

    Serum protein electrophoresis (research of M component)

HIV, HCV, HBV testing because of the prognostic and therapeutic implications if positive

Figure 1-6. Full pretreatment work-up for lymphoma patients. As soon as the diagnosis of lymphoma is confirmed, a full pretreatment work-up is mandatory to determine performance status and to screen for concomitant disease potentially affecting management. ECOG—Eastern Cooperative Oncology Group; FDG-PET—fluorodeoxyglucose positron emission tomography; HBV—hepatitis B virus; HCV—hepatitis C virus; LDH—lactate dehydrogenase.

Classification of Lymphoproliferative Syndromes

B-cell neoplasms

Lymphoma/leukemia	Precursor B-lymphoblastic leukemia/lymphoma
	Chronic lymphocytic leukemia*/small lymphocytic lymphoma
	B-cell prolymphocytic leukemia*
	Hairy cell leukemia*
	Lymphoplasmacytic lymphoma (Waldenström macroglobulinemia)
Indolent nodal or extranodal lymphomas	Marginal zone B-cell lymphoma
	MALT-type lymphomas
	Splenic marginal zone lymphoma
	Nodal marginal zone lymphomas
	Follicular lymphomas
	Mantle cell lymphoma
Aggressive nodal or extranodal lymphomas	Diffuse large B-cell lymphoma
	Subtypes:
	Mediastinal lymphoma
	Intravascular lymphoma
	Primary effusion lymphoma
	Lymphomatoid granulomatosis
	Burkitt's lymphoma/leukemia*

(Table Continued)

Classification of Lymphoproliferative Syndromes *(Continued)*

T-cell neoplasms	
Lymphoma/leukemia	Precursor T-lymphoblastic lymphoma/leukemia*
	T-cell prolymphocytic leukemia*
	T-cell large granular lymphocyte leukemia*
	NK-cell leukemia
Nodal or extranodal lymphomas	Adult T-cell leukemia/lymphoma
	Mycosis fungoides and Sézary syndrome
	Extranodal NK/T-cell lymphoma, nasal type
	Enteropathy-type T-cell lymphoma
	Hepatosplenic γ/δ T-cell lymphoma
	Subcutaneous panniculitis-like T-cell lymphoma
	Angioimmunoblastic T-cell lymphoma
	Peripheral T-cell lymphomas, unspecified
	Anaplastic large cell lymphoma
	Cutaneous CD30+ T-cell lymphoproliferative disorders
Hodgkin lymphoma	
Nodular lymphocyte predominant Hodgkin lymphoma	
Classic Hodgkin lymphoma*	
Plasma cell diseases*	
Monoclonal component of uncertain significance*	
Plasmocytoma*	
Extra-osseous plasmocytoma	
Multiple myeloma*	
Plasma cell sarcoma*	
Plasma cell leukemia*	
Immunodeficiency-associated lymphoproliferative disorders	
Lymphomas associated with hereditary immunodeficiency	
Post-transplant lymphoproliferative disorders	
Lymphomas associated with HIV infection	
Methotrexate-associated lymphoproliferative disorders	

*Not discussed in this chapter.

Figure 1-7. Classification of lymphoproliferative syndromes. Since Rappaport's classification in 1956, many classifications have been proposed; however, only two—the Kiel classification and the Working Formulation For Clinical Usage (1982)—have actually been in use for many years in Europe and the United States. These classifications were based on cell morphology and its prognostic implications (small cell lymphoma was synonymous to a good prognosis, large cell to a poor prognosis). In 1994 the International Lymphoma Study Group proposed a classification based on the morphology, immunology, genetics, and clinical presentation of the various disease entities. This Revised European-American Lymphoma (REAL) classification was recently modified to become the World Health Organization (WHO) classification [1,2]. Although this classification has minor defects, it forms the basis of the day-to-day classification of a patient's lymphoma in order to define the treatment. MALT—mucosa-associated lymphoid tissue; NK—natural killer.

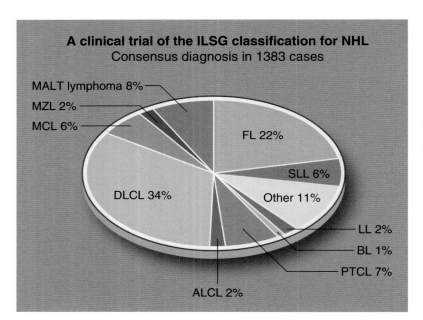

A clinical trial of the ILSG classification for NHL
Consensus diagnosis in 1383 cases

MALT lymphoma 8%
MZL 2%
MCL 6%
FL 22%
SLL 6%
DLCL 34%
Other 11%
LL 2%
BL 1%
PTCL 7%
ALCL 2%

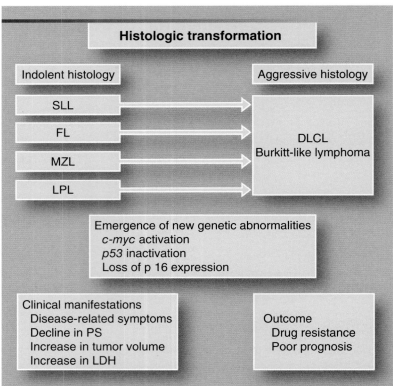

Histologic transformation

Indolent histology
Aggressive histology

SLL
FL
MZL
LPL

DLCL
Burkitt-like lymphoma

Emergence of new genetic abnormalities
c-myc activation
p53 inactivation
Loss of p 16 expression

Clinical manifestations
Disease-related symptoms
Decline in PS
Increase in tumor volume
Increase in LDH

Outcome
Drug resistance
Poor prognosis

Figure 1-8. A clinical trial of the International Lymphoma Study Group classification for non-Hodgkin lymphoma. This figure shows the incidence of each lymphoma category as defined in the review by five internationally recognized hematopathologists of 1383 cases of lymphomas seen in eight centers around the world [10].

Compared with the incidence found in our center in a larger population of patients, there are very few differences. The most important differences are the high incidence of unclassified cases and the lower frequency of marginal zone lymphoma (MZL). ALCL—anaplastic T-cell lymphoma; BL—Burkitt lymphoma; DLCL—diffuse large B-cell lymphoma; FL—follicular lymphoma; LL—lymphoblastic lymphoma; MALT— mucosa-associated lymphoid tissue lymphoma; MCL—mantle cell lymphoma; PTCL—peripheral T-cell lymphoma; SLL—small lymphocytic lymphoma.

Figure 1-9. Histologic transformation. A feature shared by all lymphomas is their potential for tumor progression or transformation at each relapse or as end-stage evolution. Examples include the transformation of small lymphocytic lymphoma (SLL), follicular lymphoma (FL), or marginal zone lymphoma (MZL) into large-cell or Burkitt-like proliferation or an increase in mitosis or in the number of cells in S phase in diffuse large B-cell lymphoma (DLCL) or peripheral T-cell lymphoma (PTCL). Transformation is usually associated with clinical deterioration. It generally follows the emergence of additional genetic abnormalities. Transformation is also commonly associated with drug resistance and an adverse outcome. LDH—lactate dehydrogenase; PS—performance status.

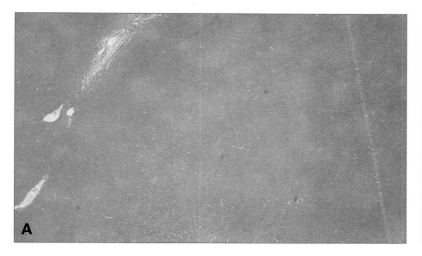
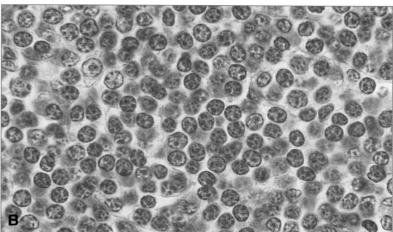
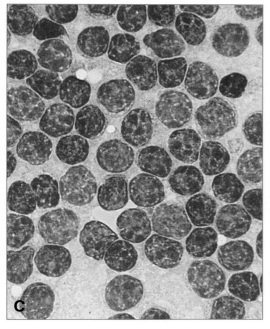
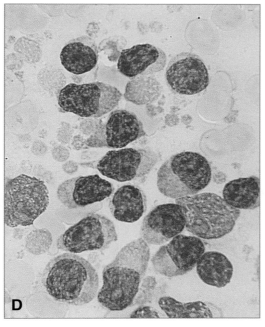

Figure 1-10. Small lymphocytic lymphoma (SLL). SLL and its plasmacytoid variant represent the lymphoma counterpart of chronic lymphocytic leukemia (CLL), which is a much more frequent disease. The term *SLL* is what remains of the Working Formulation lymphocytic subtype after describing the other recently characterized lymphomas (described later). SLL accounts for 4% to 5% of all lymphomas. Some cases show plasmacytoid differentiation. This lymphoma is highly heterogeneous with respect to clinical presentation, treatment response, and outcome, probably because it is made up of several as-yet-unidentified subtypes featuring specific genetic or cytogenetic abnormalities.

Small lymphocytic lymphoma features nodal or extranodal masses combined with infiltration of the spleen, bone marrow, and blood. By definition, infiltration of the blood must be minimal (< 5000 lymphocytes); otherwise the condition becomes CLL. A monoclonal component is often present and may be predominant, as in Waldenström macroglobulinemia.

The tumor consists of a diffuse infiltration predominantly by small lymphocytes, which appear slightly larger than normal lymphocytes, or by lymphoplasmocytes, which have a slightly more abundant and basophilic cytoplasm with clumped chromatin (**A** and **C**). There are usually some large lymphoid cells (prolymphocytes and paraimmunoblasts) that are grouped together in growth nodules (**B**). The lymphoplasmacytic cells are easily seen on smears with a more abundant basophilic cytoplasm (**D**). Few mitoses are seen. The tumor cells express the various B-cell antigens and display a CD5+, CD23±, CD43±, FMC7-, and CD10- phenotype.

Immunophenotyping

Lymphoma	CD5	CD10	CD23	CD43	sIg/cIg	Other
MCL	+	-	-	+	M(D)	Cyclin D1+
SLL/B-CLL	+	-	+	+	M(D) low	
					cIg low	
FL	-	+	±	-	M (G)	Bc16+
MZL	-	-	-	±	M (D, G, A)	
					cIg ±	

Figure 1-11. Immunophenotyping. In patients with small cell proliferation, atypical aspects are frequent and the only way to distinguish small lymphocytic lymphoma (SLL) from other lymphoid disorders is by the immunophenotype, looking at CD5, CD10, CD23, and CD43 antigens. B-CLL—B-cell lymphocytic lymphoma; FL—follicular lymphoma; MCL—mantle cell lymphoma; MZL—marginal zone lymphoma.

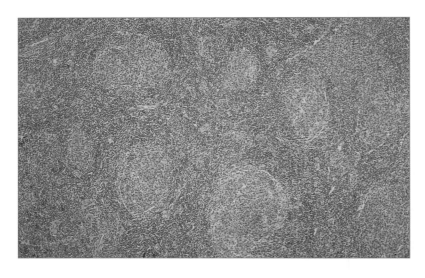

Figure 1-12. Follicular lymphoma (FL). FL accounts for 20% to 25% of all lymphomas in adults and consists of a mixture of centrocytes (cleaved, centrofollicular, small to large cells) and centroblasts (noncleaved large cells), interspersed with follicular dendritic cells. Centrocytes usually predominate and centroblasts are less numerous. Proliferation is usually follicular in appearance but diffuse proliferation is found in 20% to 25% of cases and may even predominate.

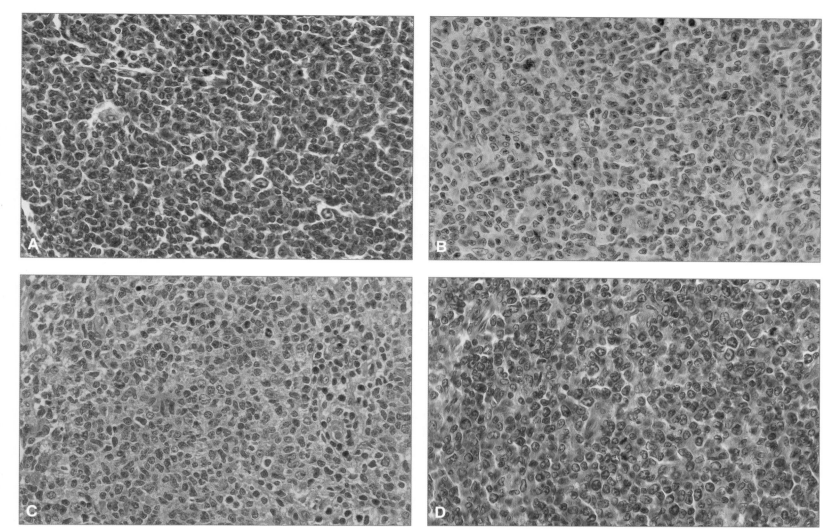

Figure 1-13. Grades of follicular lymphoma. Even if centroblasts vary in proportion, and centrocytes in size, from one node to another in the same patient, grades have been defined based on the proportion of each cell type. Attempts have been made to correlate these grades to differences in outcome. However, these differences remain unconfirmed and it has proved very difficult to reproduce grading among different groups of hematopathologists. The World Health Organization classification recognizes three grades based on counting the absolute number of centroblasts in 10 neoplastic follicles, expressed per 403 high-power microscopic field (hpf) [2]. Grade 1 cases have zero to five centroblasts per hpf (**A**); grade 2 cases have six to 15 centroblasts per hpf (**B**); grade 3 cases have more than15 centroblasts per hpf and are further divided into 3a (**C**) if centrocytes persist or 3b (**D**) with solid sheets of centroblasts. Most patients have generalized disease at diagnosis. Occasionally, peripheral blood or extranodal infiltration may be detected at diagnosis, associated with much more aggressive disease or histologic transformation.

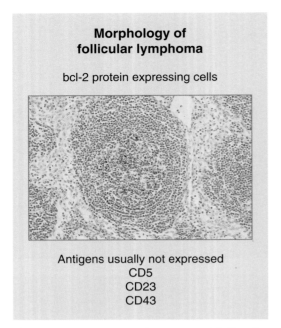

Morphology of follicular lymphoma

bcl-2 protein expressing cells

Antigens usually not expressed
CD5
CD23
CD43

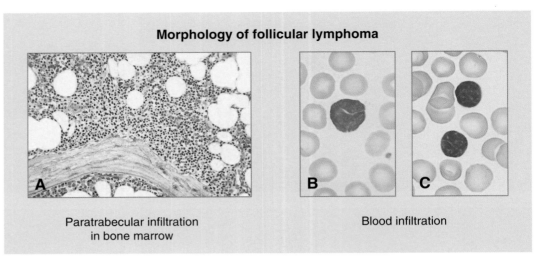

Morphology of follicular lymphoma

A

Paratrabecular infiltration
in bone marrow

B   C

Blood infiltration

Figure 1-14. Immunophenotype of follicular lymphoma. The tumor cells usually express B-cell antigens (CD19, CD20, and CD22) and surface immunoglobulins, and are CD10+, CD5-, CD23-, and CD43-; bcl-2 and bcl-6 proteins are usually expressed.

Figure 1-15. Bone marrow and blood involvement in follicular lymphoma. Morphologic bone marrow involvement is present in more than 75% of cases and blood involvement in less than 30% of the patients. However, the rearranged *bcl-2* gene is present in blood and bone marrow at diagnosis in nearly 100% of the patients with detectable rearrangement in pathologic lymph nodes. Bone marrow involvement usually shows a paratrabecular pattern of involvement. This involvement is better seen in a core biopsy than in marrow smears. **A,** Paratrabecular infiltration in bone marrow. **B** and **C,** Blood involvement.

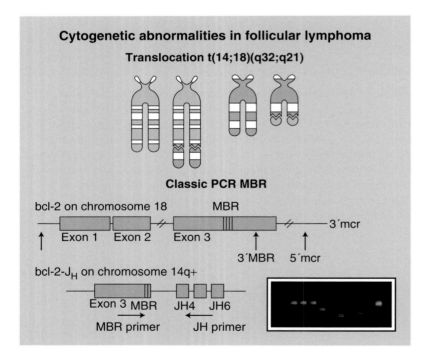

Cytogenetic abnormalities in follicular lymphoma

Translocation t(14;18)(q32;q21)

Classic PCR MBR

bcl-2 on chromosome 18   MBR

Exon 1   Exon 2   Exon 3   3′mcr

3′MBR   5′mcr

bcl-2-J$_H$ on chromosome 14q+

Exon 3   MBR   JH4   JH6

MBR primer   JH primer

Figure 1-16. Cytogenetic abnormalities in follicular lymphoma (FL). Translocation t(14;18)(q32;q21) is a recurrent cytogenetic abnormality in FL that is present in at least 80% of cases. The coding part of the *bcl-2* gene is translocated from chromosome 18 to chromosome 14 within the locus of genes coding for the immunoglobulin heavy chain. PCR MBR—polymerase chain reaction of major breakpoint region.

Histologic progression and transformation

Diffuse large B-cell aspect

Burkitt-like aspect

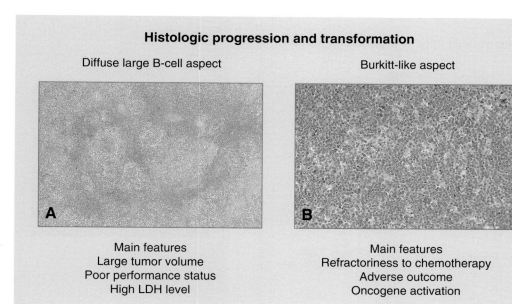

Main features
Large tumor volume
Poor performance status
High LDH level

Main features
Refractoriness to chemotherapy
Adverse outcome
Oncogene activation

Mantle cell lymphoma

Typical aspect

Cytology

Large cell variant

Cyclin D1 positivity

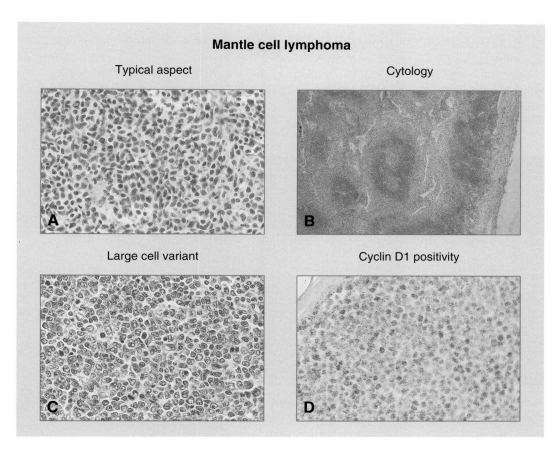

Figure 1-17. **A** and **B**, Histologic progression in follicular lymphoma (FL). Histologic transformation occurs at a rate of 3% per year. Histologic progression is always associated with a clinical picture of a highly proliferative tumor with a rapid increase in tumor volume, poor performance status, and increasing lactate dehydrogenase (LDH) level, along with disease-related symptoms.

Chemotherapy usually fails in these patients and they have a poor outcome. Transformation is attributable to an accumulation of additional gene alterations, often deletion of the *p16* gene or inactivation of *p53*.

Figure 1-18. Mantle cell lymphoma (MCL). MCL accounts for approximately 5% to 8% of all lymphomas. The tumor consists of small or medium-sized lymphoid cells with dispersed chromatin, scanty clear cytoplasm, and indistinct nucleoli (**A** and **B**).

The nucleus is often irregular or cleaved but may be round. Mitoses are usually infrequent, but may be present. The large cell, blastoid variant has a larger nucleus with more dispersed chromatin and a higher proliferation fraction (**C**). Proliferation is usually diffuse or vaguely nodular. More rarely, it is confined to the mantle zone.

The tumor cells express surface immunoglobulins, generally IgM, often combined with IgD, together with B-cell antigens (CD19, CD20, CD22). The phenotype is CD5+, CD10-, CD23-, and CD43+. The t(11;14) translocation between the immunoglobulin heavy chain loci and the *bcl-1* locus is present in 70% of cases and results in hyperexpression of the *PRAD1/CCND1* gene, the gene for cyclin D1, a cell-cycle regulatory protein (**D**). The diagnosis of MCL should be confirmed by the immunohistochemical expression of cyclin D1.

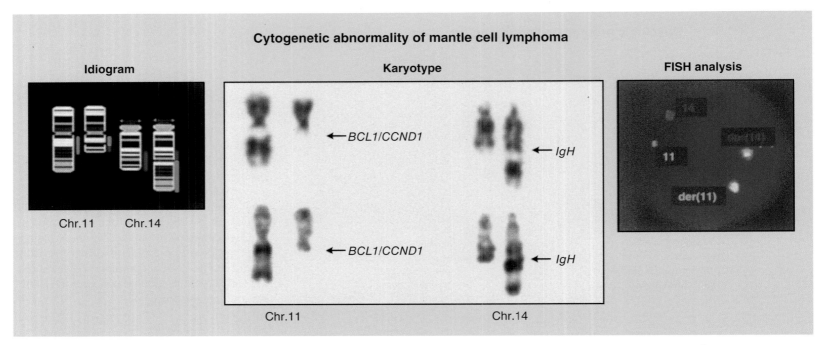

Cytogenetic abnormality of mantle cell lymphoma

Idiogram

Chr.11   Chr.14

Karyotype

← BCL1/CCND1

← IgH

← BCL1/CCND1

← IgH

Chr.11   Chr.14

FISH analysis

11

der(11)

Figure 1-19. Mantle cell lymphoma (MCL). MCL is characterized by the translocation t(11;14)(q13;q32) that colocalizes the cyclin D1 (*CCND1/BCL1*) (11q13) and the immunoglobulin heavy chain (IgH) (14q32) genes (*left*). Karyotypic analysis (*middle*) demonstrates 70% to 75% cases with t(11;14) whereas virtually all cases show this translocation using fluorescent in situ hybridization (FISH) studies (*right*).

Although recurrent in MCL, the t(11;14) translocation can also be observed in other lymphoid malignancies such as chronic lymphocytic leukemia/lymphocytic lymphoma (2% to 5%), multiple myeloma (8% to 10%), marginal zone B-cell lymphoma (15% to 20%), and B-cell prolymphocytic leukemia (20%).

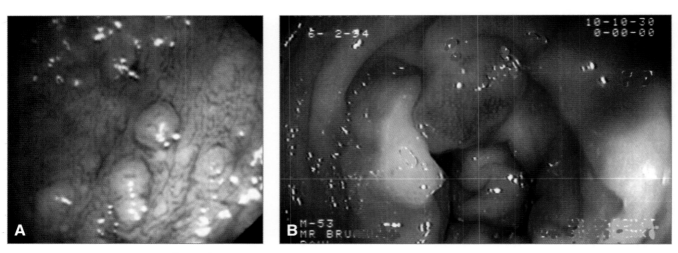

Figure 1-20. Gastrointestinal involvement in mantle cell lymphoma (MCL). MCL is more frequent in patients over 60 years of age, and in men. MCL is generally widespread at diagnosis, with extensive hypertrophy of lymph nodes and spleen, infiltration of the bone marrow and blood, and extranodal sites of involvement, particularly in the gastrointestinal tract with lymphomatoid

polyposis. **A**, Accumulation of small polyps may grow, obstructing the colon (**B**).

Although MCL is initially responsive to chemotherapy, relapse is inevitable and the median survival is 3.5 to 4 years.

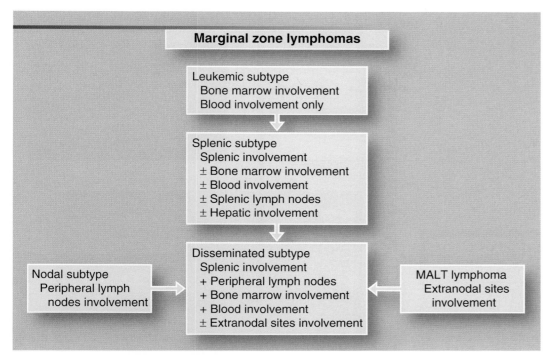

Figure 1-21. Marginal zone lymphoma (MZL). MZLs are categorized as extranodal lymphomas of mucosa-associated lymphoid tissue (MALT), splenic lymphomas (with or without villous lymphocytes), or nodal lymphomas (with or without monocytoid B cells).

Three clinical presentations have been described in the World Health Organization classification: extranodal or MALT lymphomas, nodal involvement, and splenic lymphoma. However, more disseminated presentations may occur. Similarly, the disease may exist with only blood and bone marrow involvement. In the splenic subtype, sites of involvement include the spleen and frequently the bone marrow and peripheral blood. Patients with leukemic subtype may present with bone marrow and peripheral blood involvement only. They often progress to the splenic subtype. The nodal subtype is characterized by localized or disseminated lymph nodes with rare blood involvement. In some cases the disease is too disseminated at presentation to identify the initial site of the disease [20–22].

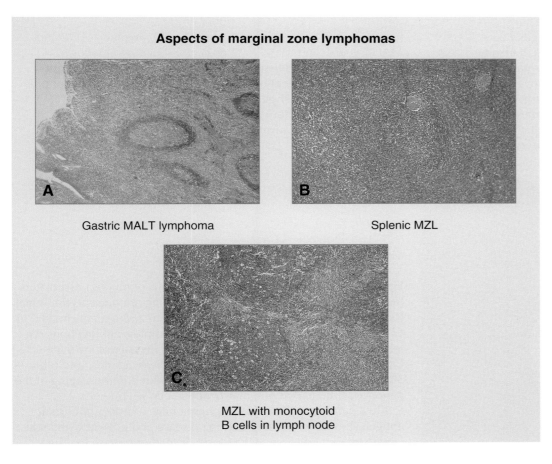

Gastric MALT lymphoma

Splenic MZL

MZL with monocytoid
B cells in lymph node

Figure 1-22. A–C, Various aspects of marginal zone lymphomas (MZLs). These lymphomas are characterized by cellular heterogeneity, comprising centrocyte-like marginal zone cells, monocytoid B cells, small lymphocytes, and plasma cells. Large cells may be present in some cases. Reactive follicles may persist within the tumor, in which the tumor cells are localized in the marginal zone of the follicles or in the interfollicular zones. In epithelial tissues, tumor infiltrates the epithelium, forming lymphoepithelial lesions. The tumor cells express surface immunoglobulin, cytoplasmic immunoglobulin in many cases, and B-cell antigens; however, most do not express CD5, CD10, CD23, or CD43. Rearrangement of the *bcl-1* and *bcl-2* genes is not seen. As in the other indolent lymphomas, transformation to a more aggressive lymphoma with large cell proliferation may occur at relapse or sometimes at the time of diagnosis.

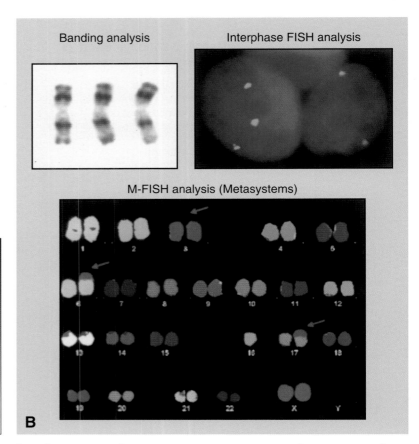

Banding analysis   Interphase FISH analysis

M-FISH analysis (Metasystems)

A	Chromosomal Abnormalities in Marginal Zone Lymphomas	
Chromosomal Abnormality	**Incidence, %**	
+3/+3q	40–80	
18	28–40	
12	18–20	
7q deletion	10–30	Splenic MZL
t(11;18)(q21;q21)	25–50	MALT MZL
t(1;14)(p22;q32)	Rare cases	MALT MZL

B

Figure 1-23. Chromosomal abnormalities in marginal zone B-cell lymphomas (MZLs). **A**, Spectrum of abnormalities. If trisomy 3 (+3) occurs as the most frequent aberration, this abnormality can be identified either as a complete +3 or as a partial trisomy 3 (trisomy 3q, tetrasomy 3q). These findings suggest that the long arm of chromosome 3 is likely of particular importance in the pathogenesis of the disease.

Other cytogenetic abnormalities are nonspecific: if they are encountered frequently in MZL, they may be observed in other lymphomas. Translocation (11;18)(q21;q21), involving *API2* and *MALT1* genes, and t(1;14)(p22;q32), are specific to mucosa-associated lymphoid tissue (MALT) lymphoma. The translocation (14;18)(q32;q21), identical to the one seen in follicular lymphoma but involving the *MLT* gene and not the *bcl-2* gene, is seen in 20% of MALT lymphomas. **B**, Various analyses of MZLs. FISH—fluorescence in situ hybridization.

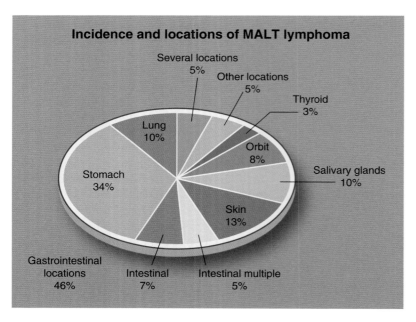

Incidence and locations of MALT lymphoma

Figure 1-24. Incidence of different locations of mucosa-associated lymphoid tissue (MALT) lymphoma. This diagram presents the initial locations of MALT lymphoma as observed in 258 patients treated in CH Lyon-Sud. In all reported studies, gastrointestinal locations represent half of the cases, stomach being the first site of involvement. Other frequent locations are skin, lung, salivary glands, and orbit. In 30% of the cases, other locations may be found in the staging of the patients, particularly bone marrow or spleen [21].

Most patients with MALT lymphoma have a history of chronic antigen stimulation or autoimmune disease and present with localized extranodal disease at diagnosis. Spread of disease to other extranodal sites, spleen, or bone marrow is found in 30% of cases at diagnosis, but can be much more frequent at relapse.

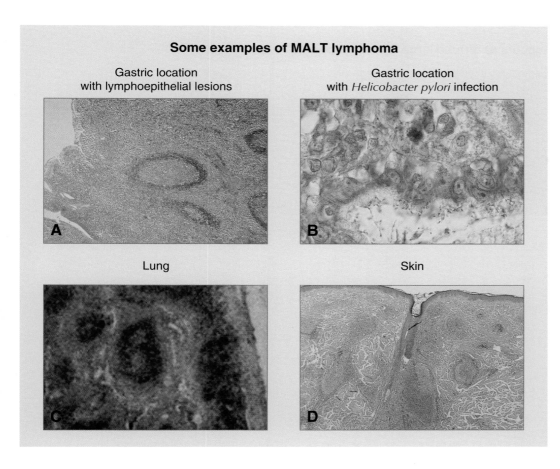

Some examples of MALT lymphoma

Gastric location
with lymphoepithelial lesions

Gastric location
with *Helicobacter pylori* infection

Lung

Skin

Figure 1-25. Examples of mucosa-associated lymphoid tissue (MALT) lymphomas. MALT lymphomas comprise various aspects according to the extranodal location. **A**, A typical gastric location with lymphoepithelioid lesions. **B**, Gastric infestation with *Helicobacter pylori* along the cryptic epithelium (Giemsa stain). **C**, Nodular lymphoid infiltrates in the lung. **D**, Dermal periannexial and perivascular lymphoid infiltrates in the skin.

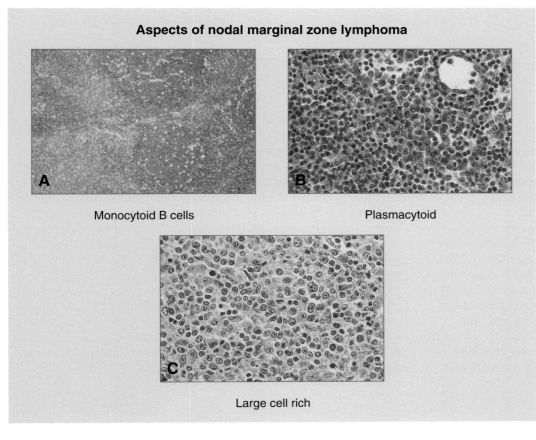

Aspects of nodal marginal zone lymphoma

Monocytoid B cells

Plasmacytoid

Large cell rich

Figure 1-26. Aspects of primary nodal marginal zone lymphoma (MZL). A large proportion of nodal MZL is observed in patients with mucosa-associated lymphomatoid tissue (MALT) lymphoma and nodal dissemination. However, lymphomas with the same histology and phenotype have been reported in purely nodal disease. In these cases, this aspect was often described as a proliferation rich in monocytoid B cells (**A**).

However, these cells are not specific to MZL and may be encountered in other B-cell lymphomas. A proliferation rich in lymphoplasmocytes or plasma cells may lead to the diagnosis of lymphoplasmacytic lymphoma (**B**). A proliferation rich in large cells may lead to the diagnosis of diffuse large B-cell lymphoma (**C**).

In the presence of centrocytic-like or monocytoid cells, the marginal zone topography of the infiltration, the frequent involvement of bone marrow with small cells, the typical phenotype, or the presence of typical cytogenetic abnormality confirms the diagnosis of MZL. These patients, particularly those with large-cell proliferation, often have more aggressive disease than MALT lymphoma or splenic MZL.

Aspects of diffuse large B-cell lymphoma

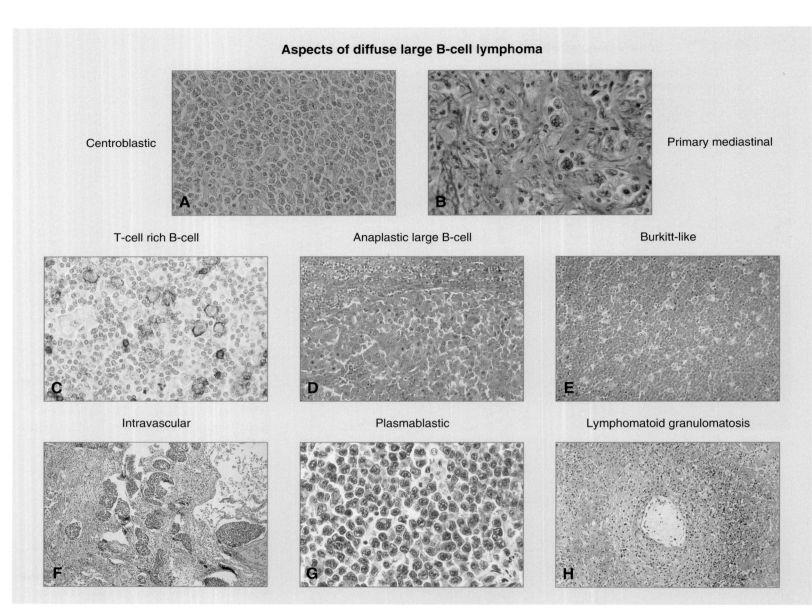

Figure 1-27. Diffuse large B-cell lymphoma (DLCL). **A**, Centro-blastic. **B**, Primary mediastinal. **C**, T-cell rich B-cell lymphoma. **D**, Anaplastic large B-cell lymphoma. **E**, Burkitt-like lymphoma. **F**, Intravascular lymphoma. **G**, Plasmablastic lymphoma. **H**, Lymphomatoid granulomatosis.

Diffuse large B-cell lymphoma encompasses various histologic subtypes, none of which are optimally defined, and is often hetero-geneous in morphology, genetics, and clinical presentation. They consist of large B cells with a round or variably cleaved nucleus, often with basophilic cytoplasm, and fairly marked mitotic activity. In most cases, the large cells are described as centroblasts (large cleaved cells) (**A**). Other cell types are observed, such as large cleaved or multilobated cells, large anaplastic B cells (**D**), or small noncleaved non-Burkitt cells (Burkitt-like lymphoma) (**E**). Some of these lymphomas may show abundant small reactive T cells and

histiocytes (**C**) or intravascular proliferation (**F**), which can cause diagnostic problems. Primary mediastinal lymphomas contain large cells with nuclei of variable appearance but clear cytoplasm sur-rounded by fibrosis (**B**). In most cases it is difficult if not impossible to subclassify these large cell lymphomas. The tumor cells often have surface immunoglobulins and cytoplasmic immunoglobulins, as well as B-cell antigens, and are CD45+, CD5+, and CD10+; *bcl-2* gene rearrangement is seen in fewer than 20% of cases and *c-myc* gene rearrangement in an even smaller proportion.

The DLCL accounts for 40% of all lymphomas. Patients generally present with rapidly expanding nodal or extranodal tumors. Approx-imately 40% present with extranodal tumors confined to one or more organs, some sites being fairly typical. The disease is localized in approximately 20% of cases. Mediastinal and abdominal involve-ment often presents as bulky tumor masses.

The Main Recurrent, Nonrandom Chromosomal Changes Observed in Diffuse Large B-cell Lymphomas	
Chromosomal Aberration	Incidence, %
BCL2: t(14;18Xq32;q21)	30
BCL6: t(3;14)q27;q32)	25
6q deletion	20
+7, +12	17
+X	13
MYC: t(8;14)(q24.1;q32)	10
BCL8: t(14;15)(q32;q11-13)	< 4

Figure 1-28. The main recurrent, nonrandom chromosomal changes observed in diffuse large B-cell lymphomas (DLCLs). DLCLs are characterized by a heterogeneous cytogenetic presentation. Most cases display complex karyotypes with hyperdiploidy (47 to 57 chromosomes) or tetraploidy (4 x N chromosomes).

Burkitt lymphoma

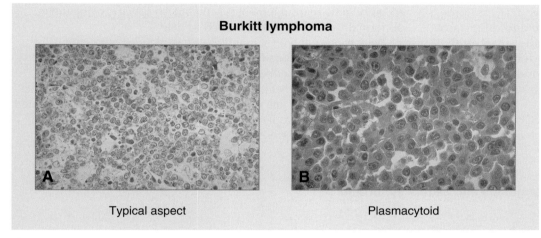

Typical aspect   Plasmacytoid

Figure 1-29. Burkitt lymphoma (BL). **A**, Typical aspect. **B**, Plasmacytoid aspect. BL consists of medium-sized monomorphic cells with a round nucleus, multiple nucleoli, and basophilic cytoplasm (**A**). Cytoplasmic lipid vacuoles are generally present. The tumor is highly proliferative with multiple mitoses. The cells are positive for surface IgM (sIgM+), express B antigens, and are CD5-, CD10+, and *bcl-6*+. Most cases show translocation of the *c-myc* gene on chromosome 8 to the immunoglobulin heavy chain region on chromosome 14, t(8;14), or to the light chain region on chromosome 2, t(2;8), or chromosome 22, t(8;22).

Burkitt lymphoma is more common in children (40% of all child lymphomas) but accounts for 5% of cases in adults. Most patients present with an abdominal tumor involving the cecum and mesentery but in some cases tumors develop in ovary, breast, testis, or peripheral lymph node. Bone marrow or meningeal involvement carries a very poor prognosis.

Cases observed in endemic zones of Africa are associated with Epstein-Barr virus (EBV) infection in 100% of cases, compared with the sporadic cases seen in Europe or the United States, where EBV infection is found in 20% of the cases. AIDS-associated cases are also different and usually have the plasmacytoid form.

B-cell lymphoblastic lymphoma

Main presentation: acute lymphoblastic leukemia

Clinical presentation as a lymphoma (solid tumor): very rare: often a transformation of an indolent lymphoma

Figure 1-30. B-cell lymphoblastic lymphoma (LL). B-cell LLs generally present like leukemia, with infiltration of the bone marrow, blood, and central nervous system. A lymphoma presentation with predominantly nodal or extranodal infiltration, with or without bone marrow infiltration, is found in fewer than 1% of cases. LL comprises lymphoblasts, which are cells slightly larger than small lymphocytes, with a B phenotype (CD19+, CD79a+, sIg+ and varying in their positivity for B-cell antigens). The immunoglobulin heavy chain gene is usually rearranged and rearrangement of the light chain gene is seen in some cases. Various cytogenetic abnormalities have been reported. B-cell LL is a rare, poorly characterized tumor, generally seen in elderly patients and often caused by transformation of a previously nondiagnosed small-cell lymphoma.

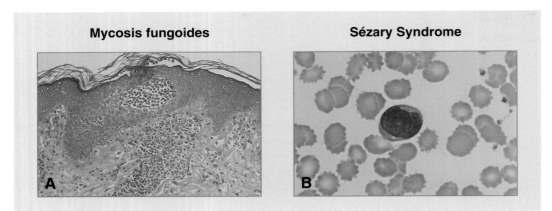

Mycosis fungoides

Sézary Syndrome

Figure 1-31. The cutaneous T cell lymphomas (CTCLs) comprise mycosis fungoides and Sézary syndrome and other rarer T-cell lymphomas. The tumor cells are generally small, with a cerebriform nucleus; large cells are seen in a few cases. These cells infiltrate the epidermis and often the blood. Langerhans cells and interdigitating cells are frequently found in the infiltrating tumor.

The tumor cells express T-cell antigens, CD2, CD3, and CD5, and in some cases CD7. Most are CD4+ but some are CD8+. T-cell receptor gene rearrangement is seen but no specific cytogenetic abnormalities have been described to date.

Patients present with skin infiltration in plaques or multiple nodules, which are localized in some cases (*see* Fig. 1-32), or with generalized erythroderma. Infiltration of the blood is present, but can be minimal, or marked as in Sézary syndrome. Infiltration of the nodes or viscera is a late event in the disease course, often associated with transformation to large cell lymphoma. The two clinical forms shown in **A** and **B** represent most, but not all, T-cell lymphomas.

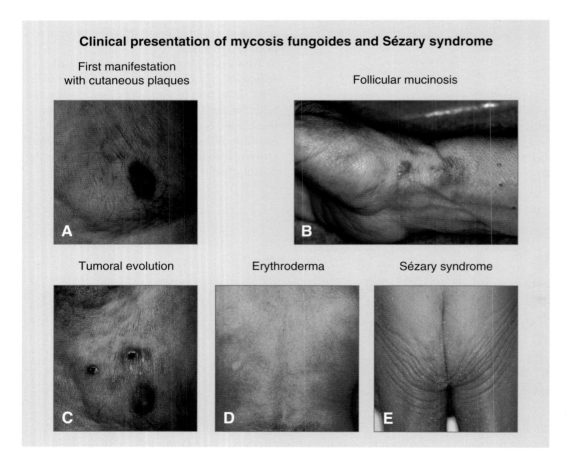

Clinical presentation of mycosis fungoides and Sézary syndrome

First manifestation with cutaneous plaques

Follicular mucinosis

Tumoral evolution

Erythroderma

Sézary syndrome

Figure 1-32. Clinical aspects of mycosis fungoides and Sézary syndrome with pruritic erythroderma. **A**, First manifestation with plaques and patches. **B**, Follicular mucinosis. **C**, Evolution with tumors. **D**, Erythroderma in mycosis fungoides. **E**, Sézary syndrome with pruritic erythroderma.

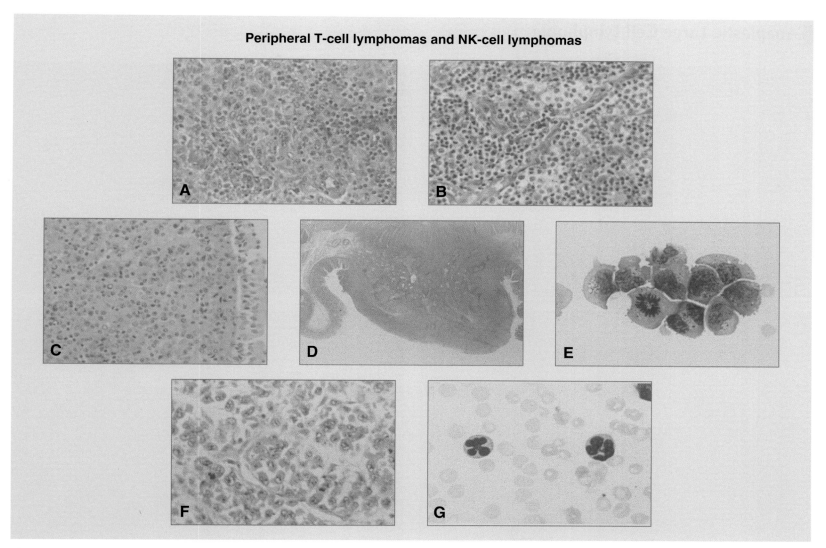

Figure 1-33. Peripheral T-cell lymphomas (PTCLs) and natural killer (NK) cell lymphomas. **A,** Interfollicular proliferation of mixed atypical cells. **B,** Angioimmunoblastic T-cell lymphoma. **C,** Extranodal NK and T-cell lymphoma, nasal type. **D** and **E,** Hepatosplenic γδ T-cell lymphoma. **F,** Subcutaneous panniculitis-like T-cell lymphoma. **G,** Human T-cell leukemia/lymphoma virus 1 (HTLV)–related lymphoma.

Peripheral T-cell lymphoma is a proliferation of atypical small and large cells. Its heterogeneity, and the difficulties in differentiating between reactive and lymphomatous cells, often make PTCL difficult to describe and classify. Several clinical or histologic syndromes have been described, such as angioimmunoblastic T-cell lymphoma (**B**), extranodal NK/T-cell lymphoma, nasal type (**C**), enteropathy-type T-cell lymphoma (**D,E**), hepatosplenic γδ T-cell lymphoma, subcutaneous panniculitis-like T-cell lymphoma, anaplastic large cell lymphoma (**F**), CD30⁺ cutaneous proliferations, and HTLV-1–related lymphoma (**G**). Although some of these variants have been conclusively defined, most have been identified on a provisional basis only. In addition, many such lymphomas present with an interfollicular proliferation of mixed atypical cells with nuclei that are small to moderate or large and cannot be assigned to a specific type (**A**).

T-cell antigens are usually present, but the pattern is variable: the cells are CD3⁺, CD2⁺, CD5⁺, and CD7⁺. The cells are more often

CD4⁺ than CD8⁺ but may be CD4⁻ CD8⁻; no B-cell antigen is present. The γδ T-cells are TiA⁺, granzyme⁺, perforin⁺, CD3⁺, and CD8⁺, and NK cells are CD2⁺, CD3⁻, CD16⁺, CD56⁺, and often Epstein-Barr virus positive. T-cell receptor gene rearrangement is generally present but not in all cases. There is no immunoglobulin gene rearrangement.

These lymphomas account for 10% to 15% of all lymphomas in Europe and the United States but are more frequent elsewhere, eg, Japan. Patients generally present with disseminated disease, comprising variably sized lymph nodes and involvement of the skin, liver, spleen, and other extranodal sites. B symptoms are often present (fever, weight loss, night sweats). Patients with angioimmunoblastic T-cell lymphoma generally present with generalized lymph node hypertrophy, fever, cutaneous reactions, and polyclonal hypergammaglobulinemia. NK and T-cell lymphomas are rare and present with predominantly extranodal involvement, particularly in the nose, palate, or skin. Gastrointestinal T-cell lymphomas often occur in adults with a history of gluten enteropathy but can occur as a primary event. In fact the feature common to all such lymphomas is the variability in presentation, with some cases being sufficiently atypical to suggest diseases other than lymphoma, resulting in diagnostic delay.

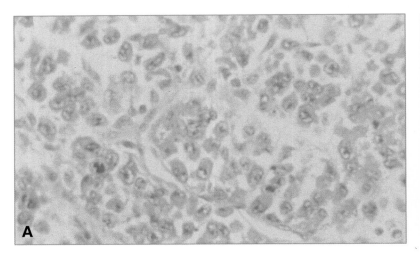

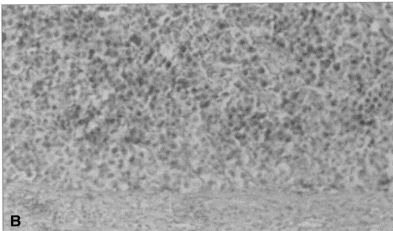

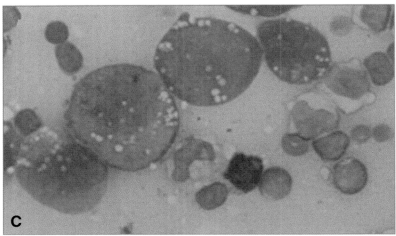

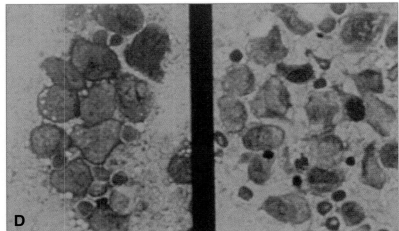

Figure 1-34. Anaplastic large cell lymphoma (ALCL). ALCL features large cells having a pleomorphic multilobed nucleus, multiple or large isolated nucleoli, and an abundant cytoplasm (**A,C**). Lymphohistiocytic and small cell variants have been described (**B**). Proliferation of these cells has a cohesive appearance and an affinity for lymph node sinuses. The tumor cells are CD30+, CD45+, EMA+ (**D**), CD15-, CD3+, and most cases are Alk1+; they are variably positive for T-cell antigens. A t(2;5) translocation is generally present; 40% show no evidence of gene rearrangement, whereas 60% only show T-cell receptor gene rearrangement.

Two clinical presentations of ALCL are encountered: the first is systemic, with nodal and/or extranodal (sometimes cutaneous) involvement; the second is exclusively cutaneous, forming a continuum from lymphomatoid papulosis (not necessarily neoplastic despite being clonal) through lymphoma. The cutaneous variant may regress spontaneously over long periods before re-emerging.

In clinical presentation and course, the systemic ALCL are fairly similar to large B-cell lymphoma, but the outcome is superior to most peripheral or T-cell lymphomas. In some cases, clinical manifestations may differ very little from those of mediastinal Hodgkin disease with a large tumor, and immunophenotyping is essential to distinguish the two entities.

Adult T-cell leukemia/lymphoma

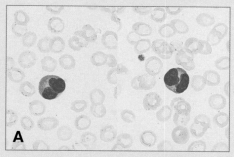

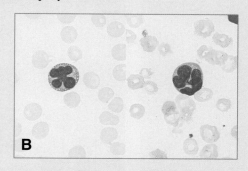

	Smoldering	Chronic	Acute
White blood cells	Normal	Increased	Increased (++)
ATLL cells in blood	< 3%	> 10%	> 30%
Increased lymph nodes	No	Yes, mild	Generalized
Skin rash	Erythema	Positive papules	Present
Hepatosplenomegaly	No	Yes	Yes
Lactate dehydrogenase	Normal	Increased	Increased
Calcium	Normal	Normal	High

Figure 1-35. Human T-cell leukemia/lymphoma virus (HTLV)-1 associated leukemia and lymphoma (**A** and **B**).In adult T-cell leukemia/lymphoma (ATLL), proliferation is secondary to HTLV-1 infection. The tumor cells express T-cell antigens (CD2, CD3, and CD5) but are usually CD7⁻ and CD4⁺. The T-cell receptor genes are rearranged and clonal incorporation of the HTLV-1 genome is found in all cases.

Most cases are seen in Japan, but the disease is endemic in the Caribbean and episodic cases are observed elsewhere. There are several clinical presentations: a leukemic presentation comprising hepato-splenomegaly, hypercalcemia, and osteolysis; a lymphomatous presentation with disseminated lymph node hypertrophy without infiltration of the blood; a chronic presentation with isolated hyperlymphocytosis and skin involvement; and slowly progressive lesions characterized by clinically silent lymphocytosis.

Immunodeficiency-associated Lymphomas

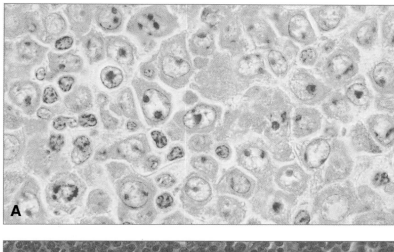

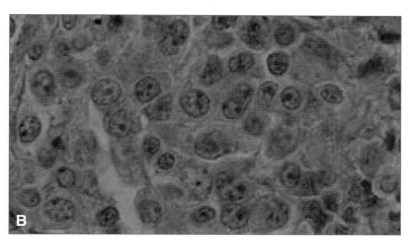

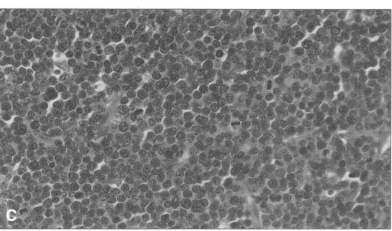

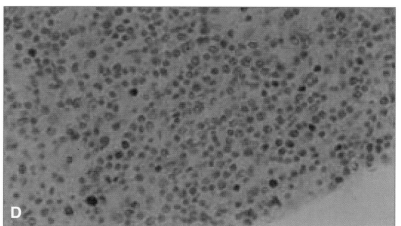

Figure 1-36. Immunodeficiency-associated lymphomas. Lymphomas occurring in patients with immunodeficiency include primary immunodeficiency syndrome such as ataxia telangiectasia, Wiskott-Aldrich syndrome, severe combined immunodeficiency, or autoimmune lymphoproliferative disorders; HIV infection (**A** and **B**); or iatrogenic immunosuppression associated with transplantation (**C**) or methotrexate treatment. These lymphomas have been attributed to deficient immune surveillance of oncogenic virus such as Epstein-Barr virus (EBV) or human herpesvirus-8. In the case of EBV-induced lymphoma, EBV latency-associated RNA is present in the majority of the cells (**D**).

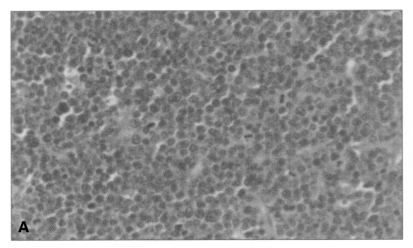

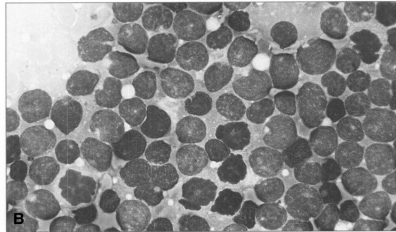

Figure 1-37. A and **B**, T-cell lymphoblastic lymphoma (LL). LLs have lymphoblastic cells slightly larger than the small lymphocytes, with a round convoluted nucleus, delicate chromatin, nearly invisible nucleoli, and scanty, slightly basophilic cytoplasm. Mitoses are frequent. The tumors share a T-cell phenotype (CD7+, CD3+, CD1α+, TdT+), and are variably positive for the other T-cell antigens. T-cell receptor gene rearrangement is sometimes present, and immunoglobulin heavy chain gene rearrangement rather less frequent. A range of cytogenetic abnormalities has been reported.

The leukemic presentation is common in children. The nodal presentation is seen in adolescents and young men. LL accounts for 40% of all childhood lymphomas but for less than 5% of adult lymphomas. Patients generally present with a rapidly expanding mediastinal tumor. Infiltration of the bone marrow and nervous system carries a very adverse prognosis.

PROGNOSTIC FACTORS

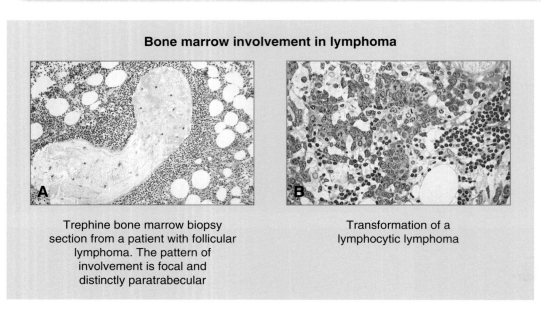

Bone marrow involvement in lymphoma

Trephine bone marrow biopsy section from a patient with follicular lymphoma. The pattern of involvement is focal and distinctly paratrabecular

Transformation of a lymphocytic lymphoma

Figure 1-38. Bone marrow involvement in lymphoma. Lymphoma cells may infiltrate any organ or lymph node. Although retrospective studies associate some sites with a poorer prognosis, most multiparametric analyses show that these locations are statistically related to the other prognostic factors already described, and that the most important factor remains the number rather than the location of extranodal sites.

Bone marrow infiltration usually carries a poor prognosis. However, it is present in over 70% of patients with follicular, small lymphocytic or mantle cell lymphomas, where it has only a moderate impact on prognosis (**A**). Conversely, in patients with Burkitt or lymphoblastic lymphoma, those with bone marrow infiltration have a considerably poorer outcome.

Only 20% to 25% of patients with diffuse large B-cell lymphoma show marrow infiltration at diagnosis, and they have a poorer treatment response and shorter survival than those without marrow infiltration; infiltration may be due to large cells similar to those found in the lymph nodes but also to small cells, in which case it probably reflects the transformation of a previously undetected indolent lymphoma (**B**). Patients with small-cell marrow infiltration have a higher risk of relapse but longer survival than those with purely large-cell infiltration.

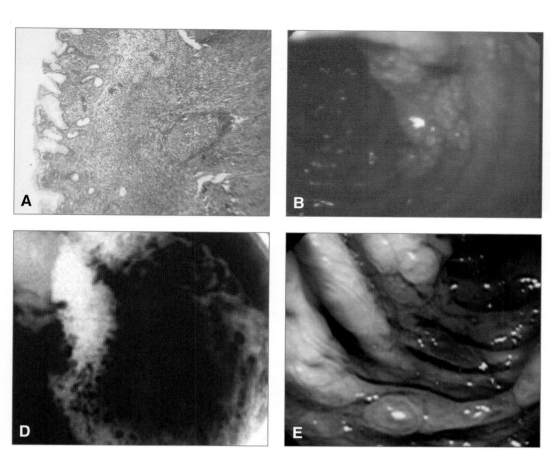

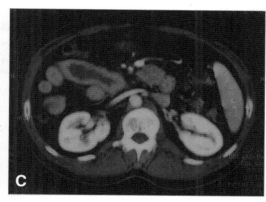

Figure 1-39. Gastrointestinal locations. The gastrointestinal tract is the most frequent location for extranodal disease, stomach being the most frequent (representing 75% of all digestive locations). Patients with gastrointestinal location are thought to have a better outcome, but at least two thirds of them have a mucosa-associated lymphoma tissue (MALT) lymphoma. One or more gastrointestinal sites are found in many types of lymphoma, in particular MALT lymphoma and large-cell lymphoma, but also Burkitt lymphoma and mantle cell lymphoma, all of which differ in prognosis. **A**, Histologic aspect of MALT gastric lymphoma. **B**, Endoscopic view of follicular lymphoma in duodenum. **C** and **D**, CT scan and barium imaging views of MALT lymphoma of small intestine. **E**, Endoscopic view of mantle cell lymphoma in the sigmoid.

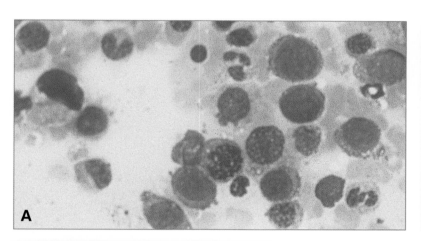

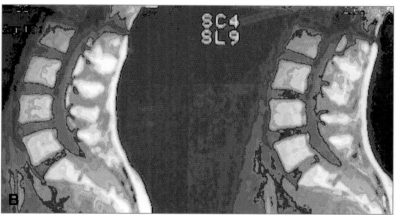

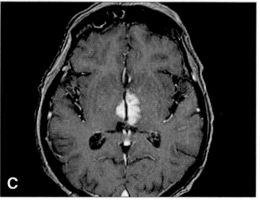

Figure 1-40. Central nervous system locations. Neurologic involvement corresponds to four syndromes: meningeal location (**A**), extradural disease with cord compression (**B**), encephalic location (**C**), and the lesions typical of immunodeficiency, in particular with HIV-positive patients.

Parameters Associated with Ability to Tolerate Treatment

Parameter	Definition	Elderly Subjects
Age	Median age of lymphoma patients	> 60–65
Occupational status	Retirement age	> 60–65
Performance status	Activities of daily living	> 75
Disease	Functional impairment of various organs	> 65
Renal function	Decrease < 50% in glomerular filtration and tubule secretion	> 70
Hormonal status	Menopause in women	> 50–55
Health	Presence of concomitant diseases	See index
Treatment	Ability to tolerate allogeneic bone marrow transplantation	> 50
Treatment	Ability to tolerate autologous stem cell transplantation	> 65
Prognosis	Change in International Prognostic Index survival curves	> 60–65

Figure 1-41. Parameters associated with ability to tolerate treatment. Outcome in lymphoma varies with the characteristics of both tumor and patient, particularly patient age and the impact of other serious diseases on the ability to tolerate treatment. It is usually thought that elderly patients do not tolerate standard chemotherapy, particularly for aggressive lymphomas. In a Southwest Oncology Group study, elderly patient survival was poor because treatment response was poorer and relapse more frequent. However, both these results were due to lower dose chemotherapy administered to elderly patients. In other studies, the oldest patients had a much higher death rate during treatment, whereas those in complete remission after treatment had a relapse rate identical to that of younger patients. The conclusion of these various studies is that elderly subjects are at greater risk of complications from chemotherapy due to concomitant disease and more frequent morbidity with advancing age.

Age Group Differences in Prognostic Factors and Lymphoma Disease Sites

Characteristic and Disease Sites	Patients, n	Patients, % per age group				
		< 35	35–49	50–59	60–69	≥ 70
Gender						
Male	662	64	51	50	53	45
Female	621	36	49	50	47	55
Stage						
I	238	22	17	15	20	22
II	259	28	18	21	20	19
III, IV	746	50	65	64	60	59
Systemic symptoms	234	20	14	17	14	30
> 1 extranodal sites	396	29	33	34	29	30
Tumor mass ≥ 10 cm	295	26	23	26	23	20
LDH > upper limit of normal	518	47	37	47	47	49
Bone marrow	417	19	35	38	36	30
Spleen	229	13	20	24	18	14
Gastrointestinal tract	178	14	12	12	14	15
Head and neck	122	12	8	11	7	10
Skin	104	7	7	7	9	9
Liver	103	8	11	10	7	5
Pleura	73	7	6	7	5	4
Lung	54	5	3	4	5	4
Bone	38	3	4	1	3	4
Central nervous system	33	5	3	2	2	2
Orbit	17	2	1	—	1	2
Thyroid	10	—	—	< 1	< 1	2
Testis/ovary	8/5	—/1	1/2	< 1/—	< 1/< 1	1/< 1
International Prognostic Index Score	1050					
0–1	412	61	61	56	24	18
2	289	22	28	29	31	26
3	174	5	4	5	26	29
4–5	175	12	7	9	19	27
Age-adjusted International Prognostic Index Score	1108					
0	250	29	24	21	23	20
1	435	37	45	40	39	36
2	301	20	22	29	32	29
3	122	14	8	10	6	16

Figure 1-42. Age-group differences in prognostic factors and lymphoma disease sites [23]. All these studies define elderly as age over 60 or 65 years. However, although treatment tolerance may decrease with age, this correlates less with chronologic age than with physiologic age. In a recent review, elderly lymphoma patients were mainly women, with poorer performance status, but their other lymphoma characteristics were the same as in younger patients, in particular stage, number of extranodal disease sites, and lactate dehydrogenase (LDH) levels.

International Prognostic Index

Parameter	Threshold	IPI	Age-adjusted IPI
Age	< 60 vs ≥ 60	+	−
PS	0–1 vs ≥ 2	+	+
Disease stage	Localized (I–II) vs disseminated (III–IV)	+	+
LDH level	Normal vs > normal	+	+
Extranodal disease sites, n	0–1 vs ≥ 2	+	−

Figure 1-43. International Prognostic Index (IPI). Given the multiplicity of prognostic parameters even in multivariate studies, an IPI was designed for aggressive lymphomas. It incorporates five factors: age, stage, lactate dehydrogenase (LDH) level, performance status (PS), and number of extranodal disease sites. In young patients, a simplified index—the age-adjusted index—was developed.

The Follicular Lymphoma International Prognostic Index

Risk Group	Adverse Parameters, n	Patients, %	5-y Survival, %	10-y Survival, %
Good	0–1	36	91	71
Intermediate	2	37	78	51
Poor	≥ 3	27	53	36

Figure 1-44. The Follicular Lymphoma International Prognostic Index (FLIPI). Although the International Prognostic Index was designed for patients with aggressive lymphomas, it has been applied to other lymphoma subtypes. However, it may not be the best index for patients with indolent lymphoma. Therefore, an international study defined parameters associated with a worse outcome in follicular lymphoma patients. These parameters were age (< 60 vs 60), disease stage (Ann Arbor I–II vs III–IV), number of nodal sites (< 4 vs > 4), lactate dehydrogenase level (below normal vs elevated), and hemoglobin level (> 12 vs < 12 g/dL). This table defines the specific index for these patients, divided into three groups.

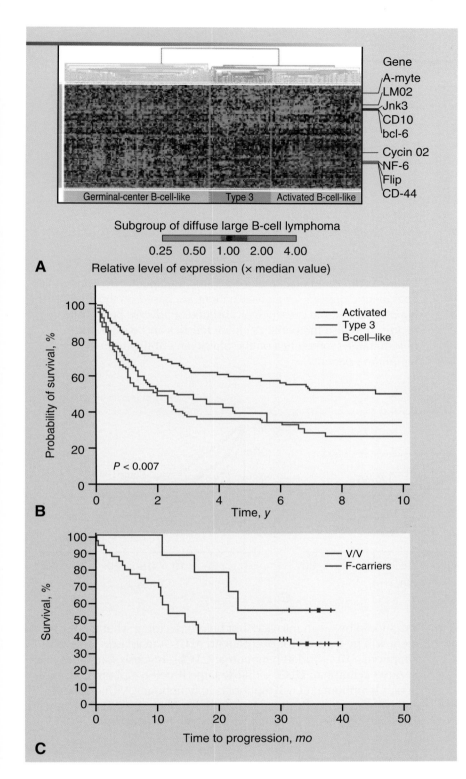

A Relative level of expression (× median value)

Gene
A-myte
LM02
Jnk3
CD10
bcl-6
Cycin 02
NF-6
Flip
CD-44

Germinal-center B-cell-like   Type 3   Activated B-cell-like

Subgroup of diffuse large B-cell lymphoma

0.25 0.50 1.00 2.00 4.00

B

Activated
Type 3
B-cell–like

$P < 0.007$

Probability of survival, %

Time, *y*

C

V/V
F-carriers

Survival, %

Time to progression, *mo*

Figure 1-45. New prognostic factors. Recently defined prognostic factors include markers of profound changes in the nature of lymphoma cells, particularly those involving the mechanisms of control of mitosis, and in the mechanisms of host response to cancer. In the near future, these biologic and genetic markers will replace the traditional International Prognostic Index parameters. They are likely to comprise changes in the genes for cell-cycle proteins (bcl-2, p53, Rb, p16, p21), cytokines (tumor necrosis factor, interleukin-10), adhesion molecules (CD44, intercellular adhesion molecule-1), angiogenic peptides (vascular endothelial growth factor), and intracellular signaling factors.

Gene expression profiling in diffuse large B-cell lymphomas allows the definition of three subgroups (**A**) with different survival (**B**) [24]. FcgRIIIa receptor 158V homozygosity is associated with a better response to rituximab in follicular patients and a longer response rate than heterozygosity (**C**) [25].

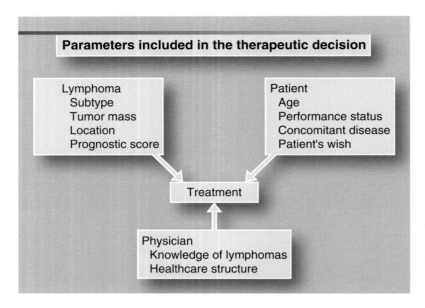

Parameters included in the therapeutic decision

Lymphoma
Subtype
Tumor mass
Location
Prognostic score

Patient
Age
Performance status
Concomitant disease
Patient's wish

Treatment

Physician
Knowledge of lymphomas
Healthcare structure

Figure 1-46. Parameters included in the therapeutic decision. Therapeutic options for a given patient are based on the type of lymphoma and the presence or absence of adverse prognostic factors, and also the patient's characteristics and wishes, and, unfortunately, sometimes on the physician's ability to treat lymphoma patients.

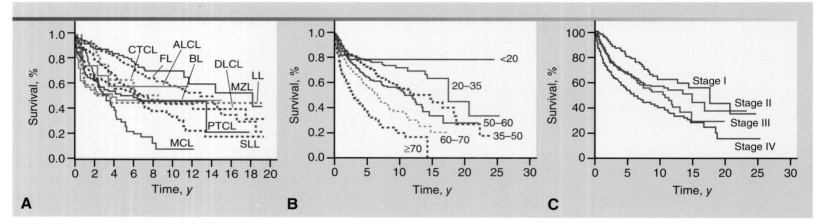

Figure 1-47. Survival data for different types of lymphoma treated in our department. These data clearly demonstrate that survival is not similar in the different types of lymphoma (**A**).

These 3000 patients were treated according to the usual standards or included in prospective studies. Survival is also plotted according to patient age (**B**) and disease stage (**C**). The message here is that histology cannot summarize outcome and that other parame-

ters should be taken into account before deciding what type of treatment will be the best for one patient. ALCL—anaplastic large cell lymphoma; BL—Burkitt lymphoma; CTCL—mycosis fungoides and Sézary's syndrome; DLCL—diffuse large B-cell lymphoma; FL—follicular lymphoma; LL—lymphoblastic lymphoma; MCL—mantle cell lymphoma; MZL—marginal zone lymphoma; PTCL—peripheral T-cell lymphoma; SLL—small lymphocytic lymphoma.

The Standard CHOP Regimen

Drug	Dose	Day of Treatment*
Cyclophosphamide	750 mg/m^2	d1
Doxorubicin	50 mg/m^2	d1
Vincristine	1.4 mg/m^2 (topped to 2 mg)	d1
Prednisone	40 to 60 mg/m^2 or 100 mg	d1–5

Every 3 weeks for six to eight cycles.

Figure 1-48. The standard CHOP (cyclophosphamide, doxorubicin, vincristine, and prednisone) regimen. CHOP combination therapy has been used for over 25 years in lymphoma therapy [26–28].

Standard Treatments for Patients with Follicular and Small Lymphocytic Lymphoma

Regimen	Standard Doses
Chlorambucil	16 mg/m²/d x 5 d/mo
	6 mg/d every day
CVP + rituximab	Several regimens described with different doses of cyclophosphamide (intravenously for 1 d, orally for 5 d, and so on) + rituximab 375 mg/m²
Fludarabine + rituximab	25 mg/m²/d x 5 d/mo + rituximab 375 mg/m²
Fludarabine–cyclophospha-mide–rituximab	Fludarabine, 25 mg/m²/d 3 x d; cyclophosphamide, 250 mg/m²/d x 3 d; rituximab, 375 mg/m²
CHOP + rituximab	see Figure 1-48 + rituximab 375 mg/m²

Figure 1-49. Standard treatment for follicular and low-grade lymphocytic lymphoma. The usual treatment of patients is either single-agent chemotherapy with chlorambucil, cyclophosphamide, or fludarabine, or a multidrug regimen such as CVP (cyclophosphamide, vincristine, prednisone), CHOP, or FC (fludarabine plus cyclophosphamide) [29]. However, few prospective studies have been conducted in these lymphomas and optimal therapy for these patients has yet to be identified. These lymphomas are CD20+ but the intensity of the expression of CD20 or other antigens is usually weak. Thus, the putative role of rituximab or other anti-CD20 monoclonal antibodies is not fully determined [30]. Currently, follicular and low-grade lymphocytic lymphoma is considered as a nodal presentation of classic chronic lymphocytic leukemia and thus must be treated according to the same recommendations.

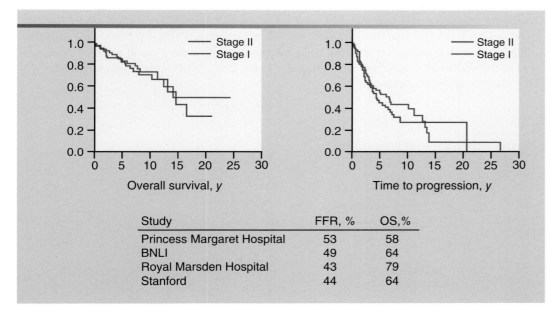

Study	FFR, %	OS,%
Princess Margaret Hospital	53	58
BNLI	49	64
Royal Marsden Hospital	43	79
Stanford	44	64

Figure 1-50. Treatment of localized follicular lymphoma (FL). Approximately 20% of FL patients have localized disease with no bulky tumor mass. In such patients, targeted radiotherapy achieves complete remission in over 95% of cases and relapse-free 10-year survival in 50%. However, the probability of cure is very low because there is no plateau in the survival curve and most of the patients tend to relapse.

This figure shows long-term survival observed in large centers and our personal results with 154 patients with stage I or II FL. If the 10-year survival reflects what was observed in other centers, the time to progression showed that 60% of our patients had progressed at 10 years after initial treatment. Thus, these results may be improved and chemotherapy or monoclonal antibodies have to be included in the treatment of these patients. No randomized data exist to support adjuvant chemotherapy, and only one trial of low-intensity chemotherapy was sufficiently powerful to address the question. Nevertheless, data from a large phase II study from the MD Anderson Cancer Center, Dallas, suggest that combined chemo- and radiotherapy can produce progression-free survival results that are far superior to historical series, with survival at 10 years approximately 20% better than radiation alone [31]. BNLI—British National Lymphoma Investigation; FFR—frequency following response; OS—overall survival.

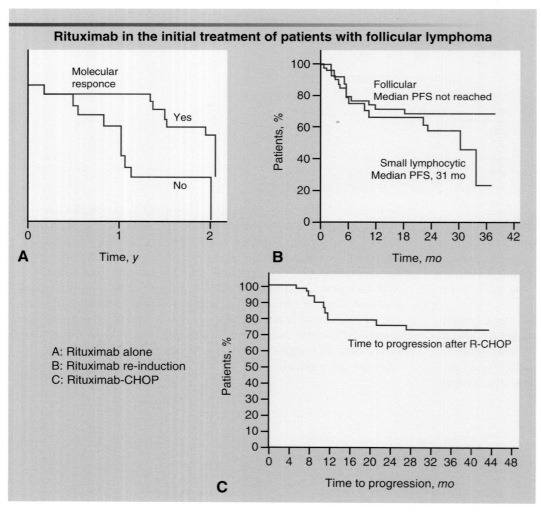

Considerations regarding patients with follicular lymphoma

Disseminated disease without adverse prognostic parameters

Criteria of low tumor burden:
Good performance status
No B symptoms
Diameter of the largest mass < 7 cm (5, 10?)
Normal LDH or β_2-microglobulin levels
No extranodal involvement but bone marrow

GELF-86 study
Overall survival
193 patients with low tumor burden

Failure, %

— Intron A
— No initial treatment
— Chlorambucil

Time, y

Figure 1-51. Treatment of disseminated disease. Treatment of disseminated disease must be based on the presence or absence of adverse prognostic factors. In the absence of adverse prognostic factors at diagnosis, treatment is not mandatory and can be deferred until there is evidence of progression, *ie*, when adverse prognostic factors become apparent.

Spontaneous complete regression occurs in approximately 5% of cases and most other patients may have stable disease for 1 to 4 years depending on the proportion of large cells. However, the disease eventually progresses in most patients, resulting in death (40% to 70% of cases after histologic transformation) after a median survival of 8 to 10 years.

Prospective studies have shown that treatment at diagnosis did not prolong survival in these patients with low tumor burden [32]. For this reason, we recommend that these patients do not start treatment at diagnosis, and that they be monitored until they develop progressive disease with emergence of adverse prognostic factors, and only then treated as described later. Several randomized trials have failed to show a survival benefit for patients with a low tumor burden as a result of early intervention. However, none of these studies were in the rituximab era. GELF-86—Groupe d'Etude des Lymphomes Folliculaires (study); LDH—lactate dehydrogenase.

Rituximab in the initial treatment of patients with follicular lymphoma

Molecular responce

Yes

No

A

Time, y

100
80
60
40
20
0

Patients, %

Follicular
Median PFS not reached

Small lymphocytic
Median PFS, 31 mo

B

Time, mo

A: Rituximab alone
B: Rituximab re-induction
C: Rituximab-CHOP

100
90
80
70
60
50
40
30
20
10
0

Patients, %

Time to progression after R-CHOP

C

Time to progression, mo

Figure 1-52. Rituximab (R) in the initial treatment of patients with follicular lymphoma. When used alone in patients with low tumor burden, rituximab yielded a good response rate (75% with 50% complete response) but was not associated with a long progression-free survival, even in patients with a molecular response (**A**) [33].

Re-induction every 6 months prolonged progression-free survival (PFS) in these patients (**B**) [30]. The combination of rituximab with six cycles of CHOP was associated with the best outcome (**C**) [34]. However, all these studies were phase II, and a direct comparison is not possible because the patients probably had different characteristics. CHOP—cyclophosphamide, doxorubicin, vincristine, prednisone.

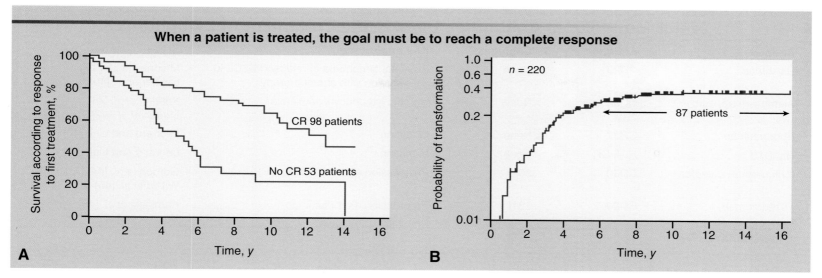

Figure 1-53. When a patient with follicular lymphoma (FL) needs to be treated. **A**, Survival according to first treatment. **B**, Probability of histologic transformation. At least 50% of FL patients require treatment at time of progression or shortly after diagnosis because of the presence of adverse prognostic factors or high tumor bulk. The choice of treatment has long been debated, and prospective randomized studies designed to compare treatments failed to respond because they often included patients with other indolent lymphomas in addition to FL or enrolled patients with and without adverse prognostic factors. Patients with FL, who are often considered incurable, have been treated with nonintensive, nonaggressive therapies such as chlorambucil or cyclophosphamide, vincristine, prednisone. However, it has been shown that achieving complete remission (CR) with the initial treatment results in longer overall and progression-free survival and a lower risk of histologic transformation at relapse [35]. Complete CR must therefore be the aim of first-line treatment, in particular for young patients.

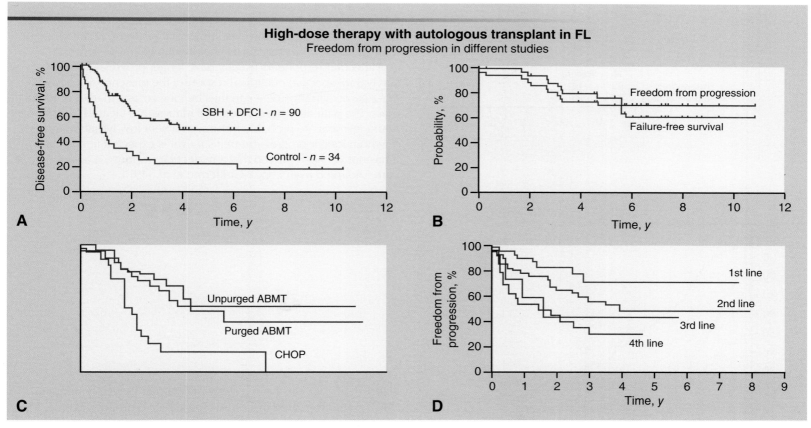

Figure 1-54. High-dose therapy with autologous transplant in follicular lymphoma (FL). For several years, intensive chemotherapy has been combined with autologous stem cell transplantation in the treatment of relapsed FL, using either purged marrow cells or unpurged peripheral cells (**A–C**), and also in first-line patients [36–38]. This treatment significantly prolongs progression-free survival compared with standard chemotherapy regimens (**A**). It has been demonstrated as the best treatment for relapsing patients (**C**), but the ex vivo purging did not decrease the failure rate after transplant. **D**, Data from our center showing that results were better in patients in partial response after first-line or in first relapse than later.

However, efficacy has not been demonstrated in prospective studies and several questions remain, eg, the nature of the intensive therapy, in particular the place of total body irradiation, the place of rituximab, and the optimal timing of intensification.

Although this regimen is probably the most efficacious in relapsing patients, it is not recommended as a first-line therapy, except in prospective therapeutic trials, on account of its potential toxicity. ABMT—autologous bone marrow transplantation; DFCI—Dana Farber Cancer Institute; SBH—St. Bartholomew's Hospital.

Major Monoclonal Antibodies Used in the Treatment of Lymphoma

Antibody	Antigen	Conjugate	Proven Efficacy	Study
Rituximab	CD20	None	Follicular lymphoma in relapsed DLCL in combination with chemotherapy	Maloney *et al.* [39], Coiffier *et al.* [40]
Alemtuzumab	CD52	None	Chronic lymphocytic leukemia	Keating *et al.* [41], Lundin *et al.* [42]
Epratuzumab	CD22	None	In testing	Leonard and Link [43]
Hu1D10	HLA-DR	None	In testing	Leonard and Link [43]
Ibritumomab* tiuxetan	CD20	90Y	Progression after rituximab	Gordon *et al.* [44], Witzig *et al.* [45]
Tositumomab*	CD20	131I	Progression after rituximab	Kaminski *et al.* [46], Vose *et al.* [47]

*Radiolabeled antibodies.

Figure 1-55. Although rituximab is the monoclonal antibody primarily used in patients with follicular lymphoma, others have shown efficacy, particularly the radiolabeled antibodies ^{131}I-tositumomab and ^{90}Y-ibritumomab tiuxetan in follicular lymphoma after failure of rituximab [48]. IL-2R—interleukin-2 receptor; DLCL—diffuse large cell lymphoma.

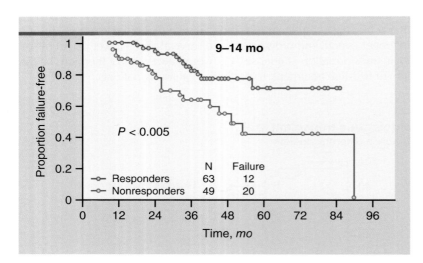

Figure 1-56. Failure-free survival (FFS) of patients with follicular lymphoma (FL) according to molecular response (polymerase chain reaction status in responders: negative; in nonresponders: positive) assessed in peripheral blood at 9 to 14 months after the onset of therapy ($P < 0.005$).

Follicular lymphoma displays *bcl-2* gene rearrangement in more than 80% of cases. Some studies have suggested that complete remission is longer when molecular markers of rearrangement disappear (molecular response). However, molecular response in the blood or marrow does not always correlate with clinical remission.

Molecular responders usually have longer progression-free survival irrespective of clinical response; the presence of cells with *bcl-2* gene rearrangement can thus be viewed as a marker of tumor mass. The patients whose blood and marrow are cleared of *bcl-2* gene rearrangement are probably those with a very low lymphoma mass, in whom longer progression-free survival is expected in any case. It has not yet been proved that a molecular response is a surrogate of cure. (*Adapted from* Lopez-Guillermo *et al.* [49].)

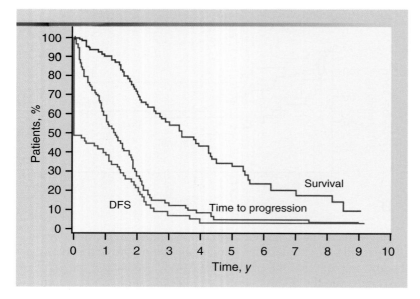

Figure 1-57. Results from a study of 119 mantle cell lymphoma (MCL) patients treated in Centre Hospitalier Lyon-Sud, France. MCL is usually resistant to currently available treatment options. Treatment generally achieves incomplete regression at best, and only for a brief 6 to 18 months; progression then occurs with at best partial response to any therapy, and then death after a median survival of 3 to 4 years [50]. DFS—disease-free survival.

A — Rituximab Alone in Relapsing Mantle Cell Lymphoma Patients

Study	Patients, n	OR, n (%)
Coiffier et al. 1998	12	4 (33)
Nguyen et al. 1999	10	2 (20)
Foran et al. 2000	50	19 (37)
Ghielmini et al. 2000	39	9 (22)
Total	111	34 (31)

B — FCM versus R-FCM in Mantle Cell Lymphoma*

	FCM	R-FCM
Complete response, %	0	29
Partial response, %	46	29
PD, %	42	29
EX, %	13	0
Complete and partial response, %	46	58

*Fludarabine, 25 mg/m² d1–3; cyclophosphamide, 200 mg/m² d1–3; mitoxantrone, 8 mg/m² d1; rituximab, 375 mg/m² d0–1.

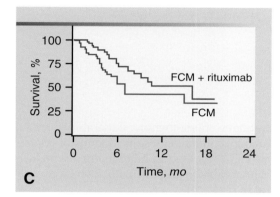

C

Figure 1-58. Rituximab in relapsing mantle cell lymphoma (MCL) patients. **A–C,** Standard chemotherapy regimens failed to improve survival but most investigators believe that CHOP or a combination with high-dose aracytine secures a higher response rate, with no clear difference in terms of overall survival. Fludarabine failed to improve on these results, but rituximab achieved a 30% to 40% response in relapsing patients. A recent trial showed that rituximab combined with the FCM (fludarabine, cyclophosphamide, mitoxantrone) regimen allowed a better response and a longer duration of response [51]. Bortezomib has recently been approved for patients with relapsed MCL based on response rates of 35% to 50%

In a recent presentation, the combination of CHOP plus rituximab (R-CHOP) allowed a greater than 90% response rate with 50% of the patients in complete remission for previously untreated patients. However, patients relapsed with event-free survival (EFS) similar to that commonly reported. If a clearing of blood and bone marrow involvement was observed in 50% of the responding patients, these patients did not have longer EFS [52].

First-line treatment with intensive chemotherapy combined with autologous stem cell transplantation (ASCT) gave remarkable results in one study, but unfortunately the results were unconfirmed in two other studies [53]. The combination of rituximab with chemotherapy before harvesting the peripheral blood stem cell (in vivo purge) and ASCT with total body irradiation may be the most promising treatment, but long-term results are not yet known [54].

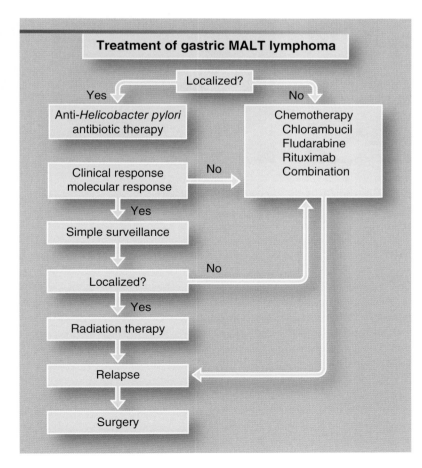

Figure 1-59. Gastric mucosa-associated lymphoid tissue (MALT) lymphomas may regress after anti-*Helicobacter pylori* antibiotic therapy. Ongoing prospective studies are evaluating the survival benefit of this treatment, which must be confined to gastric lymphoma patients without intra-abdominal lymph node involvement. A 2-week combination of two antibiotics, generally amoxicillin and metronidazole, plus an antacid such as omeprazole or bismuth, eliminates *H. pylori* in 90% of cases and achieves complete regression of the lymphoma in 60%, although this may take several weeks or months. What may be left is either a nonlymphomatous lymphocytic gastritis or a few lymphomatous cells detectable only by the presence of immunoglobulin gene rearrangement. Although it has not been shown that this treatment prolongs progression-free survival, the low-grade potential of this lymphoma means that this conservative approach should be recommended in the majority of cases.

For patients responding only partially to antibiotic therapy and in relapsing patients, radiation therapy is the best treatment choice [26]. In patients with more advanced disease, chemotherapy with chlorambucil, fludarabine, or rituximab achieves a good response. In some cases with extensive persistent tumor or resistance to standard treatment, the lymphoma can be resected by total gastrectomy because the lesions are multifocal. However, given the operative morbidity and postoperative impact on quality of life, gastrectomy should be confined to disease failing to respond to correctly administered previous therapy.

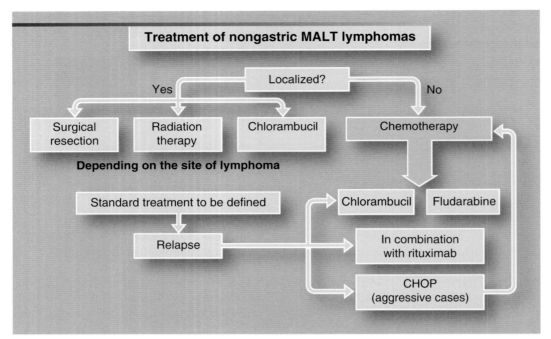

Treatment of nongastric MALT lymphomas

Figure 1-60. Treatment of nongastric mucosa-associated lymphoid tissue (MALT) lymphomas. Patients with localized nongastric MALT lymphoma can be treated by surgical resection, local radiotherapy, or chlorambucil, depending of the site of the lymphoma, the demand of the patient, and the opinion of the physician, although few prospective studies have been performed to confirm the validity of these options. Given the late complications of radiotherapy and the sequelae of surgical resection, chlorambucil (16 mg/m^2/d for 5 days per month for 6 to 12 months) is the ideal treatment in most of the patients.

Disseminated disease requires chemotherapy: fludarabine, chlorambucil, and rituximab give identical results in terms of complete response. However, CHOP (cyclophosphamide, doxorubicin, vincristine, prednisone) is preferable in patients with extensive tumor or a high contingent of large cells.

Relapse may occur either at the initial site or in other extranodal sites. Chemotherapy with chlorambucil or multidrug regimens has achieved identical results in patients with more disseminated disease.

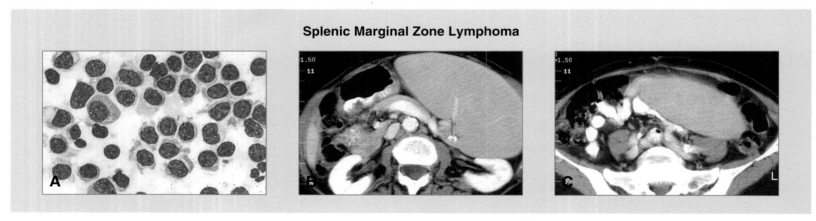

Splenic Marginal Zone Lymphoma

Figure 1-61. Splenic marginal zone lymphoma. This figure shows the characteristics of splenic marginal zone lymphoma, with the large splenomegaly, the blood and bone marrow involvement, and the absence of location in lymph nodes or extranodal sites. **A**, Cytology. **B** and **C**, Spleen.

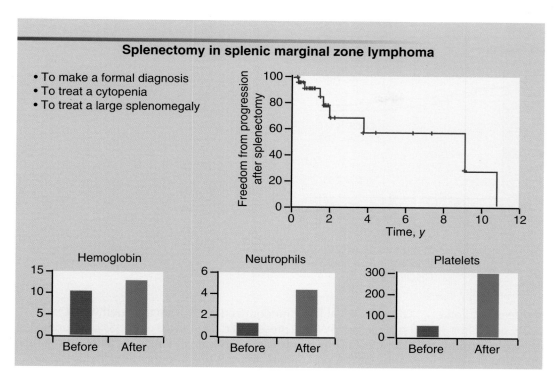

Figure 1-62. Splenectomy in splenic marginal zone lymphoma (MZL). Patients with splenic MZL, with or without villous lymphocytes, are often elderly and have a long history before diagnosis. In this nonaggressive disease with marked splenomegaly, delayed treatment may initially be offered to patients with limited splenomegaly; however, splenectomy is certainly the treatment of choice. Splenectomy is indicated when the diagnosis is uncertain because of the absence of blood or bone marrow involvement, because of a cytopenia, or because of a large splenomegaly and discomfort or pain [55].

Splenectomy is associated with a long response even it only is a partial response [56]. Bone marrow infiltration may decrease, but in all cases, patients improved their performance status and their hemoglobin, neutrophil, and platelet levels. Lymphocytosis may develop after but usually takes time to reach alarming levels. Chemotherapy, including rituximab, should be reserved for relapse after splenectomy and transformation into a more aggressive lymphoma.

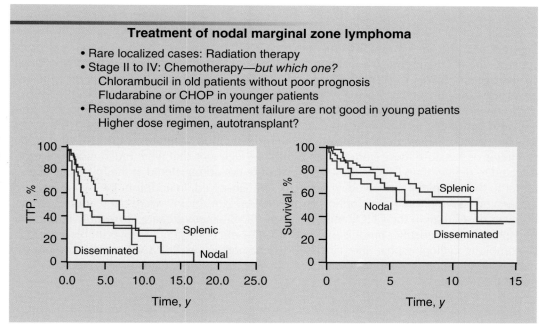

Figure 1-63. Treatment of nodal marginal zone lymphoma (MZL). Young patients with nodal MZL require prompt treatment given the progression potential of the disease, but no prospective study has defined the most appropriate treatment. In our experience, progression-free survival is fairly short in such patients, but overall survival tends to be long. This suggests that there could be successive responses to the different treatments used.

Local radiotherapy can be used for highly localized disease and R-CHOP (rituximab plus cyclophosphamide, doxorubicin, vincristine, prednisone) for more disseminated disease. However, no prospective study exists for such patients and the best treatment is not known. Intensive chemotherapy with autologous stem cell transplantation should only be considered in these patients if they are refractory to the standard treatments or have a high contingent of transformed cells. TTP—time to progression.

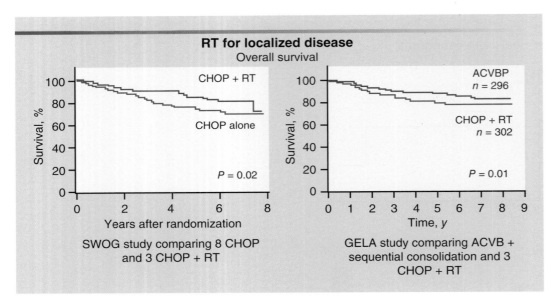

Figure 1-64. Radiation therapy (RT) for localized disease. Patients with the best prognosis have highly localized disease and a normal lactate dehydrogenase (LDH) or β_2-microglobulin levels and no adverse prognostic factor. Such patients can be cured using standard treatments, *ie*, three cycles of CHOP (cyclophosphamide, doxorubicin, vincristine, prednisone) followed by local RT for stage I patients, or six to eight cycles of CHOP for those with more aggressive disease. The most intensive treatments should be reserved for patients failing to achieve complete remission or relapsing on standard treatment. The aim of current ongoing studies is to determine the optimal number of chemotherapy cycles and evaluate the need for local RT. A randomized study from the Southwest Oncology Group (SWOG) presented data in favor of RT [57]. An update of these data showed the same survival with a longer follow-up in both arms [58]. A preliminary analysis of a Groupe d'Etude des Lymphomes de l'Adulte (GELA) trial showed equally the same survival with or without radiation therapy [59].

Currently, there has been no demonstration of the advantage of radiotherapy in standard patients with aggressive localized lymphoma, but if radiotherapy is not used, at least four cycles of chemotherapy must be administered to the patient. ACVBP—doxorubicin, cyclophosphamide, vindesine, bleomycin, prednisolone.

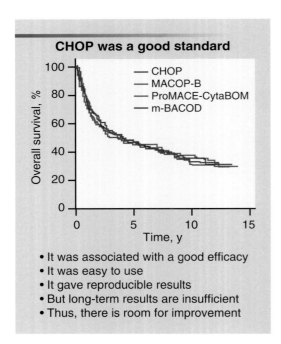

- It was associated with a good efficacy
- It was easy to use
- It gave reproducible results
- But long-term results are insufficient
- Thus, there is room for improvement

Figure 1-65. The need for improvement in the CHOP regimen (cyclophosphamide, doxorubicin, vincristine, prednisone). Patients with more disseminated disease, elevated lactate dehydrogenase levels, or β_2-microglobulin levels or B symptoms, *ie*, one of the recognized adverse prognostic factors, have a worse outcome than the group designed in Figure 1-66. These patients may require more intensive treatment than CHOP to achieve complete remission and cure, but this has not been conclusively demonstrated—several randomized studies have failed to show greater efficacy by "third-generation" chemotherapy [28].

However, because these studies used multidrug regimens that were much more complicated to deliver than CHOP, they were probably not administered at the full dose, due either to the complexity involved or to the toxicity observed. In addition, the two drugs most active against lymphoma—cyclophosphamide and doxorubicin—were often administered at lower doses than in the CHOP regimen. MACOP-B—methotrexate, doxorubicin, cyclophosphamide, vincristine, prednisone; m-BACOD—methotrexate, leucovorin, bleomycin, doxorubicin, cyclophosphamide, vincristine, dexamethasone; ProMACE-cytaBOM—prednisone, doxorubicin, cyclophosphamide, etoposide, cytarabine, bleomycin, vincristine, methotrexate, leucovorin.

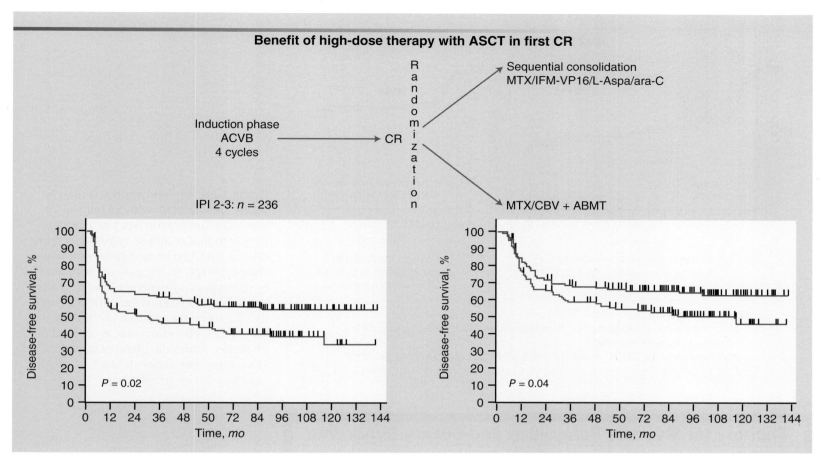

Benefit of high-dose therapy with ASCT in first CR

Figure 1-66. Benefit of high-dose therapy with autologous stem cell transplantation (ASCT). Patients with more than one adverse prognostic factor have a lower response rate to chemotherapy and a higher relapse rate. In such patients, high-dose therapy followed by ASCT has achieved longer progression-free and overall survival than standard treatments in different randomized studies [60–62]. However, these results were not confirmed in other studies differing slightly in design and patient population. Consequently, the jury at the most recent Consensus Conference on Intensive Chemotherapy and ASCT concluded that intensification as first-line therapy could not be recommended in these patients but suggested that it may be of utility for patients with high-risk aggressive lymphoma who respond to their first chemotherapy [63].

Some centers, including the Groupe d'Etude des Lymphomes de l'Adulte (GELA), believe that currently available results are conclusive and consider that first-line intensification should be the standard treatment for young patients with more than one adverse prognostic factor and who reach a complete or good response to standard chemotherapy. It has been demonstrated that performing ASCT early in patients who are still not in good response was not associated with any benefit [64,65]. ABMT—autologous bone marrow transplantation; MTX—methotrexate.

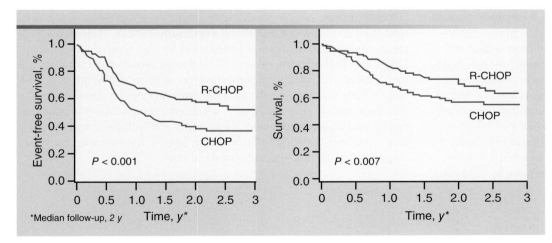

Figure 1-67. Results of the first randomized study with rituximab therapy for lymphoma. In this study, the Groupe d'Etude des Lymphomes de l'Adulte (GELA) showed that adding a monoclonal antibody to standard chemotherapy improved survival of elderly patients with diffuse large cell lymphoma [66]. Although several monoclonal antibodies have efficacy in the treatment of lymphoma patients, rituximab was the only one that has proven this efficacy in a randomized study. CHOP—cyclophosphamide, doxorubicin, vincristine, prednisone. R-CHOP—CHOP+rituximab.

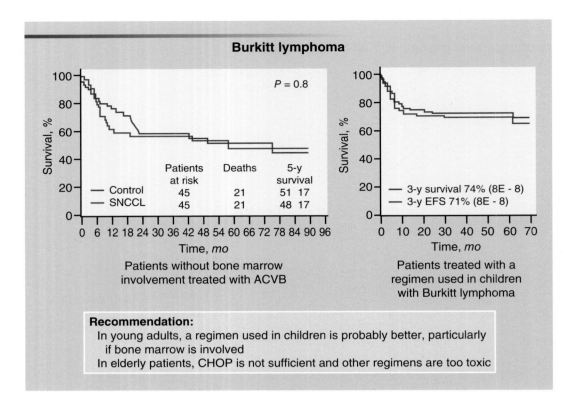

Figure 1-68. Burkitt lymphoma (BL). In adults, localized BL without marrow or meningeal infiltration has a prognosis similar to that of diffuse large B-cell lymphoma (DLCL) if treated with combination chemotherapy. Young patients with marrow or meningeal involvement have a poorer prognosis and require the same regimens that have proved effective in children [70,71]. ACVB—doxorubicin, cyclophosphamide, vindesine, bleomycin, prednisone. EFS—event-free survival; SNCCL—small noncleaved cell lymphomas.

Therapy for Mycosis Fungoides and Sézary Syndrome

Therapy	Comments
Topical nitrogen mustard	Now largely abandoned
PUVA photochemotherapy	For low-grade nonextensive disease
PUVA + interferon	For PUVA failure, or more aggressive disease at diagnosis
Total skin electron beam therapy	—
Systemic chemotherapy (cladribine, interferon-alfa, retinoid)	After failure of combination therapy

Figure 1-69. Therapy for mycosis fungoides and Sézary syndrome. Survival is fairly long in most patients with cytotoxic T-cell lymphoma, although treatments rarely achieve complete remission. Four therapies have been found to achieve fairly long remissions: topical nitrogen mustard, now largely abandoned; psoralen photochemotherapy (PUVA); total skin electron beam therapy; and systemic chemotherapy (cladribine, interferon-alfa, or retinoid). At diagnosis, PUVA therapy alone is recommended for low-grade nonextensive disease. Combination PUVA therapy plus interferon is recommended for patients failing to respond to PUVA alone, or for patients with more aggressive disease at diagnosis. After failure of combination therapy, adding a retinoid (etretinate) to the interferon may help, but in all cases the disease eventually progresses to involve the entire skin surface where it forms tumor nodules, subsequently infiltrating the satellite nodes, deep nodes, and finally the viscera. Chemotherapy generally delays progression, but no treatment is curative. Unfortunately, most patients eventually develop large cutaneous or visceral tumors, often converting to large cell lymphoma. These are refractory to treatment and death eventually ensues. New treatment modalities are absolutely essential for this type of lymphoma. Ontak is a DAB389 interleukin (IL)-2 fusion protein that combines the cytotoxic A chain of diphtheria toxin with recombinant IL-2 and targets cells that express the IL-2 receptor. Vorinostat (suberoylanilide hydroxamic acid [SAHA]) is a histone deacetylace inhibitor and has recently been appro ved for patients with relapsed and refractory cutaneous T-cell lymphoma. Both agents achieve about a 30% response rate in heavily pretreated patients.

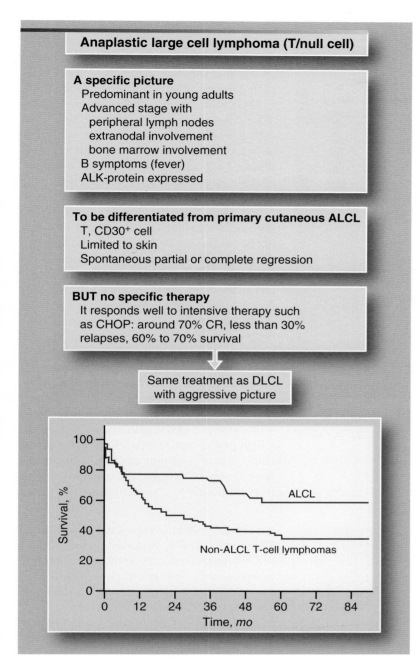

Anaplastic large cell lymphoma (T/null cell)

A specific picture
Predominant in young adults
Advanced stage with
    peripheral lymph nodes
    extranodal involvement
    bone marrow involvement
B symptoms (fever)
ALK-protein expressed

To be differentiated from primary cutaneous ALCL
T, CD30$^+$ cell
Limited to skin
Spontaneous partial or complete regression

BUT no specific therapy
It responds well to intensive therapy such as CHOP: around 70% CR, less than 30% relapses, 60% to 70% survival

Same treatment as DLCL with aggressive picture

Figure 1-70. Anaplastic large cell lymphoma. Large T or null cell anaplastic lymphomas (ALCL) are found mainly in young adults. In systemic ALCL, disease is usually aggressive with several adverse prognostic factors, but patients respond well to a high-dose chemotherapy regimen: 5-year survival in complete remission is 60% to 70%. The same treatment strategy used in diffuse large B-cell lymphoma (DLCL) is recommended in systemic ALCL [67].

Patients with primary cutaneous involvement have low-grade disease and usually require nonintensive therapy.

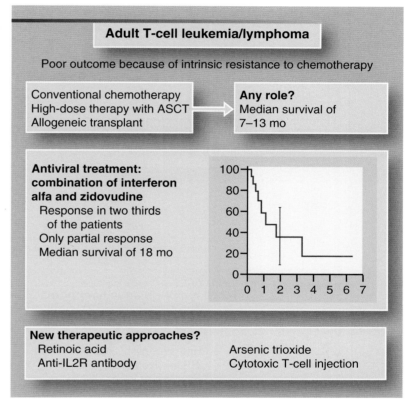

Adult T-cell leukemia/lymphoma

Poor outcome because of intrinsic resistance to chemotherapy

Conventional chemotherapy
High-dose therapy with ASCT
Allogeneic transplant

Any role?
Median survival of 7–13 mo

Antiviral treatment: combination of interferon alfa and zidovudine
Response in two thirds of the patients
Only partial response
Median survival of 18 mo

New therapeutic approaches?
Retinoic acid
Anti-IL2R antibody
Arsenic trioxide
Cytotoxic T-cell injection

Figure 1-71. Adult T-cell leukemia/lymphoma (ATL). ATL patients are normally considered refractory to CHOP (cyclophosphamide, doxorubicin, vincristine, prednisone) or other therapeutic regimens. The combination of interferon alfa plus zidovudine has been reported to achieve high response rates. These results require large-scale confirmation but appear promising [68,69]. Other modalities are currently tested but none has implemented it as a standard. ASCT—autologous stem cell transplantation.

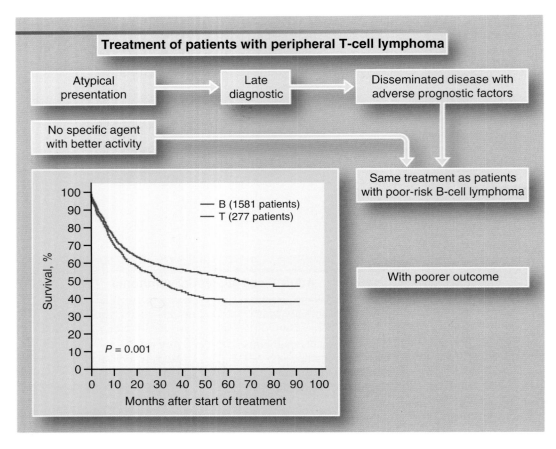

Figure 1-72. Peripheral T-cell lymphomas and T/natural killer (NK) cell lymphomas. Clinical presentations of these patients vary greatly and very few studies have identified such patients before starting treatment.

Patients usually receive the same treatment as for diffuse large cell lymphoma (DLCL) but with generally much poorer results, in particular in terms of overall survival. In retrospective studies, T-cell lymphoma always has a higher relapse rate and shorter progression-free survival than aggressive B-cell lymphoma.

However, intensification plus autologous stem cell transplantation at first remission has not been shown to lead to improved results. Although some centers treat such patients with regimens that differ from those used in DLCL, these regimens are not supported with firm evidence of improved results.

Patients with NK cell lymphoma or γδ T-cell lymphoma are usually refractory to CHOP (cyclophosphamide, doxorubicin, vincristine, prednisone), showing an initial incomplete response with very rapid progression and median survival less than 12 months. Localized radiotherapy does not greatly improve outcome.

Peripheral T-cell lymphoma patients with a high percentage of small T cells or reactive cells, as in angioimmunoblastic lymphoma, have slowly progressive disease and may respond poorly to chemotherapy.

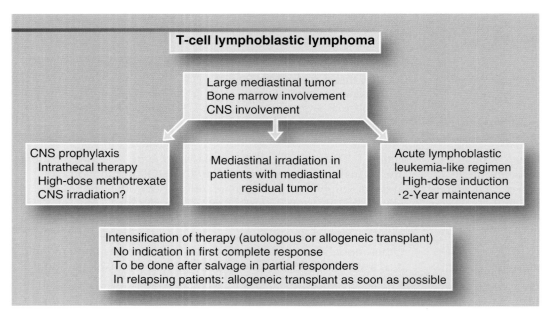

Figure 1-73. T-cell lymphoblastic lymphoma (TLL). Patients with TLL may present with localized nodal disease, particularly in the mediastinum, or disseminated disease involving lymph nodes, bone marrow, and central nervous system (CNS). The best therapeutic approach is thought to be an acute lymphoblastic leukemia (ALL) treatment [72,73]. Complete remission is achieved in 80% of patients but the relapse rate is approximately 30%, whereas only 40% to 50% of

patients achieve long-term survival in complete remission [74]. Systematic prophylaxis of CNS relapse is an important issue: it must comprise early onset of intrathecal chemotherapy and high-dose methotrexate or cytarabine. The role of CNS irradiation is less clear.

Mediastinal recurrence is frequent in persisting CT scan abnormalities and it may be prevented by intensifying the chemotherapy in patients with large mediastinal tumor and doing local irradiation at a dose of 36 Gy.

First-line intensive chemotherapy with autologous or allogeneic transplant does seem to decrease the relapse rate in adults and it should be reserved for patients with partial response. The analysis of published prognostic factors demonstrates that no convincing risk model is available. However, doing allogeneic transplant in second complete response is the only chance for long survival in these patients and they should be transplanted as soon as possible after relapse. The challenge is to develop a good salvage regimen.

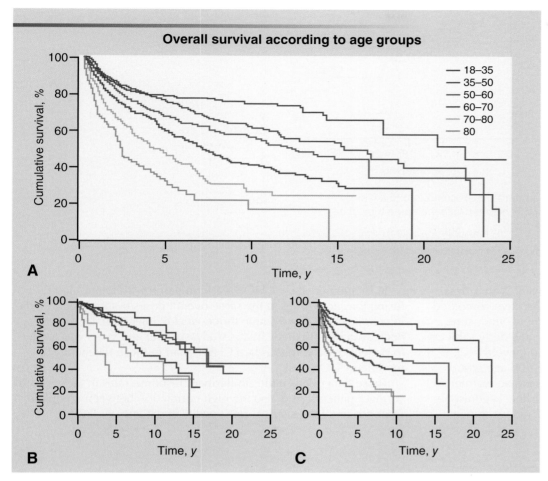

Figure 1-74. Overall survival according to age groups. Complete remission rates decline steadily with age, from 68% in the young to 45% in the elderly. Mean relapse-free and overall survival also decline with age. All studies show shorter survival in elderly versus younger patients matched for lymphoma and characteristics; the difference persists after correction for non–lymphoma-related deaths. The shorter survival has been ascribed to two main causes: a tendency by physicians to administer weaker, "better-tolerated" (hence less effective) treatment in the elderly; and poor drug tolerability in the elderly, largely due to the presence of concomitant disease.

This figure shows the overall survival of 3320 patients with lymphoma (**A**). Whatever the type of lymphoma, stage, and treatment, survival regularly decreased with age groups but was still 25% for patients 70 to 80 years of age and 20% for patients older than 80 years at 10 years. This was observed for patients with follicular lymphoma (**B**) or diffuse large B-cell lymphoma (**C**) even if the effect of age was less pronounced in follicular lymphoma.

As in young patients, therapy for elderly patients must be based on the type of lymphoma and the presence or absence of adverse prognostic factors. Given their age and above all the presence of concomitant disease, the elderly have been considered ineligible for treatment with regimens that are usually curative in the young.

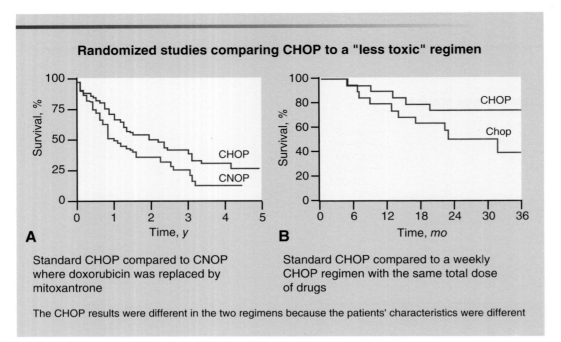

Figure 1-75. Randomized studies comparing CHOP with a "less toxic" regimen. Several recent randomized studies have compared results with CHOP (cyclophosphamide, doxorubicin, vincristine, prednisone) to those using less-intensive therapy in elderly subjects with diffuse large B-cell lymphoma (DLCL). **A**, Sonneveld et al. [75] showed that CHOP was well tolerated in the over-60 age group; toxicity did not differ from that of a reputedly less toxic regimen, CNOP (cyclophosphamide, mitoxantrone, vincristine, prednisone); the complete remission rate was also higher and survival longer with the CHOP regimen.

B, In another study, CHOP was compared with a modified CHOP (using the same drugs at the same overall doses but in three weekly injections instead of a single thrice-weekly injection), leading to decreased drug toxicity. In this study, survival at 2 years was longer in patients receiving standard CHOP than in those receiving the modified CHOP [76].

These data confirm the similarity of response rates in elderly and younger patients, and also the high correlation between complete response and long survival irrespective of patient age [77].

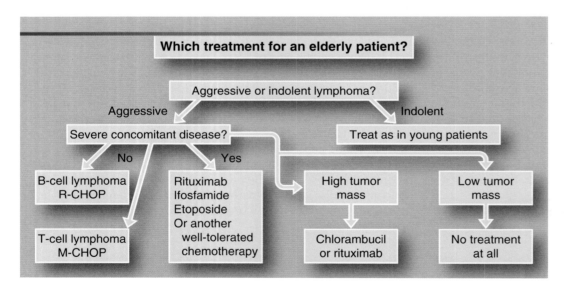

Figure 1-76. Treatment decision making for the elderly patient. Age must also be integrated in the decision process; the old elderly patients (> 80 to 85 years of age) are only proposed a palliative treatment if they have to be treated.

Epstein-Barr virus–related Subtypes and Therapy for Lymphoproliferative Disorders	
Related to Transplant Recipients and Immunodeficient Patients	
Type of LPD	Treatment
PTLD	
Benign polyclonal polymorphic B-cell hyperplasia	Antiviral drugs, *eg*, acyclovir
Early malignant transformation in polyclonal polymorphic lymphoma	Light immunosuppressive regimen plus decrease in immunosuppressive regimen
Monoclonal polymorphic B-cell lymphoma	Appropriate chemotherapy plus decrease in immunosuppressive regimen

Figure 1-77. Types of and therapy for lymphoproliferative disorders (LPDs) related to transplant recipients and immunodeficient patients. Epstein-Barr virus (EBV) has been implicated in the origin of a wide range of LPDs associated with organ and allogeneic marrow transplantation, congenital immunodeficiency (Wiskott-Aldrich syndrome, ataxia-telangiectasia, and severe combined immunodeficiency), and AIDS. LPDs account for almost 90% of post-transplant lymphomas. Post-transplant LPD (PTLD) have been classified into three groups, as listed in this table. The first PTLD is an infectious disease and can often be cured using antiviral drugs such as acyclovir. The second group may respond to a lighter immunosuppressive regimen. Patients with monoclonal polymorphic lymphoma, on the other hand, require appropriate chemotherapy combined with a decrease in immunosuppressive regimen. The ProMACE-CytaBOM protocol—combining prednisone, doxorubicin, cyclophosphamide and etoposide, followed by cytarabine, bleomycin, vincristine, methotrexate, and folinic acid—has given the best therapeutic results. Rituximab has recently been used in PTLD, with remission in 50% of cases. Late-onset PTLD tends to be less associated with EBV and requires standard chemotherapy.

Epstein-Barr virus–related lymphoma has been described in patients receiving long-term immunosuppressive therapy, *eg*, methotrexate for rheumatoid arthritis. Withdrawal of the immunosuppression has been followed by regression of the lymphoma in some cases.

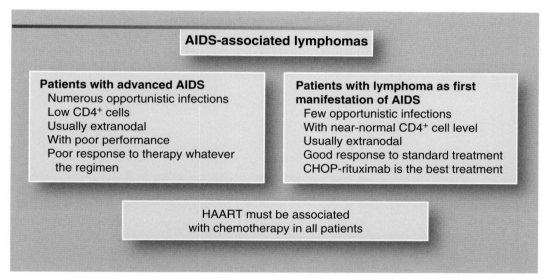

Figure 1-78. Five lymphoma types have been described in AIDS: DLCL, with and without plasma cell differentiation; Burkitt lymphoma; ALCL; and EBV-related LPD. Lymphoma may develop in an HIV-positive subject as the first sign of AIDS or in patients with advanced AIDS and a history of multiple opportunistic infections, in which case it tends to be extranodal and often cerebral, although atypical sites may well be involved. Treatment cannot be curative in such patients, who usually die from an infectious complication, sometimes as a result of the chemotherapy. The impact of highly active antiretroviral therapy (HAART) on the incidence of these lymphomas remains a matter of debate.

Lymphoma as a presentation of AIDS occurs in patients previously free of infectious manifestations of the disease, at low risk of opportunistic infection, and who have maintained a high CD4+ lymphocyte count. Although such patients have a relatively poor prognosis, they need treatment with an appropriate chemotherapy regimen to avoid early death from lymphoma. The lymphoma is usually disseminated, involving the bone marrow or brain. Standard treatments achieve the best results. CHOP— cyclophosphamide, doxorubicin, vincristine, prednisone

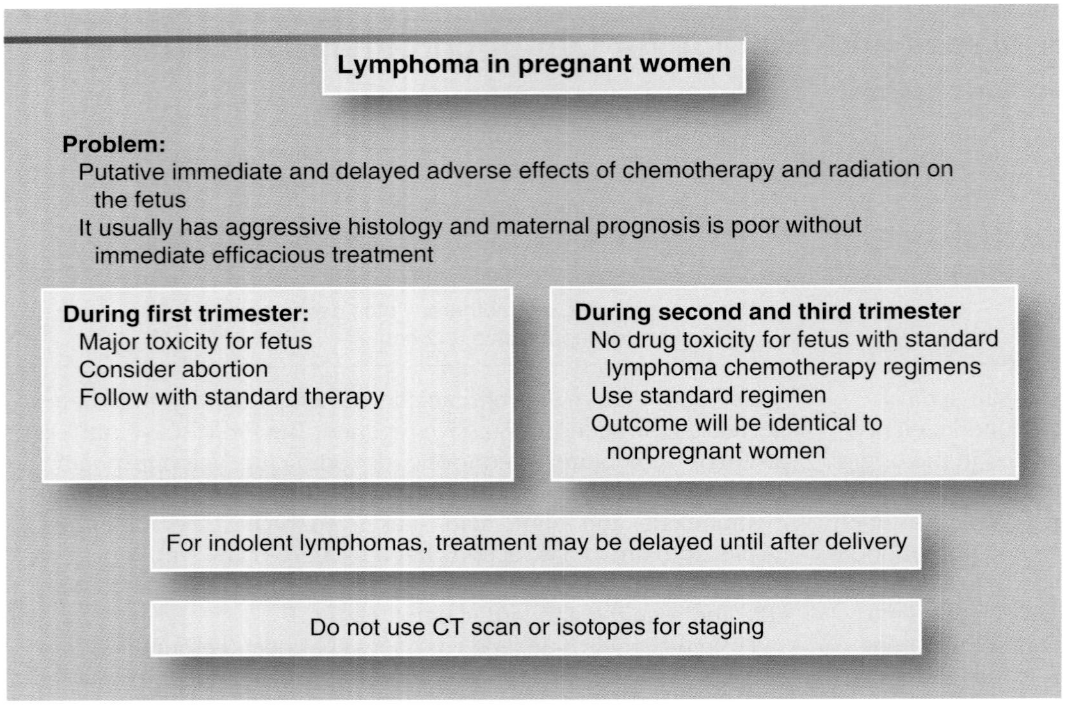

Lymphoma in pregnant women

Problem:
Putative immediate and delayed adverse effects of chemotherapy and radiation on the fetus
It usually has aggressive histology and maternal prognosis is poor without immediate efficacious treatment

During first trimester:
Major toxicity for fetus
Consider abortion
Follow with standard therapy

During second and third trimester
No drug toxicity for fetus with standard lymphoma chemotherapy regimens
Use standard regimen
Outcome will be identical to nonpregnant women

For indolent lymphomas, treatment may be delayed until after delivery

Do not use CT scan or isotopes for staging

Figure 1-79. The occurrence of a lymphoma during pregnancy is rare. To protect the fetus, staging procedures require noninvasive radiologic examinations. Most lymphomas occurring during pregnancy are of disseminated stage. Treatment choices during pregnancy raise difficult problems because of the putative immediate and delayed adverse effects of chemotherapy and radiation on the fetus. Lymphomas associated with pregnancy usually have an aggressive histology, and maternal prognosis is poor without an efficacious treatment administered as soon as possible. Treatment with a multi-drug regimen may allow the achievement of high complete remission rates and long survival. These regimens have been used in the second and third trimester without apparent deleterious effect to the fetus. Women with an aggressive lymphoma during the first trimester should be considered for a therapeutic abortion and immediate treatment with a multidrug regimen.

Gastrointestinal Tract Lymphomas

Site	Entity	Incidence*	Treatment	Outcome
Esophagus	All	Very rare	See other	See other
Stomach	MALT	50%	Antibiotics then chemotherapy or RT	Very good
	Other indolent	Very rare	As other DLCL	Good
	DLCL	20%	As other Burkitt	Good
	Burkitt	< 1%	As other PTCL	Good
	PTCL	< 1%		Poor
Duodenum	Follicular	Rare	As other FL	Good
	MALT	Rare	As other MALT	Good
Small intestine	MALT	10%	Chemotherapy	Very good
	Follicular	< 1%	Chemotherapy	Good
	DLCL	5%	As other DLCL	Good
	PTCL	Rare	No good treatment	Poor
Colon	MCL	5% rare	Chemotherapy	Poor
	DLCL	5% rare	As other DLCL	Good
Rectum	MALT	< 1% rare	Chemotherapy	Very good
	DLCL		As other DLCL	Good

*Incidence is given as the percentage of all gastrointestinal lymphomas.

Figure 1-80. Gastrointestinal tract lymphomas. Just over 50% of gastrointestinal lymphomas are of the mucosa-associated lymphoid tissue (MALT) variety; they are usually localized and associated with high long-term survival. The second largest entity comprises large cell lymphomas and Burkitt lymphoma, which carry a much poorer prognosis, even if localized. However, large cell lymphomas are often transformations of previously undetected MALT lymphomas, as shown by the presence of residual small cell infiltration. There is no consensus defining either the grading of gastric MALT lymphoma, the percentage of large cells required to diagnose transformation, the prognostic significance of such transformation, or the therapeutic implication of finding foci of large cells in a gastric MALT lymphoma.

Diagnosis is relatively easy following endoscopy of the stomach or colon, but often requires laparotomy for small intestine lymphoma. Small intestine diffuse large B-cell lymphoma (DLCL) is typically insidious in onset, presenting as acute intestinal obstruction. No robust study has shown a difference in results between total or partial resection in gastrointestinal DLCL. Wide resection must be avoided in all cases, appropriate and effective chemotherapy being used to present the surgical complications of hemorrhage and perforation. Except for the early treatment with antibiotics in gastric MALT lymphoma, treatment should be identical to that for nongastrointestinal lymphomas similar in histology and severity. FL—follicular lymphoma; MCL—mantle cell lymphoma; PTCL—peripheral T-cell lymphoma; RT—radiation therapy.

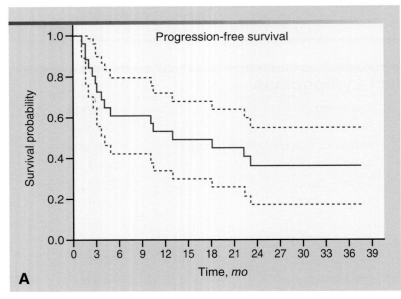

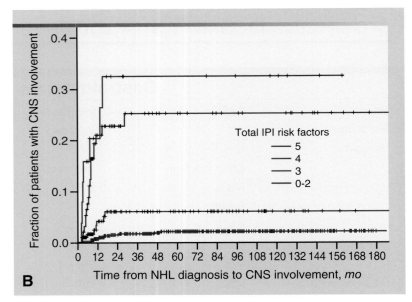

Figure 1-81. Central nervous system lymphomas are usually localized diffuse large B-cell lymphoma (DLCL). Surgery is of no clinical benefit and should therefore be reserved for diagnostic biopsy. Radiotherapy carries a median survival of 12 months and is noncurative, with local relapse in 90% of cases. Chemotherapy regimens with high-dose and intrathecal methotrexate usually achieve complete remission. In combination with radiotherapy, chemotherapy achieves a median survival of 30 months, but the local relapse rate remains high. The optimal chemotherapy regimen and requirement for adjuvant radiotherapy remain to be defined. Prospective studies in such patients are essential. **A,** Progression-free survival for patients treated with high-dose methotrexate (*dots* represent 95% CI) [78].

B, Central nervous system relapse occurs in 5% of DLCL or peripheral T-cell lymphoma (PTCL), more frequently in lymphoblastic lymphoma or Burkitt's lymphoma, and rarely (probably only after transformation) in indolent lymphoma. Meningeal prophylaxis is mandatory in patients with a Burkitt or lymphoblastic lymphoma. For those with DLCL or PTCL, the role of cerebrospinal fluid examination at diagnosis is controversial. Higher risk patients are those with bone marrow and multiple extranodal involvements. Prophylaxis is useful in bone marrow involvement, poor International Prognostic Index (IPI) score, or high lactate dehydrogenase level [79].

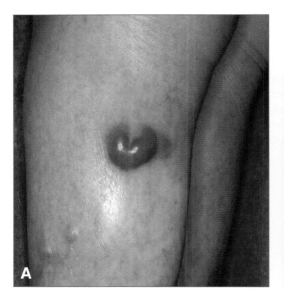

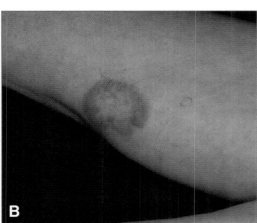

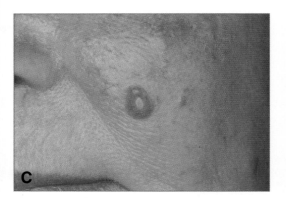

Figure 1-82. Cutaneous involvement occurs as an ancillary feature in most types of lymphoma, and as the primary presenting feature in cutaneous T-cell lymphoma, cutaneous diffuse large B-cell lymphoma (DLCL), and CD30+ cutaneous lymphoproliferative disorder, a benign condition that can regress spontaneously.

In cutaneous anaplastic T-cell lymphoma (ALCL), spread beyond the skin occurs only at a late stage and such presentations should not be confused with nodal ALCL. The disease is usually localized and simple nodule excision achieves remission. Patients with several cutaneous foci can be treated with chlorambucil.

Primary cutaneous DLCL may be localized for a long period, but usually spreads to noncutaneous sites eventually. Location on the

legs is associated with a much poorer outcome and should probably be treated at diagnosis (**A**). The appropriate treatment for such patients is unknown: local radiotherapy or CHOP chemotherapy (cyclophosphamide, doxorubicin, vincristine, prednisone).

Follicular lymphoma and marginal zone lymphoma account for a substantial proportion of primary cutaneous DLCL (**B** and **C**). If the disease is localized, it can be treated with local therapy, radiotherapy or surgery, but the lymphoma is usually disseminated at presentation, in which case it responds to the same treatments as for the noncutaneous forms.

Aspects of Bone Lymphoma
Localized
Disseminated in several bone sites
Associated with nonbone sites
Treatment as for nonosseous lymphomas of similar histology

Figure 1-83. Aspects of bone lymphoma. Bone lymphoma can be localized, disseminated in several bone sites, or associated with nonbone sites. Diffuse large B-cell lymphoma (DLCL) is more often responsible than other lymphomas. Such patients should be treated as for nonosseous lymphomas of similar histology. The specificity of these lymphomas is that the radiologic bone abnormalities persist long after the infiltrating lymphoma has disappeared, making it difficult to determine when complete remission has been achieved. The utility of local radiotherapy has not been demonstrated.

TREATMENT STRATEGIES BASED ON THE INITIAL TREATMENT RESPONSE

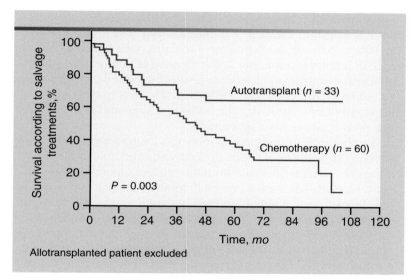

Allotransplanted patient excluded

Figure 1-84. Autologous transplantation versus conventional salvage therapy in aggressive non-Hodgkin lymphoma partially responding to first-line chemotherapy: a study of 94 patients enrolled in the LNH87-2 protocol. Fewer than 70% of lymphoma patients achieve complete remission with their initial therapy, and approximately 40% relapse. Patients who fail to respond to their initial treatment will eventually die of their disease unless a complete response is achieved with salvage therapy. If such therapy consists of chemotherapy only, fewer than 5% of these patients are likely to be free of further progression. Salvage therapy must therefore comprise intensive chemotherapy autologous stem cell transplantation (ASCT), with immunotherapy in some cases.

Approximately 5% to 10% of patients do not respond to their initial therapy, and 5% to 25% only show an incomplete response. However, outcome in nonresponders is much poorer than in partial responders. Nonresponders to initial therapy do not usually respond to subsequent treatment and die fairly rapidly. Such patients should be included in new-drug or new-strategy phase II studies. Long-term survival is also poor in partial responders, in particular those with an aggressive lymphoma—5% to 25% 5-year survival. Although encouraging results have been reported with intensification and ASCT in such patients, the term *partial response* has been defined differently in the literature. It should be interpreted solely as the persistence of ongoing disease in the form of lymphomatous cells in either marrow or lymph nodes in a treatment responder. In these patients with ongoing disease, no definite conclusion can be drawn as to the role of intensification.

In patients too old to tolerate treatment intensification with ASCT, local radiotherapy may be of value for localized persistent masses. However, the better strategy in terms of quality of life is probably to wait for clear evidence of progression, associated with clinical symptoms, before initiating palliative chemotherapy.

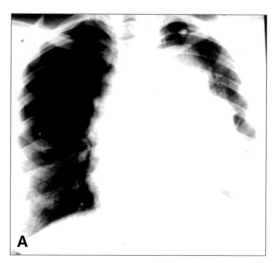
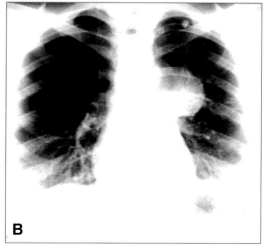
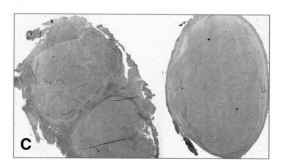

Figure 1-85. Fibronecrotic disease in a patient with mediastinal lymphoma. **A**, Thoracic radiography before treatment. **B**, Thoracic radiograph after treatment. **C**, Biopsy of the large residual mass showing fibronecrotic aspect.

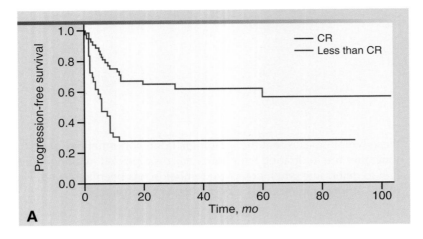

A

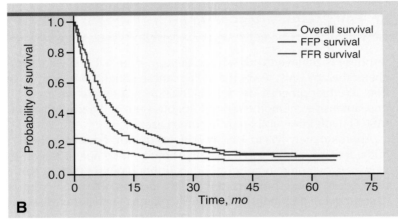

B

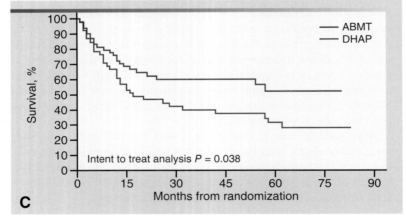

C

Figure 1-86. Survival after relapse in aggressive lymphoma.
A, Importance of complete response (CR) before intensification.
B, Prognosis of patients after relapse in aggressive lymphoma.
C, High-dose therapy followed by stem cell transplantation is superior to conventional chemotherapy.

Approximately 40% of patients in complete remission relapse. In indolent lymphoma, follicular lymphoma (FL), marginal zone lymphoma, or small lymphocytic lymphoma, this percentage is even higher. Relapse tends to occur within 2 years of completing treatment, but can occur more than 10 years later. In relapsed patients the main prognostic factor is their response to salvage treatment,

the other factors being the same as at diagnosis. Multidrug regimens have been proposed but none have proved superior to the others. Although 70% of patients respond to salvage therapy, only 20% to 35% achieve a second complete remission, and its duration is usually less than 12 months, with fewer than 10% of patients experiencing progression-free survival longer than 3 year. It is difficult to interpret the various therapeutic studies that have used chemotherapy regimens of variable complexity, because many patients with relapsing lymphoma die before treatment or are not included in prospective studies.

The encouraging results observed in phase II studies with intensive chemotherapy followed by autologous stem cell transplantation (ASCT) were confirmed by analysis of the patients in the LNH-84 study and by the final analysis of the randomized Parma trial. Intensive chemotherapy followed by ASCT has become the standard therapy for patients under 65 years of age with relapsing aggressive lymphoma responding to salvage therapy, since this is the only treatment which secures 30% to 50% progression-free survival 5 years postrelapse. Conversely, the benefit of intensification in patients refractory to salvage chemotherapy also remains open to question, because it achieves satisfactory results in only 5% to 10% of patients. Such treatment remains open to question in the case of indolent lymphoma in the absence of randomized studies, although it appears to give better results than standard chemotherapy. Although this treatment is effective, it has yet to be codified in all its modalities: in particular, the optimal salvage and intensification regimens have not been determined.

Another major question regarding this treatment concerns the need to purge the hematopoietic stem cells and how to do so. Although relapse may result from the reinjection of pathologic cells, no study has shown benefit in terms of relapse rate or progression-free survival in patients whose harvest underwent positive or negative CD34+ cell selection. Studies are ongoing with new and increasingly effective selection modalities, including the possibility of purging the patient in vivo using an antibody such as rituximab prior to stem cell harvest. First results with the latter strategy show a decrease in pathologic cells in the stem cell harvest for patients with FL or mantle cell lymphoma, but no relapse data are as yet available. Stem cell expansion in vitro appears a purely experimental possibility at this time. Another approach for consolidating the response achieved with intensification is immunotherapy: several ongoing studies are testing interleukin-2, interferon, and rituximab.

Intensive chemotherapy with ASCT should be offered to all patients irrespective of histology whose first progression responds to salvage therapy. With further relapses, malignant cells will become increasingly treatment-resistant. Response is less frequent and shorter in duration in patients receiving third-line therapy. Patients with refractory lymphoma have response rates less than 15% to any salvage therapy, and fewer than 5% of them are likely to have a favorable response to ASCT. Various studies have shown that intensification therapy can be undertaken in such patients but that the risk of further progression increases markedly. Late relapses have the same prognosis as early relapses and thus also require intensive chemotherapy with ASCT. ABMT—autologous bone marrow transplantation; FFP—freedom from progression; FFR—freedom from relapse.

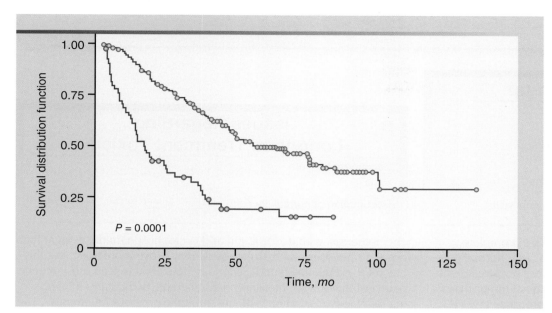

Figure 1-87. The GELF-86 trial (Groupe d' Etude des Lymphomes Folliculaire): overall survival after the first progression according to the presence of histologic transformation. Progression in indolent lymphoma, small lymphocytic lymphoma, marginal zone lymphoma, follicular lymphoma, and cutaneous T-cell lymphoma tends to involve transformation to more aggressive disease, *eg,* large cell or Burkitt-like lymphoma, expressed clinically by bulky tumor mass, elevated lactate dehydrogenase, levels, and frequently impaired performance status. Survival in patients with histologic transformation is usually short, less than 12 months. They require standard or high-dose CHOP (cyclophosphamide, doxorubicin, vincristine, prednisone) followed by intensive chemotherapy with autologous stem cell transplantation.

Palliation
Good quality of life is priority
Optimal regimen should not reduce quality of life

Figure 1-88. Palliation. Although the aim of lymphoma therapy is to achieve complete remission and cure, some patients cannot be offered regimens consistent with such strategies. These patients require palliative treatment, either at the time of diagnosis owing to advanced age or to concomitant incapacitating conditions, or at a later stage following unsuccessful curative treatment. They should be treated only for symptoms impairing their quality of life, for the remainder of their life expectancy. The persistence of tumor cells, even in bulk, or infiltration of the blood, are not in themselves reasons for reinitiating a new, toxic and minimally effective treatment, provided the patient has good quality of life. Various palliative chemotherapy regimens have been proposed. The criteria of an optimal regimen are compatibility with minimal inpatient stay, minimal toxicity (especially hematologic toxicity), and some evidence of efficacy.

FOLLOW-UP

A	Post-treatment Follow-up
Regularly monitor original tumor masses by CT	
CBC for complications	
Monitoring intervals:	
3-monthly in first year	
4-monthly in second year	
6-monthly for 2–5 years, followed by yearly/biannual visits	

B	Issues Regarding Long-term Treatment Toxicity
Secondary cancers	
Fertility	
Resumption of normal life	

Figure 1-89. A, Post-treatment follow-up. A patient in complete remission will be normal on clinical examination, with normal performance status. These two parameters require close post-treatment monitoring in order to detect progression. The original tumor masses should be monitored by CT scan or other site-appropriate investigation at 3 months, 6 months, and 1 year. Subsequent intervals between specialized investigations are determined on a clinical basis. There is currently no defined role for routine surveillance FDG-PET scans. If all clinical parameters are normal, specialized investigations provide no useful supplementary information and should not be repeated on a routine basis. Obviously, if the patient is symptomatic, the cause must be determined. Few laboratory tests are important for monitoring purposes. Lactate dehydrogenase and β_2-microglobulin are late markers, becoming abnormal only in advanced disease. The complete blood count (CBC) is useful for detecting complications.

Monitoring intervals are determined by the nature of the disease at presentation. The general guideline is provided in this table.

B, Issues involved in long-term treatment effects. Given the steady increase in the percentage of cured patients, the study of treatment side effects, in terms of management and prevention, must include those that can occur several years later. Because most lymphoma patients will have been cured by chemotherapy alone, most of the toxic effects observed after cure in Hodgkin disease (which are mainly caused by radiotherapy) are not seen after lymphoma therapy. These cured patients, particularly those included in prospective studies, must be monitored over many years for late toxicity but also for late relapse.

Secondary myelodysplastic syndrome and leukemia are seen in fewer than 2% of cured patients or those alive at 10 years after chemotherapy with doxorubicin and cyclophosphamide, even at high doses. Other drugs such as etoposide may prove more toxic, but this has yet to be demonstrated. Secondary leukemia is seen most often in patients treated with intensive chemotherapy, particularly if involving total body irradiation (TBI) and multiple previous treatments. However, it may be secondary to previous therapies received by the patient and not the intensive regimen preceding autologous stem cell transplantation. The incidence of this complication in patients receiving first-line intensification chemotherapy is not yet known.

Secondary solid tumors tend to be rare. A number of patients develop one or more cancers after chemotherapy but such is the heterogeneity in time of diagnosis, tumor types, and treatments received that coincidence is the most likely explanation in most cases. However, the incidence of second cancers is steadily increasing in cured patients.

One third of patients under 35 years of age wish to have children if cured. This is possible in the great majority of cases because CHOP chemotherapy and its variants do not interfere with the menstrual cycle or cause azoospermia. Most patients encounter no difficulty in post-therapy family planning. Problems may arise in older patients, those who have received repeated treatments for relapse, and those who have undergone TBI.

Young cured patients can resume their normal lives 6 months to 1 year after completing treatment. They are fit to work and should be encouraged to resume their previous activities. The over-50 age group, on the other hand, tend to remain chronically fatigued, and have difficulty in sustaining either a level of concentration compatible with work or normal sexual relationships.

CONCLUSIONS

Lymphomas are a group of cancers that consist of numerous subgroups, some of which can be cured with conventional therapy, while others require more experimental treatments. Treatment is guided by lymphoma subgroup and the presence or absence of adverse prognostic factors. Cure is the aim of initial therapy for certain histologies and can be achieved in 50% of cases if the appropriate treatment is chosen. Salvage therapy with intensive chemotherapy and autologous stem cell transplantation cures one third of the patients with diffuse large B-cell lymphoma who are not cured by their initial therapy. Optimal treatment strategies have not been determined in all cases, in particular for the most aggressive lymphomas. New possibilities are associated with the development of monoclonal antibodies. To include such patients in prospective studies is a requirement of good clinical practice. All lymphoma patients should be monitored for treatment toxicity, relapse, and intercurrent events.

ACKNOWLEDGMENT

This work was prepared with the collaboration of Françoise Berger, Paul-André Bryon, Pascale Felman, Evelyne Callet-Bauchu, and Gilles Salles. Histologic slides were kindly provided by Françoise Berger and Paul-André Bryon, cytologic slides by Pascale Felman, cytogenetic material by Evelyne Callet-Bauchu, and genetic material by Gilles Salles and Catherine Thieblemont.

REFERENCES

1. Harris NL, Jaffe ES, Stein H, et al.: A revised European-American classification of lymphoid neoplasms: a proposal from the International Lymphoma Study Group. *Blood* 1994, 84:1361–1392.

2. Jaffe ES, Harris NL, Stein H, Vardiman JW: World Health Organization Classification of Tumours: pathology and genetics of tumours of haematopoietic and lymphoid tissues. Lyon: IARC; 2001.

3. Coiffier B, Lepage E: Prognosis of aggressive lymphoma: a study of five prognostic models with patients included in the LNH-84 regimen. *Blood* 1989, 74:558–564.

4. The International Non-Hodgkin's Lymphoma Prognostic Factors Project: A predictive model for aggressive non-Hodgkin's lymphoma. *N Engl J Med* 1993, 329:987–994.

5. Shipp MA: Prognostic factors in aggressive non-Hodgkin's lymphoma: who has "high-risk" disease? *Blood* 1994, 83:1165–1173.

6. Salles G, Shipp MA, Coiffier B: Chemotherapy of non-Hodgkin's aggressive lymphomas. *Semin Hematol* 1994, 31:46–69.

7. Coiffier B: Treatment of Non-Hodgkin's lymphomas in 1996: a risk-adapted strategy. In *Textbook of Medical Oncology*. Edited by Cavalli F, Hansen H, Kaye S. London: Martin Dunitz; 1996.

8. Shipp MA, Abeloff MD, Antman KH, et al.: International consensus conference on high-dose therapy with hematopoietic stem cell transplantation in aggressive non-Hodgkin's lymphomas: report of the jury. *J Clin Oncol* 1999, 17:423–429.

9. Clarke CA, Glaser SL: Changing incidence of non-Hodgkin lymphomas in the United States. *Cancer* 2002, 94:2015–2023.

10. The Non-Hodgkin's Lymphoma Classification Project: A clinical evaluation of the International Lymphoma Study Group Classification of Non-Hodgkins Lymphoma. *Blood* 1997, 89:3909–3918.

11. Bower M: Acquired immunodeficiency syndrome-related systemic non-Hodgkin's lymphoma. *Br J Haematol* 2001, 112:863–873.

12. Carbone A: Emerging pathways in the development of AIDS-related lymphomas. *Lancet Oncol* 2003, 4:22–29.

13. Hatta Y, Koeffler HP: Role of tumor suppressor genes in the development of adult T cell leukemia/lymphoma (ATLL). *Leukemia* 2002, 16:1069–1085.

14. Ferri C, Caracciolo F, Zignego AL, et al.: Hepatitis C virus infection in patients with non-Hodgkin's lymphoma. *Br J Haematol* 1994, 88:392–394.

15. Hausfater P, Cacoub P, Sterkers Y, et al.: Hepatitis C virus infection and lymphoproliferative diseases: prospective study on 1,576 patients in France. *Am J Hematol* 2001, 67:168–171.

16. Malkin D: Simian virus 40 and non-Hodgkin lymphoma. *Lancet Oncol* 2002, 359:812–813.

17. Isaacson PG: Mucosa-associated lymphoid tissue lymphoma. *Semin Hematol* 1999, 36:139–147.

18. Cavalli F, Isaacson PG, Gascoyne RD, Zucca E: MALT lymphomas. *Hematology (Am Soc Hematol Educ Program)* 2001, 241–258.

19. Garbe C, Stein H, Dienmann D, Orfanos CE: *Borrelia burgdorferi*-associated cutaneous B-cell lymphoma: clinical and immunohistologic characterization of four cases. *J Am Acad Dermatol* 1991, 24:584–590.

20. Thieblemont C, Felman P, Callet-Bauchu E, et al.: Splenic marginal-zone lymphoma: a distinct clinical and pathological entity. *Lancet Oncol* 2003, 4:95–103.

21. Thieblemont C, Berger F, Dumontet C, et al.: Mucosa-associated lymphoid tissue lymphoma is a disseminated disease in one third of 158 patients analyzed. *Blood* 2000, 95:802–806.

22. Thieblemont C, Felman P, Berger F, et al.: Treatment of splenic marginal zone B-cell lymphoma: an analysis of 81 patients. *Clin Lymphoma* 2002, 3:41–47.

23. The NHL Classification Project: Effect of age on the characteristics and clinical behavior of non-Hodgkins lymphoma patients. *Ann Oncol* 1997, 8:973–978.

24. Rosenwald A, Wright G, Chan WC, et al.: The use of molecular profiling to predict survival after chemotherapy for diffuse large-B-cell lymphoma. *N Engl J Med* 2002, 346:1937–1947.

25. Cartron G, Dacheux L, Salles G, et al.: Therapeutic activity of humanized anti-CD20 monoclonal antibody and polymorphism in IgG Fc receptor Fc gamma RIIIa gene. *Blood* 2002, 99:754–758.

26. DeVita VT, Canellos GP, Chabner B, et al.: Advanced diffuse histiocytic lymphoma, a potentially curable disease. *Lancet* 1975, i:248–250.

27. Fisher RI, Miller T, Dana B, et al.: SouthWest Oncology Group clinical trials for intermediate- and high-grade non-Hodgkin's lymphomas. *Semin Hematol* 1987, 24:S1, 21–25.

28. Fisher RI, Gaynor ER, Dahlberg S, et al.: Comparison of a standard regimen (CHOP) with three intensive chemotherapy regimens for advanced non-Hodgkin's lymphoma. *N Engl J Med* 1993, 328:1002–1006.

29. Frewin R, Turner D, Tighe M, et al.: Combination therapy with fludarabine and cyclophosphamide as salvage treatment in lymphoproliferative disorders. *Br J Haematol* 1999, 104:612–613.

30. Hainsworth JD, Litchy S, Burris HA, et al.: Rituximab as first-line and maintenance therapy for patients with indolent non-Hodgkin's lymphoma. *J Clin Oncol* 2002, 20:4261–4267.

31. McLaughlin P, Fuller LM, Velasquez WS, et al.: Stage I-II follicular lymphoma: treatment results for 76 patients. *Cancer* 1986, 58:1596–1602.

32. Brice P, Bastion Y, Lepage E, et al.: Comparison in low-tumor-burden follicular lymphomas between an initial no-treatment policy, prednimustine, or interferon alfa: a randomized study from the Groupe d'Etude des Lymphomes Folliculaires. *J Clin Oncol* 1997, 15:1110–1117.

33. Colombat P, Salles G, Brousse N, et al.: Rituximab (anti-CD20 monoclonal antibody) as single first-line therapy for patients with follicular lymphoma with a low tumor burden: clinical and molecular evaluation. *Blood* 2001, 97:101–106.

34. Czuczman MS, Grillo-Lopez AJ, White CA, et al.: Treatment of patients with low-grade B-cell lymphoma with the combination of chimeric anti-CD20 monoclonal antibody and CHOP chemotherapy. *J Clin Oncol* 1999, 17:268–276.

35. Bastion Y, Berger F, Bryon PA, et al.: Follicular lymphomas: assessment of prognostic factors in 127 patients followed for 10 years. *Ann Oncol* 1991, 9:123–129.

36. Rohatiner A, Johnson P, Price C, et al.: Myeloablative therapy with autologous bone marrow transplantation as consolidation therapy for recurrent follicular lymphoma. *J Clin Oncol* 1994, 12:1177–1184.

37. Schouten HC, Kvaloy S, Sydes M, et al.: The CUP trial: a randomized study analyzing the efficacy of high dose therapy and purging in low-grade non-Hodgkin's lymphoma (NHL). *Ann Oncol* 2000, 11(suppl 1):91–94.

38. Horning SJ, Negrin RS, Hoppe RT, et al.: High-dose therapy and autologous bone marrow transplantation for follicular lymphoma in first complete or partial remission: results of a phase II clinical trial. *Blood* 2001, 97:404–409.

39. Maloney DG, Liles TM, Czerwinski DK, et al.: Phase I clinical trial using escalating single-dose infusion of chimeric anti-CD20 monoclonal antibody (IDEC-C2B8) in patients with recurrent B-cell lymphoma. *Blood* 1994, 84:2457–2466.

40. Coiffier B, Lepage E, Brière J, et al.: CHOP chemotherapy plus rituximab compared with CHOP alone in elderly patients with diffuse large B-cell lymphoma. *N Engl J Med* 2002, 346:235–242.

41. Keating MJ, Flinn I, Jain V, et al.: Therapeutic role of alemtuzumab (Campath-1H) in patients who have failed fludarabine: results of a large international study. *Blood* 2002, 99:3554–3561.

42. Lundin J, Kimby E, Bjorkholm M, et al.: Phase II trial of subcutaneous anti-CD52 monoclonal antibody alemtuzumab (Campath-1H) as first-line treatment for patients with B-cell chronic lymphocytic leukemia (B-CLL). *Blood* 2002, 100:768–773.

43. Leonard JP, Link BK: Immunotherapy of non-Hodgkin's lymphoma with hLL2 (epratuzumab, an anti-CD22 monoclonal antibody) and Hu1D10 (apolizumab). *Semin Oncol* 2002, 29:81–86.

44. Gordon LI, Witzig TE, Wiseman GA, et al.: Yttrium 90 ibritumomab tiuxetan radioimmunotherapy for relapsed or refractory low-grade non-Hodgkin's lymphoma. *Semin Oncol* 2002, 29:87–92.

45. Witzig TE, Gordon LI, Cabanillas F, et al.: Randomized controlled trial of yttrium-90-labeled ibritumomab tiuxetan radioimmunotherapy versus rituximab immunotherapy for patients with relapsed or refractory low-grade, follicular, or transformed B-cell non-Hodgkin's lymphoma. *J Clin Oncol* 2002, 20:2453–2463.

46. Kaminski MS, Estes J, Zasadny KR, et al.: Radioimmunotherapy with iodine I-131 tositumomab for relapsed or refractory B-cell non-Hodgkin lymphoma: updated results and long-term follow-up of the University of Michigan experience. *Blood* 2000, 96:1259–1266.

47. Vose JM, Wahl RL, Saleh M, et al.: Multicenter phase II study of iodine-131 tositumomab for chemotherapy-relapsed/refractory low-grade and transformed low-grade B-cell non-Hodgkin's lymphomas. *J Clin Oncol* 2000, 18:1316–1323.

48. Coiffier B: Monoclonal antibodies combined to chemotherapy for the treatment of patients with lymphoma. *Blood Rev* 2003, 17:25–31.

49. Lopez-Guillermo A, Cabanillas F, McLaughlin P, et al.: The clinical significance of molecular response in indolent follicular lymphomas. *Blood* 1998, 91:2955–2960.

50. Samaha H, Dumontet C, Ketterer N, et al.: Mantle cell lymphoma: a retrospective study of 121 cases. *Leukemia* 1998, 12:1281–1287.

51. Forstpointner R, Hanel A, Repp R, et al.: Increased response rate with rituximab in relapsed and refractory follicular and mantle cell lymphomas: results of a prospective randomized study of the German Low-Grade Lymphoma Study Group. *Dtsch Med Wochenschr* 2002, 127:2253–2258.

52. Howard OM, Gribben JG, Neuberg DS, et al.: Rituximab and CHOP induction therapy for newly diagnosed mantle-cell lymphoma: molecular complete responses are not predictive of progression-free survival. *J Clin Oncol* 2002, 20:1288–1294.

53. Ketterer N, Salles G, Espinouse D, et al.: Intensive therapy with peripheral stem cell transplantation in 16 patients with mantle cell lymphoma. *Ann Oncol* 1997, 8:701–704.

54. Hiddemann W, Unterhalt M, Dreyling M, et al.: The addition of rituximab (R) to combination chemotherapy (CT) significantly improves the treatment of mantle cell lymphomas (MCL): results of two prospective randomized studies by the German Low Grade Lymphoma Study Group. *Blood* 2002, 100:92a.

55. Thieblemont C, Felman P, Callet-Bauchu E, et al.: Splenic marginal-zone lymphoma: a distinct clinical and pathological entity. *Lancet Oncol* 2003, 4:95–103.

56. Thieblemont C, Felman P, Berger F, et al.: Treatment of splenic marginal zone B-cell lymphoma: an analysis of 81 patients. *Clin Lymphoma* 2002, 3:41–47.

57. Miller TP, Dahlberg S, Cassady JR, et al.: Chemotherapy alone compared with chemotherapy plus radiotherapy for localized intermediate-and high-grade non-Hodgkin's lymphoma. *N Engl J Med* 1998, 339:21–26.

58. Schmits R, Trumper L: 4. Report on workshop: UICC workshop "Therapy of NHL in early stages." Part 2: Aggressive lymphomas. *Ann Hematol* 2001, 80:B16–B19.

59. Reyes F, Lepage E, Munck JN, et al.: Superiority of the ACVBP regimen over a combined treatment with three cycles of CHOP followed by involved field radiotherapy in patients with low risk localized aggressive non Hodgkin's lymphoma: results of the LNH93-1 study. *Blood* 2000, 96:832a.

60. Haioun C, Lepage E, Gisselbrecht C, et al.: Survival benefit of high-dose therapy in poor-risk aggressive non-Hodgkin's lymphoma: final analysis of the prospective LNH87-2 protocol: a Groupe d'Etude des Lymphomes de l'Adulte Study. *J Clin Oncol* 2000, 18:3025–3030.

61. Haïoun C, Lepage E, Gisselbrecht C, et al.: Benefit of autologous bone marrow transplantation over sequential chemotherapy in poor-risk aggressive non-Hodgkin's lymphoma. Updated results of the prospective study Lnh87-2. *J Clin Oncol* 1997, 15:1131–1137.

62. Haïoun C, Lepage E, Gisselbrecht C, et al.: Autologous bone marrow transplantation versus sequential chemotherapy in first complete remission aggressive non-Hodgkin's lymphoma: 1st interim analysis on 370 patients (LNH87 Protocol). 1992, 11:316.

63. Shipp MA, Abeloff MD, Antman KH, et al.: International consensus conference on high-dose therapy with hematopoietic stem cell transplantation in aggressive non-Hodgkin's lymphomas: report of the jury. *J Clin Oncol* 1999, 17:423–429.

64. Gisselbrecht C, Lepage E, Molina T, et al.: Shortened first-line high-dose chemotherapy for patients with poor-prognosis aggressive lymphoma. *J Clin Oncol* 2002, 20:2472–2479.

65. Kaiser U, Uebelacker L, Abel U, et al.: Randomized study to evaluate the use of high-dose therapy as part of primary treatment for "aggressive" lymphoma. *J Clin Oncol* 2002, 20:4413–4419.

66. Coiffier B, Lepage E, Briere J, et al.: CHOP chemotherapy plus rituximab compared with CHOP alone in elderly patients with diffuse large-B-cell lymphoma. *N Engl J Med* 2002, 346:235–242.

67. Tilly H, Gaulard P, Lepage E, et al.: Primary anaplastic large-cell lymphoma in adults: clinical presentation, immunophenotype, and outcome. *Blood* 1997, 90:3727–3734.

68. Bazarbachi A, Hermine O: Treatment of adult T-cell leukaemia/lymphoma: current strategy and future perspectives. *Virus Res* 2001, 78:79–92.

69. Matutes E, Taylor GP, Cavenagh J, et al.: Interferon alpha and zidovudine therapy in adult T-cell leukaemia lymphoma: response and outcome in 15 patients. *Br J Haematol* 2001, 113:779–784.

70. Divine M, Lepage E, Briere J, et al.: Is the small non-cleaved-cell lymphoma histologic subtype a poor prognostic factor in adult patients: a case-controlled analysis. *J Clin Oncol* 1996, 14:240–248.

71. Soussain C, Patte C, Ostronoff M, et al.: Small noncleaved cell lymphoma and leukemia in adults: a retrospective study of 65 adults treated with the LMB pediatric protocols. *Blood* 1995, 85:664–674.

72. Hoelzer D, Gokbuget N: Treatment of lymphoblastic lymphoma in adults. *Best Pract Res Clin Hematol* 2002, 15:713–728.

73. Hoelzer D, Gokbuget N, Digel W, et al.: Outcome of adult patients with T-lymphoblastic lymphoma treated according to protocols for acute lymphoblastic leukemia. *Blood* 2002, 99:4379–4385.

74. Morel P, Lepage E, Brice P, et al.: Prognosis and treatment of lymphoblastic lymphoma in adults: a report on 80 patients. *J Clin Oncol* 1992, 10:1078–1085.

75. Sonneveld P, Deridder M, Vanderlelie H, et al.: Comparison of doxorubicin and mitoxantrone in the treatment of elderly patients with advanced diffuse non-Hodgkin's lymphoma using CHOP versus CNOP chemotherapy. *J Clin Oncol* 1995, 13:2530–2539.

76. Meyer RM, Browman GP, Samosh ML, et al.: Randomized phase II comparison of standard CHOP with weekly CHOP in elderly patients with non-Hodgkin's lymphoma. *J Clin Oncol* 1995, 13:2386–2393.

77. Bastion YB, Blay JY, Divine M, et al.: Elderly patients with aggressive non-Hodgkin's lymphoma: disease presentation, response to treatment, and survival. A Groupe d'Etude des Lymphomes de l'Adulte study on 453 patients older than 69 years. *J Clin Oncol* 1997, 15:2945–2953.

78. Batchelor T, Carson K, O'Neill A, et al.: Treatment of primary CNS lymphoma with methotrexate and deferred radiotherapy: a report of NABTT 96-07. *J Clin Oncol* 2003, 15:1044–1049.

79. Hollender A, Kvaloy S, Nome O, et al.: Central nervous system involvement following diagnosis of non-Hodgkin's lymphoma: a risk model. *Ann Oncol* 2002, 13:1099—1107.

CHAPTER 2

Hodgkin Lymphoma

Joseph M. Connors and Randy D. Gascoyne

Hodgkin lymphoma, originally "Hodgkin's disease," was initially described in the mid-19th century by the physician and humanitarian Thomas Hodgkin, one of the first to publish on the concept of primary tumors of the lymph nodes and spleen. The combined clinical and pathologic criteria for the diagnosis have gradually evolved over more than a century and a half into a precisely defined entity, which can now be quite accurately diagnosed in the hands of an experienced hematopathologist [1]. In the past decade, the underlying cell of origin, a B cell with profound impairment of normal apoptosis, has been tightly defined, although many questions about fundamental biology remain to be answered.

The importance of careful disease staging; input from a team of multidisciplinary specialists, including hematopathologists, diagnostic imaging experts, medical oncologists and hematologists, radiation specialists, and nurses and technologists; the critical need to base conclusions about treatment on formal clinical trials; and the necessity to observe patients for decades of follow-up to appreciate the full impact, both positive and negative, of effective treatment have served as a paradigm for the entire field of modern oncology. Today all clinicians managing this highly curable neoplasm must understand the necessity of balancing potency of treatment with minimization of late side effects.

PATHOLOGY

Hodgkin Lymphoma Subtypes and Typical Frequencies

Subtype	Frequency, %
Classical	> 90
Nodular sclerosis	65
Mixed cellularity	20
Lymphocyte-rich classical	5
Lymphocyte depletion	2
Lymphocyte predominant, nodular	5
Not classifiable	3

Figure 2-1. Hodgkin lymphoma subtypes and typical frequencies. Most cases fit into one of the classical subtypes. In the developed countries, the majority of cases, especially in younger patients, fall into the nodular sclerosing subtype. Nodular lymphocyte predominant Hodgkin lymphoma is now recognized in a special separate category with its own unique immunophenotypic characteristics, clinical presentation, response to treatment, and natural history [1].

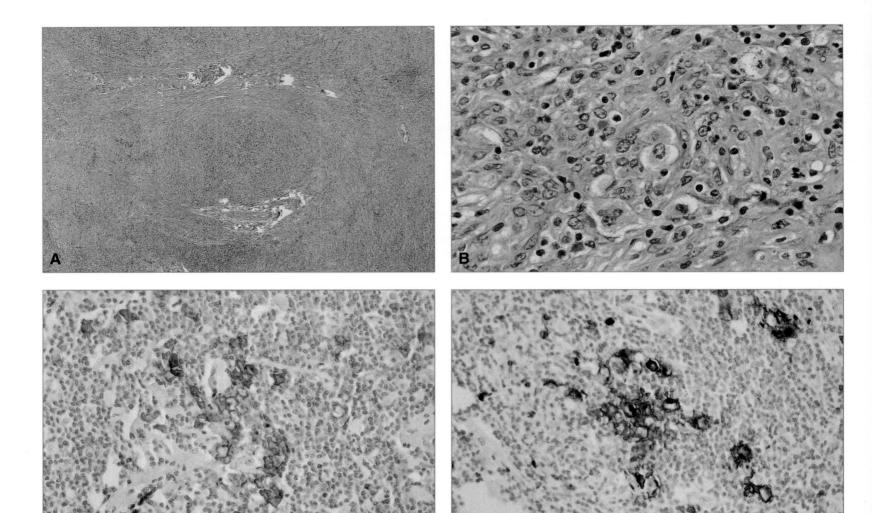

Figure 2-2. Nodular sclerosis Hodgkin lymphoma (NSHL). NSHL is characterized by bands of sclerosis surrounding clusters of Reed-Sternberg (RS) cell variants called lacunar cells, named for their propensity to sit in lacuna-like spaces that are an artifact of formalin fixation. These mononuclear RS cell variants have large nuclei with prominent nucleoli and abundant clear cytoplasm. Clustering of these cells is common, and areas of central necrosis are sometimes present. These cells are set in the background of mixed inflammatory cell infiltrate composed of neutrophils, eosinophils, plasma cells, lymphocytes, and histiocytes. Typical RS cells are uncommonly seen. **A**, Section stained with hematoxylin and eosin showing a nodular infiltrate with coarse bands of sclerosis. **B**, High magnification showing scattered large atypical RS variants termed *lacunar cells*. These cells have large nuclei, variably prominent nucleoli, and abundant pale cytoplasm. **C**, CD30 immunostain highlighting the lacunar cells. **D**, CD15 immunostain is also positive in these cells.

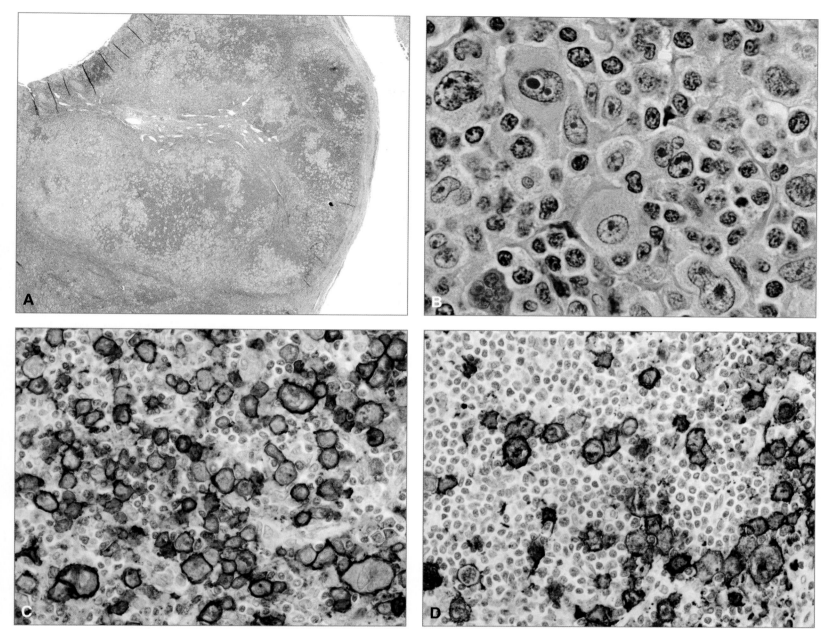

Figure 2-3. A, Low-power appearance of typical nodular sclerosis Hodgkin lymphoma (NSHL). The cellular areas form macronodules separated by intranodal collagen bands. This case has large numbers of lacunar cells that impart a moth-eaten appearance to the section. **B,** High-power magnification of diagnostic Reed-Sternberg (RS) cells. Classic diagnostic RS cells have eosinophilic nucleoli and are binucleated. Several of the other large cells in this section are RS cell variants. **C,** Case of NSHL with abundant RS cells stained with anti-CD30. The classic staining pattern is membranous with accentuation of the Golgi apparatus, the latter imparting a dot-like cytoplasmic staining pattern. Note the large number of cells lacking the typical quality of diagnostic RS cells that strongly express CD30 antigen. **D,** Another case of NSHL stained with anti-CD15. Note that the staining pattern (membrane and Golgi) is similar to that of CD30.

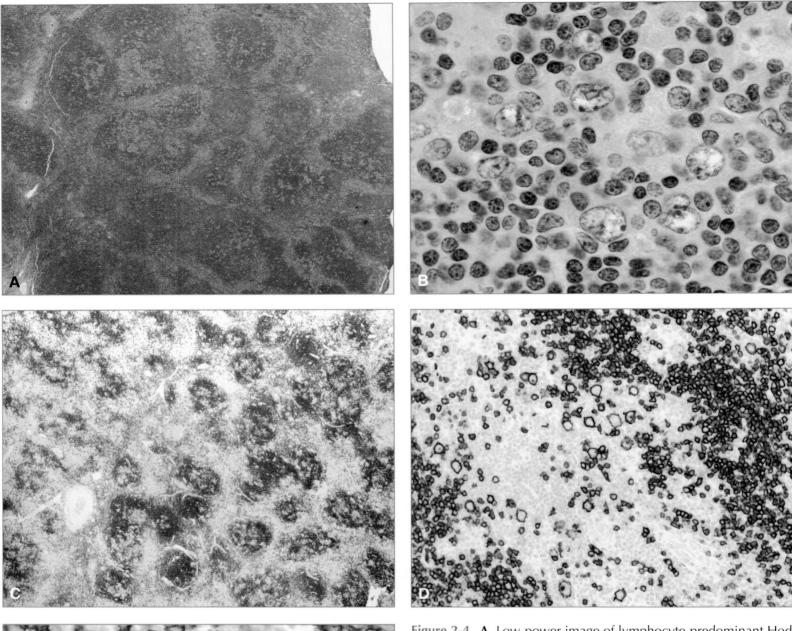

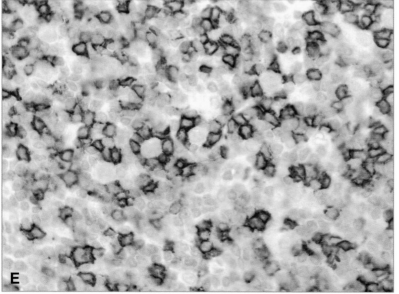

Figure 2-4. **A,** Low-power image of lymphocyte-predominant Hodg-kin lymphoma (LPHL). The infiltrate is macronodular, with abundant small lymphocytes and numerous histiocytes. **B,** High-power image of the neoplastic cells of nodular LPHL. These cells typically show multilobulated nuclei, often referred to as popcorn cells. These cells express B cell markers (CD20, CD79a) and the germinal center marker Bcl-6, and often express epithelial membrane antigen. **C,** Low-power magnification of a lymph node with involvement by nodular LPHL stained with anti-CD20. This stain highlights the nodular pattern of infiltration and reveals that many of the posi-tive-staining lymphoid cells are small reactive B cells. **D,** Higher magnification showing the characteristic staining pattern seen with anti-CD20 in nodular LPHL. Virtually no other disease produces this appearance when stained with anti-CD20. In addition to many small benign B cells, the characteristic popcorn cells strongly express CD20 and are easily seen because of their larger size and more abundant cytoplasm. **E,** High-power magnification of a case of nodular LPHL stained with anti-CD57. Some of the popcorn cells in nodular LPHL are surrounded by small reactive T cells. These latter cells express CD3, a pan–T cell antigen, but a subset also expresses the natural killer cell antigen CD57. Some popcorn cells are com-pletely surrounded by these T cells, producing collarettes.

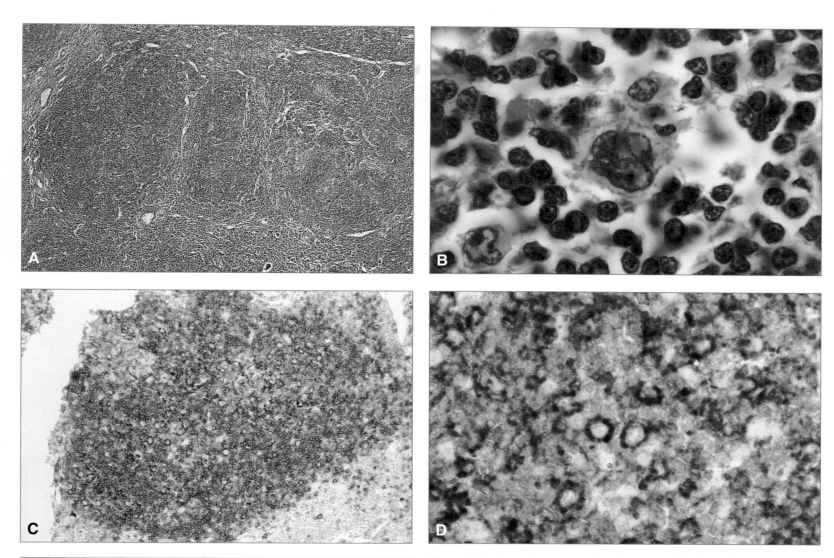

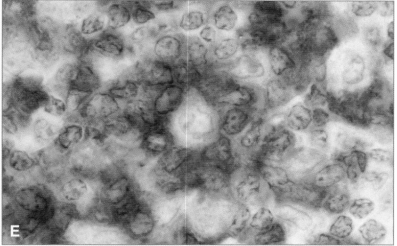

Figure 2-5. Lymphocyte-predominant Hodgkin lymphoma (LPHL). LPHL contains Reed-Sternberg (RS) cells and variants in a generally diffuse background of small lymphocytes with a paucity of other inflammatory cells. Lymphocyte-depleted Hodgkin lymphoma (LDHL) is very uncommon and consists of sheets of RS cells and variants with little of the inflammatory cell infiltrate seen in the other subtypes. It is subdivided into diffuse fibrosis and reticular types. The former shows a prominent fibrous connective tissue background with few lymphocytes. Scattered RS cells are present and are sometimes numerous. The reticular type shows increased numbers of RS cells that are pleomorphic and may also mimic a pleomorphic sarcoma. The typical immunophenotype of classic Hodgkin lymphoma is CD3⁻, CD20⁻/⁺, CD45RB⁻, CD30⁺, and CD15⁺. The small lymphocytes are predominantly T cells. Recent single-cell studies using polymerase chain reaction have demonstrated monoclonal immunoglobulin gene rearrangement in RS cells, confirming the monoclonal B-cell nature of this lymphoma. No specific structural abnormalities have been identified. **A**, Hematoxylin and eosin section showing a macronodular pattern with small lymphocytes and scattered histiocytes. **B**, High magnification showing a large, multilobulated (popcorn) cell. **C**, CD20 immunostain showing that, characteristically, many of the small cells are B cells. **D**, CD20 immunostain showing that the large popcorn cells are CD20⁺ cells. **E**, CD3 immunostain showing a popcorn cell surrounded by a rim of small positive T cells.

Diagnostic and Staging Evaluation of a Patient With Hodgkin Lymphoma

Pathology review	
Complete history searching for B symptoms or other symptomatic problems suggesting more advanced disease	
Physical examination for lymphadenopathy or organomegaly	
Complete blood count plus erythrocyte sedimentation rate	
Serum creatinine, alkaline phosphatase, lactate dehydrogenase, bilirubin, calcium, AST, serum protein electrophoresis (including albumin level)	
Chest radiograph, PA and lateral views	
CT scan of the neck, thorax, abdomen, and pelvis	
Certain special tests, such as bone marrow examination or ENT examination, are required only for specific Hodgkin lymphoma presentations	

Special Test	Presentation/Condition
Bone marrow biopsy and aspiration	B symptoms or WBC < 4.0 x 10^9/L; or Hgb < 120 g/L (women) or < 130 g/L (men); or platelets < 125 x 10^9/L
ENT examination	Stage IA or IIA disease with upper cervical lymph node involvement (suprahyoid)

Figure 2-6. Diagnostic and staging evaluation of a patient with Hodgkin lymphoma. The purpose of these tests is to determine the apparent extent of disease and to estimate the overall tumor burden, a strong predictor of outcome. History and physical examination are complemented by screening blood tests, diagnostic imaging, and selective biopsies to identify the extent of nodal and extra-nodal disease; to assess the impact of the lymphoma and comorbid conditions on the function of bone marrow, liver, kidneys, and body metabolism; and to catalogue findings of proven prognostic importance. AST—aspartate aminotransferase; ENT—ear, nose, and throat; Hgb—hemoglobin; PA—posteroanterior; WBC—white blood cells.

The Cotswolds Modification of the Ann Arbor Staging System

Stage	Description
Stage I	Involvement of a single lymph node region or lymphoid structure (eg, spleen or Waldeyer's ring) or extralymphatic site
Stage II	Involvement of two or more lymph node regions or lymphoid structures or localized single or contiguous extralymphatic sites, with all lymphoma on one side of the diaphragm
Stage III	Involvement of two or more lymph node regions or lymphoid structures or localized single or contiguous extralymphatic sites, with lymphoma on both sides of the diaphragm
Stage IV	Diffuse or disseminated involvement of one or more extralymphatic sites, with or without associated lymph node involvement
A	No B symptoms
B	B symptoms (unexplained fever, drenching night sweats, or unintentional weight loss > 10% of baseline)
X	Bulky disease (mediastinal mass with a transverse diameter greater than one third the largest transverse thoracic diameter on chest radiograph or any tumor mass > 10 cm)
E	Involvement of a single extranodal site alone or localized contiguous extension of lymphoma into extranodal tissue from a known nodal site

Figure 2-7. The Cotswolds modification of the Ann Arbor staging system. The Ann Arbor system is based on the number and location of lymph nodes or extranodal sites involved (designated by a Roman numeral), the absence or presence of B symptoms (designated by the letter A or B, respectively) [2], and, if applicable, the additional letter X to denote bulky disease (the modification added after the Cotswolds conference [3]) or E to denote localized direct spread into extranodal tissue from an involved lymph node.

Prognostic Factors for Advanced Hodgkin Lymphoma

Factor	Adverse Criteria
Sex	Male
Age	> 45 y
Stage	IV
Hemoglobin	< 105 g/L
WBC	> 15.0 x 10^9/L
Lymphocyte count	< 0.6 x 10^9/L or < 8% of the total white cell count
Serum albumin	< 40 g/L

Five-Year FFP of Patients With Advanced-Stage Hodgkin Lymphoma Treated With ABVD or an Equivalent Regimen

Factors, *n*	Frequency, %	5-y FFP, %
0–1	29	79
2–7	71	60
0–2	58	74
3–7	42	55
0–3	81	70
4–7	19	47

Figure 2-8. Prognostic factors indicating decreased probability of freedom from progression and overall survival in advanced-stage Hodgkin lymphoma treated with ABVD (doxorubicin, bleomycin, vinblastine, dacarbazine) or an equivalent regimen. In a large study of more than 5000 patients with advanced-stage Hodgkin lymphoma in which almost all patients were treated with ABVD or an equivalent regimen, seven patient or disease characteristics emerged as independent prognostic factors in this International Prognostic Factor Project for Hodgkin Lymphoma [4]. A score ranging from 0 to 7 can be constructed by adding one point for each of the factors present. WBC—white blood cells.

Figure 2-9. Impact of the number of adverse prognostic factors for advanced-stage Hodgkin lymphoma. The prognosis of patients with advanced-stage Hodgkin lymphoma treated with ABVD (doxorubicin, bleomycin, vinblastine, dacarbazine) or equivalently effective chemotherapy can be predicted based on the number of adverse prognostic factors present at diagnosis [4]. The specific impact of the number of prognostic factors is shown in the table, with patients grouped by number of prognostic factors followed by the frequency with which that score occurs and the 5-year freedom from progression (FFP) for that subgroup. The various groupings of the prognostic scores allow appreciation of the infrequency with which patients present with the most adverse prognoses. Thus, more than 80% of patients with advanced Hodgkin lymphoma present with zero to three adverse factors, and this group has a 5-year FFP of 70%. Only 19% of patients with advanced-stage Hodgkin lymphoma present with four to seven adverse prognostic factors, but this group has a markedly inferior likelihood of remaining free of disease progression, with a 5-year FFP of less than 50%.

Overall Approach to Primary Treatment of Hodgkin Lymphoma

Stage	Bulk	IPFP score	Treatment
IA, IIA	Low (< 10 cm)	Not applicable	ABVD x 4 cycles (if CR after 2 cycles) or ABVD x 2 cycles + IFRT (if < CR after 2 cycles)
Any stage with B symptoms or III or IV	Low (< 10 cm)	0–4	ABVD until 2 cycles past CR (minimum 6, maximum 8)
Any stage with B symptoms or III or IV	Low (< 10 cm)	5–7	Intensified chemotherapy (such as escalated BEACOPP)
Any stage	High (> 10 cm)	0–7	Chemotherapy as above followed by IFRT to the bulky site

Figure 2-10. Overall approach to primary treatment of Hodgkin lymphoma. A reasonable plan of treatment for patients with Hodgkin lymphoma can be advocated based on stage, presence of bulky tumor (any single tumor mass ≥10 cm in maximum diameter), and International Prognostic Factor Project (IPFP) score. Patients with limited-stage disease (stage IA or IIA) may be treated with either ABVD (doxorubicin, bleomycin, vinblastine, dacarbazine) for two cycles followed by involved field radiotherapy (IFRT) or, if an early complete response (CR) is achieved after two cycles of chemotherapy, with ABVD for four cycles [5].

Patients with advanced-stage lymphoma (stage III or IV, or any stage with B symptoms, or any stage with bulky disease [any single tumor mass ≥10 cm in maximum diameter]) may be treated with an extended course of chemotherapy, usually six to eight cycles of ABVD (minimum six, maximum eight cycles; planning to deliver at least two cycles beyond the time when the maximum response is achieved). Some authorities advise using intensified chemotherapy, such as the escalated BEACOPP (bleomycin, etoposide, doxorubicin, cyclophosphamide, vincristine, procarbazine, prednisone) program, if a patient with advanced-stage Hodgkin lymphoma presents with five or more adverse prognostic factors as defined by the IPFP score, is under the age of 60 years, and has no comorbid illnesses that would make the regimen too toxic [5].

Patients presenting with any stage and with bulky disease (any single tumor mass ≥10 cm in maximum diameter) should be considered for involved field radiation at the conclusion of chemotherapy. If a complete response by CT scanning has been achieved by the chemotherapy, there is no need for the radiation. Some authorities now advocate omission of the radiation if any residual mass detected by CT scanning is negative by fluorodeoxyglucose positron emission tomography [6].

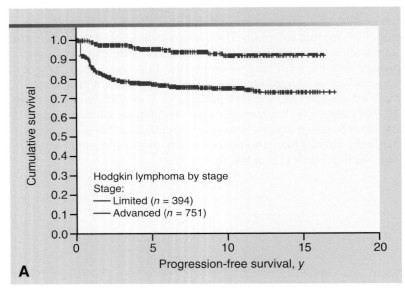

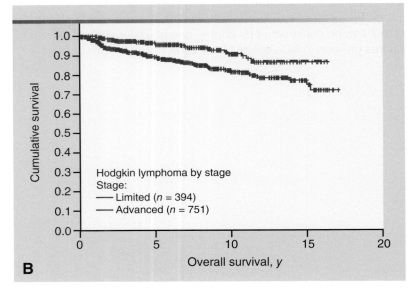

Figure 2-11. Outcomes of treatment of Hodgkin lymphoma. These two graphs show the progression-free survival (**A**) and overall survival (**B**) for adult patients (ages 16 to 70, inclusive) with Hodgkin lymphoma by stage at presentation treated at the British Columbia Cancer Agency since 1990, thus representing what can be achieved with modern chemotherapy and radiation therapy. The BC Cancer Agency provides care for the entire population of the province of British Columbia, population approximately 4 million, and thus represents what can be achieved in an unselected population. Limited stage is Ann Arbor stage IA or IIA without bulky tumor (*bulky* is defined as having any tumor from the lymphoma that is ≥10 cm in largest diameter; advanced stage is Ann Arbor stage III or IV with or without B symptoms, or any stage with B symptoms or bulky disease). Events on the progression-free survival curve are progression of lymphoma at any time after treatment was initiated, initiation of any additional treatment not planned at the time of diagnosis, or death from treatment related toxicity; patients in sustained complete remission without evidence of recurrent lymphoma at the time of death are censored on the date of death. Thus, progression-free survival indicates the likelihood of being cured by the initially planned treatment. Patients alive and free of Hodgkin lymphoma are noted with a *tick*. Overall survival counts death from any cause as an event; *ticks* indicate living patients. It is clear from these curves that the majority of patients can be cured of their Hodgkin lymphoma, especially those with limited-stage disease at presentation.

Late Effects and Follow-up of Patients Treated for Hodgkin Lymphoma

Risk/Problem	Incidence/Response
Relapse	10% to 30% of patients relapse. Careful attention should be directed to lymph node sites, especially if previously involved with disease. New persistent focal symptoms, such as bone pain, should be investigated with appropriate laboratory and imaging studies.
Dental caries	Neck or oropharyngeal irradiation may cause decreased salivation. Patients should have careful dental care follow-up and should make their dentist aware of the previous irradiation.
Hypothyroidism	After external beam thyroid irradiation to doses sufficient to cure Hodgkin lymphoma, at least 50% of patients will eventually become hypothyroid. All patients who have been exposed to neck irradiation should have an annual thyrotropin level performed. Those whose thyrotropin level becomes elevated should be treated with lifelong thyroxine replacement in dosages sufficient to suppress thyrotropin levels to low normal. This replaces thyroid function; puts the glandular tissue to rest, avoiding prolonged stimulation of the radiation-damaged thyroid tissue; and avoids the risk of osteoporosis that would accompany over-replacement.
Infertility	ABVD is not known to cause permanent gonadal toxicity, although temporary oligospermia or irregular menses may persist for 1 to 2 years after treatment. Direct or scatter radiation to gonadal tissue may cause infertility, amenorrhea, or premature menopause, but this seldom occurs with the current fields used for the treatment of Hodgkin lymphoma. Thus, with the current chemotherapy regimens and radiation fields used, most patients will not develop these problems. In general, after treatment, women who continue menstruating are fertile, but men require semen analysis to provide a specific answer.
Cardiovascular	Increased risk of arteriosclerosis and coronary artery disease follows treatment of Hodgkin lymphoma. Patients should be counseled to avoid other risk factors, such as tobacco use, lack of exercise, or a high-fat diet, and symptoms suggestive of coronary artery disease should be promptly and vigorously investigated.

Figure 2-12. Late effects and follow-up of patients treated for Hodgkin lymphoma. Most patients with Hodgkin lymphoma can be successfully treated and cured of the disease. However, the treatments employed may have lifelong effects that may affect the patient's health and quality of life. In addition, relapse of the lymphoma may occur and should be promptly investigated and appropriately treated. Monitoring for reoccurrence of the lymphoma or development of late complications of treatment is an important aspect of the follow-up care of patients treated for Hodgkin lymphoma. ABVD—doxorubicin, bleomycin, vinblastine, dacarbazine.

Second Neoplasms and Follow-up of Patients Treated for Hodgkin Lymphoma

Secondary Neoplasm	Response
Acute myelogenous leukemia	Most cases of leukemia secondary to treatment occur within 4–6 years of the treatment and will be detected on routine blood screening at planned follow-up visits
Thyroid	Palpation of neck for masses
	Thyroxine replacement if elevated thyrotropin discovered at planned follow-up visits
Breast	Breast self-examination
	Women should begin annual mammography 10 years after completing Hodgkin lymphoma treatment or at age 40 years, whichever comes first
Lung	Avoidance of tobacco use
	Careful investigation of new persistent respiratory symptoms
Gastrointestinal	Colorectal cancer screening starting at age 40 years
	Careful investigation of persistent dyspepsia, dysphagia, or unexplained weight loss
Melanoma	Careful complete skin examination at least annually, more often if dysplastic nevi present
Cervical carcinoma	Annual Papanicolaou smears

Figure 2-13. Second neoplasms and follow-up of patients treated for Hodgkin lymphoma. Although uncommon, certain secondary neoplasms occur with increased frequency in patients who have been treated for Hodgkin lymphoma. These include acute myelogenous leukemia; thyroid, breast, lung, and gastrointestinal carcinomas; and melanoma and cervical carcinoma [7,8]. It is appropriate to screen for these neoplasms for the rest of the patient's life because they may have a lengthy induction period. Patients cured of Hodgkin lymphoma have a persistent risk of developing secondary neoplasms that appears to last at least three or more decades from the conclusion of their treatment and may be lifelong. Specific counseling and screening are appropriate.

REFERENCES

1. Jaffe ES, Harris NL, Stein H, Vardiman JW, eds: *Pathology and Genetics of Tumours of Haematopoietic and Lymphoid Tissues.* Lyon: IARC Press; 2001.

2. Carbone PP, Kaplan HS, Musshoff K, *et al.*: Report of the Committee on Hodgkin's Disease Staging Classification. *Cancer Res* 1971, 31:1860–1861.

3. Lister TA, Crowther D, Sutcliffe SB, *et al.*: Report of a committee convened to discuss the evaluation and staging of patients with Hodgkin's disease: Cotswolds meeting. *J Clin Oncol* 1989, 7:1630–1636.

4. Hasenclever D, Diehl V: A prognostic score for advanced Hodgkin's disease. International Prognostic Factors Project on Advanced Hodgkin's Disease. *N Engl J Med* 1998, 339:1506–1514.

5. Connors JM: State-of-the-art therapeutics: Hodgkin's lymphoma. *J Clin Oncol* 2005, 23:6400–6408.

6. Zinzani PL, Tani M, Fanti S, *et al.*: Early positron emission tomography (PET) restaging: a predictive final response in Hodgkin's disease patients. *Ann Oncol* 2006, 17:1296–1300.

7. Franklin J, Pluetschow A, Paus M, *et al.*: Second malignancy risk associated with treatment of Hodgkin's lymphoma: meta-analysis of the randomised trials. *Ann Oncol* 2006, 17:1749–1760.

8. Ng AK, Bernardo MV, Weller E, *et al.*: Second malignancy after Hodgkin disease treated with radiation therapy with or without chemotherapy: long-term risks and risk factors. *Blood* 2002, 100:1989–1996.

CHAPTER 3

Plasma Cell Disorders

Sagar Lonial

Plasma cell dyscrasias (PCDs) represent a set of disorders united by an abnormal and clonal proliferation of plasma cells. On the benign end of the spectrum, the vast majority of PCD cases are encompassed within a group known as monoclonal gammopathy of unknown significance (MGUS), a majority of which will not progress to a true plasma cell malignancy. The other end of the spectrum is plasma cell leukemia, a highly aggressive PCD that often represents a virulent clone of cells that circulate in the peripheral blood and are independent of the usual stromal regulatory machinery. Progression between MGUS and end-stage myeloma is regulated by a series of important genetic events, but the specific sequence and genetic aberrations are only now beginning to be understood and are the focus of intense laboratory study.

Patients with PCD present with a median age of 65 and often appear with findings such as anemia or with abnormal blood counts and chemistries. African Americans have a twofold higher incidence of MGUS and myeloma compared with non–African Americans in the United States, contrasted with Asians, in whom the rate is significantly lower. Genetic predisposition is not thought to play a major role in the development of myeloma, though a few rare cases of hereditary myeloma have been reported. Overall, population-based differences in incidence remain largely unexplained.

Plasma cell disorders are typically characterized by secretion into the blood and/or urine of a monoclonal protein. The protein may be a combination of a typical immunoglobulin protein (light chain combined with an immunoglobulin heavy chain) or may be an isolated light chain. Complications of plasma cell disorders include infections (typically with encapsulated organisms), skeletal-related events (osteopenia, compression fractures, and long bone fractures), renal compromise (proteinuria, acute renal failure, urate nephropathy), electrolyte disorders (hypercalcemia), and hematologic disorders (anemia, thrombocytopenia, leucopenia), to name a few.

Prognosis has historically been determined by surrogate markers for proliferative capacity of the tumor cells. This has included lactate dehydrogenase, C-reactive protein, β_2-microglobulin, and plasma cell labeling index. These have been largely supplanted with the use of conventional cytogenetics and interphase fluorescence in situ hybridization. These latter two approaches have identified particularly high-risk patients not likely to benefit from chemotherapy-based approaches.

Treatment options for patients with myeloma have radically changed over the past 5 years. The widespread use of high-dose therapy and autologous transplantation can achieve durable remissions in certain groups of patients. For a disease in which corticosteroids and alkylate-based therapy historically have been the mainstay, novel agents such as thalidomide, bortezomib, and lenalidomide have become widely used and represent a "chemotherapy-free" approach to treatment. These agents are effective not only in myeloma, but also in other PCDs, such as Waldenström macroglobulinemia, systemic amyloidosis, and plasma cell leukemia. Allogeneic transplantation remains largely an experimental procedure that is complicated by the advanced age of patients with PCD, as well as significant treatment-related morbidity and mortality.

Future directions include the increasing use of novel targeted agents alone or in combination with one another to enhance overall responses and survival.

Screening and Diagnosis

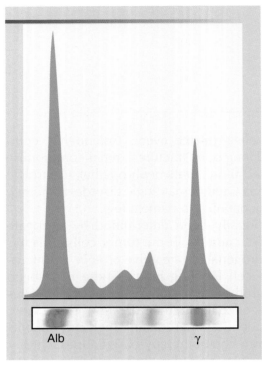

Figure 3-1. Serum protein electrophoresis. An M protein is seen as a narrow peak (like a church spire in the densitometer tracing) or as a dense, discrete band on the agarose gel. Although the immunoglobulins (IgG, IgA, IgM, IgD, and IgE) compose the γ component, they are also found in the β-γ or β region, whereas IgG may actually extend to the α_2-globulin area. An M protein may be present when the total protein concentration, β and γ globulin levels, and quantitative immunoglobulin values are all within normal limits. A small M protein may be concealed in the normal β or γ areas and be overlooked. In addition, monoclonal light chains (Bence Jones proteinemia) are rarely seen in the agarose gel. Alb—albumin.

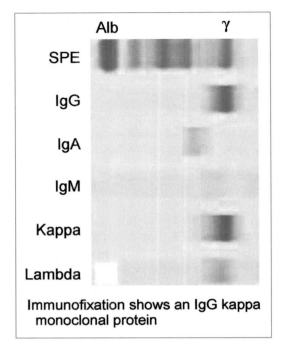

Immunofixation shows an IgG kappa monoclonal protein

Figure 3-2. Immunofixation of serum. Immunofixation should be performed when a peak or band is seen on protein electrophoresis or when multiple myeloma or a related disorder is suspected. It is particularly useful for finding a small M protein in primary (AL) amyloidosis, solitary plasmacytoma, or extramedullary plasmacytoma, or after successful treatment of multiple myeloma or macroglobulinemia. Alb—albumin; Ig—immunoglobulin; SPE—serum protein electrophoresis.

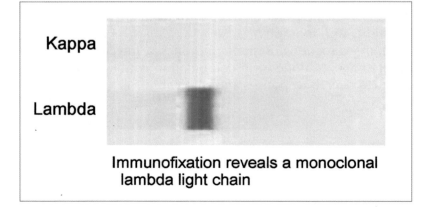

Immunofixation reveals a monoclonal lambda light chain

Figure 3-3. Immunofixation of urine. Immunofixation of urine is indicated in the presence of a serum M protein level of 1.5 g/dL or higher. Immunofixation is also recommended for every adult over 40 years of age who has a nephrotic syndrome of unknown cause. The presence of a monoclonal protein in nephrotic urine strongly suggests primary (AL) amyloidosis or light chain deposition disease.

Classification of Plasma Cell Proliferative Disorders

I. Monoclonal gammopathies of undetermined significance

  A. Benign (IgG, IgA, IgD, IgM, and, rarely, free light chains)

  B. Associated neoplasms or other diseases not known to produce monoclonal proteins

  C. Biclonal gammopathies

  D. Idiopathic Bence Jones proteinuria

II. Malignant monoclonal gammopathies

  A. Multiple myeloma (IgG, IgA, IgD, IgE, and free light chains)

    1. Overt multiple myeloma

    2. Smoldering multiple myeloma

    3. Plasma cell leukemia

    4. Nonsecretory myeloma

    5. IgD myeloma

    6. Osteosclerotic myeloma (POEMS syndrome)

    7. Solitary plasmacytoma of bone

    8. Extramedullary plasmacytoma

  B. Waldenström macroglobulinemia

    1. Other lymphoproliferative diseases

III. Heavy chain diseases

  A. γ-HCD

  B. α-HCD

  C. μ-HCD

IV. Cryoglobulinemia

V. Primary amyloidosis

Figure 3-4. Classification of plasma cell proliferative disorders. The variants of multiple myeloma include smoldering or asymptomatic multiple myeloma, plasma cell leukemia, nonsecretory myeloma, immunoglobulin (Ig)D myeloma, osteosclerotic myeloma (POEMS [polyneuropathy, organomegaly, endocrinopathy, M protein, skin changes] syndrome), solitary plasmacytoma of bone, and extramedullary plasmacytoma. The heavy chain diseases (HCDs), cryoglobulinemia, and primary (AL) amyloidosis also are included as is idiopathic Bence Jones proteinuria, which is characterized by the excretion of large amounts of monoclonal light chains without evidence of multiple myeloma, AL amyloidosis, or a related disorder. These patients should not be treated because they may remain stable for years [1]. (*Adapted from* Kyle [2].)

Epidemiology

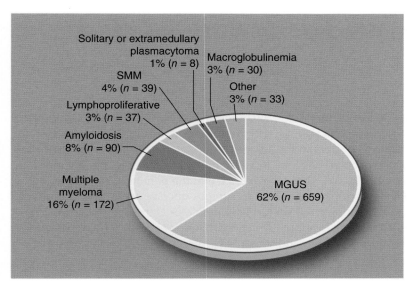

Figure 3-5. Incidence of the plasma cell proliferative disorders among 1068 patients. Monoclonal gammopathy of undetermined significance (MGUS) is the most common plasma cell disorder, accounting for more than 60% of cases. Multiple myeloma and primary (AL) amyloidosis account for one fourth of patients. The "other" category consists of the POEMS (polyneuropathy, organomegaly, endocrinopathy, M protein, skin changes) syndrome (osteosclerotic myeloma), plasma cell leukemia, γ heavy chain disease, μ heavy chain disease, light chain deposition disease, acquired Fanconi's syndrome, scleromyxedema (lichen myxedematosus), and cold agglutinin disease. SMM—smoldering multiple myeloma. (*Data from* the Mayo Clinic, Rochester, MN.)

Criteria for Diagnosis of MGUS

Serum M protein <3 g/dL
Bone marrow plasma cells <10%
No evidence of other B-cell disorder
No ROTI

Figure 3-6. Criteria for diagnosis of monoclonal gammopathy of undetermined significance (MGUS). MGUS is a condition in which there is presence of an M protein in patients without evidence of multiple myeloma, macroglobulinemia, amyloidosis, or other related disorders. MGUS is found in 1% of patients aged 50 years or older and in 3% of patients older than 70 [3]. Revised criteria from the International Myeloma Working Group defines related organ or tissue impairment (ROTI) as lack of the criteria needed for symptomatic myeloma (CRAB criteria [calcium elevation, renal insufficiency, anemia, and bone abnormalities]) [4].

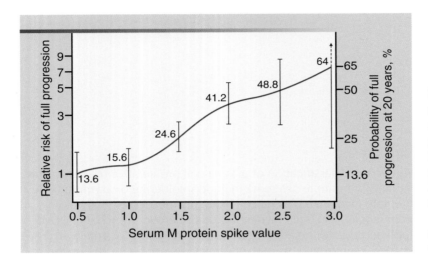

Figure 3-7. Relative risk of full progression by serum M protein–spike size. The risk of progression to multiple myeloma or a related cancer at 20 years was 14% for an initial M protein value of 0.5 g/dL or less, 25% for an initial M protein value of 1.5 g/dL, 41% for an initial M protein value of 2.0 g/dL, 49% for an initial M protein value of 2.5 g/dL, and 64% for an initial M protein value of 3.0 g/dL. The risk of progression to multiple myeloma or a related disorder at 20 years with an initial M protein value of 1.5 g/dL was 1.9 times the risk of progression with an initial value of 0.5 g/dL or less, whereas the risk was 4.6 times if the initial M protein value was 2.5 g/dL.

Follow-up

Criteria for High-Risk MGUS

Abnormal κ/λ FLC ratio (<0.26 or >1.65)
High serum monoclonal protein level (>1.5 g/dL)
Non-IgG MGUS

Figure 3-8. Criteria for high-risk monoclonal gammopathy of undetermined significance (MGUS). A recent study from the Mayo Clinic evaluated the utility of the serum free light chain (FLC) assay in combination with the magnitude of the M spike, and the type of γ-globulin, to define risk categories of MGUS. Patients with all three of these features have the highest risk of progression to myeloma or related disorders at 20 years (58%). Patients with two risk factors have a 37% risk of progression at 20 years, compared with patients with one risk factor (21%) or none of the risk factors (5%) [5]. IgG—immunoglobulin G.

MGUS Follow-up Studies

If serum M protein <2.0 g/dL
Bone marrow and bone radiography rarely necessary
Repeat SPE at 6 mo; if stable, repeat yearly
If M protein >2.0 g/dL
Repeat SPE at 3 mo; if stable, repeat every 6–12 mo

Figure 3-9. Follow-up guideline for monoclonal gammopathy of undetermined significance (MGUS). Differentiation of the patient with MGUS from one who has multiple myeloma is often difficult. The size of the M protein in the serum and urine and the number of plasma cells in the bone marrow are of some help. An increase in the plasma cell labeling index, which measures the synthesis of DNA, is good evidence that the patient has multiple myeloma or will soon develop symptomatic disease. The presence of increased numbers of circulating plasma cells in the peripheral blood usually indicates active multiple myeloma. A patient with MGUS or smoldering myeloma needs to be followed with serial measurements of the M protein level in the serum and urine. SPE—serum protein electrophoresis.

Epidemiology and Etiology

Mayo Clinic Study Results

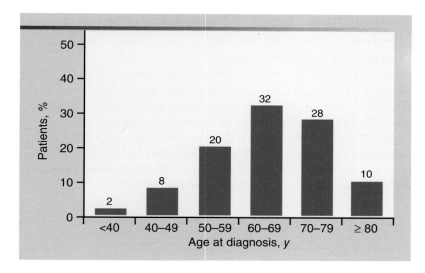

Figure 3-10. Age and gender in 1027 patients with multiple myeloma (Mayo Clinic, 1985 to 1998). Multiple myeloma is a neoplastic disorder characterized by the proliferation of a single clone of plasma cells derived from B cells. Myeloma accounts for about 1% of all types of malignancies and slightly more than 10% of hematologic malignancies. Of the 1027 patients, 59% were men and 41% were women. The actuarial risk is four per 100,000 per year, but the incidence in blacks is almost twice that in whites. The median age at the time of diagnosis is approximately 65 years (range, 20 to 92 years); only 2% of patients are younger than 40 years.

Laboratory Test Results in 1027 Patients with Multiple Myeloma					
	Patients, *n*	Median	Range	Distribution of Results	Patients, %
Hemoglobin, *g/dL*	1025	10.9	2.7–17	≤8	7
				8.1–10.0	28
				10.1–12	38
				>12	27
Creatinine, *mg/dL*	1020	1.2	0.5–18.2	<1.3	52
				1.3–1.9	29
				≥2	19
Calcium, *mg/dL*	1018	9.6	7.2–17.2	≤10.1	73
				10.2–10.9	14
				≥11	13
Cholesterol, *mg/dL*	364	173	52–433	≤100	10
				>250	9
Triglyceride, *mg/dL*	332	123	25–640	≤100	33
				>250	12
β_2-Microglobulin	735	3.9	0.8–82	≤2.7	25
				2.8–4.0	28
				4.1–6.0	21
				>6	26
C-reactive protein	285	0.4	0.01–49	<0.8	66
				>5.0	10

Figure 3-11. Laboratory test results in 1027 patients with multiple myeloma. Normocytic normochromic anemia is present initially in more than 70% of patients but eventually occurs in nearly everyone with multiple myeloma. The serum creatinine level is increased initially in almost half of patients and is 2.0 mg/dL or higher in 50%. Hypercalcemia is present in one fourth of patients at the time of diagnosis and is a treatable cause of renal insufficiency. β_2-Microglobulin is elevated in 75% and is an important prognostic factor. The serum protein electrophoretic pattern shows a peak or localized band in 80% of patients, hypogammaglobulin in almost 10%, and no apparent abnormality in the remainder; 93% have an M protein in the serum at diagnosis [6].

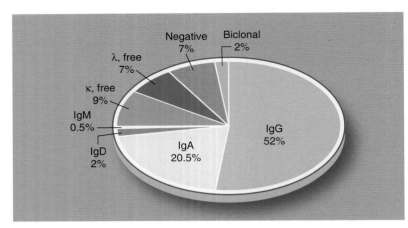

Negative 7%   Biclonal 2%

λ, free 7%

κ, free 9%

IgM 0.5%

IgD 2%

IgA 20.5%

IgG 52%

Figure 3-12. Types of serum monoclonal protein. Immunoglobulin (Ig)G accounts for one half and IgA for one fifth of monoclonal proteins. About one sixth have only a light chain (light chain myeloma). The M protein migrates in the γ range in about one half of patients, whereas the remainder migrate in the β or β-γ areas. In a group of 895 myeloma patients with a serum M protein, the M spike was 1 g/dL or lower in 18%. One or more uninvolved immunoglobulins were reduced in 90.5%, and both were reduced in 73%. The serum albumin level was less than 3.0 g/dL in 15%.

Clinical Presenting Features for Patients with Multiple Myeloma

Constitutional symptoms
Anemia
Bone pain or fracture
Hypercalcemia or other electrolyte abnormalities
Renal dysfunction/failure
Neurologic dysfunction (cord compression, neuropathy)
Immunologic dysfunction (infections)
Neutropenia and thrombocytopenia

Figure 3-13. Patients with newly diagnosed myeloma or myeloma progressing from monoclonal gammopathy of undetermined significance do so with a wide range of different symptoms. Most commonly, they present with some weakness and fatigue or bone pain. When further explored, laboratory studies may demonstrate the presence of anemia, renal dysfunction, an elevated serum protein, or the presence of a urinary monoclonal protein.

Diagnosis

Criteria for the Diagnosis of Asymptomatic Myeloma

M protein in serum >3.0 g/dL
and/or
Bone marrow with >10% clonal plasma cells
No ROTI

Figure 3-14. Criteria for the diagnosis of asymptomatic myeloma. Diagnostic criteria for myeloma from the International Myeloma Working Group define two categories of myeloma separate from monoclonal gammopathy of undetermined significance (MGUS). The first is patients with asymptomatic myeloma who exceed the criteria for MGUS but do not have any of the criteria needed for the diagnosis of symptomatic myeloma. Patients with asymptomatic myeloma do not require therapy and are observed until disease progression is noted with the development of symptomatic myeloma [4]. ROTI—related organ or tissue impairment.

Criteria for Symptomatic Myeloma

M protein in the serum and/or the urine
Clonal plasma cells in the bone marrow or a plasmacytoma
Presence of ROTI

Figure 3-15. Criteria for symptomatic myeloma. Patients with symptomatic myeloma require therapy. Treatment options depend on the location and type of symptoms, as well as overall performance status and the likelihood that a given patient can be considered for high-dose therapy and autologous transplantation. ROTI—related organ or tissue impairment.

Myeloma-Related Organ or Tissue Impairment

Hypercalcemia
Renal dysfunction
Anemia (Hgb <10 g/dL)
Bone lesions (lytic disease or osteoporosis with compression fracture)
Other: symptomatic hyperviscosity, amyloidosis, or recurrent infections

Figure 3-16. Criteria for symptomatic myeloma include the above criteria and can be remembered as the CRAB criteria (C for calcium elevation, R for renal insufficiency, A for anemia, and B for bone disease). These criteria are critical for the distinction between asymptomatic myeloma, monoclonal gammopathy of undetermined significance, and symptomatic myeloma. Patients without these criteria may be observed. Randomized trials have demonstrated poorer outcomes for patients with asymptomatic myeloma who undergo therapy early rather than waiting until they become symptomatic [4]. Hgb—hemoglobin.

Durie-Salmon Staging Criteria

Stage	Criteria	Median OS, *mo*
I (low cell mass)	Hemoglobin value >10 g/dL	62 (IA), 22 (IB)
	Serum calcium value normal or <10.5 mg/dL	
	Bone radiography, normal bone structure (scale 0) or solitary bone plasmacytoma only	
	Low M-component production rates	
	IgG value <5.0 g/dL	
	IgA value <3.0 g/dL	
	Urine light chain M-component on electrophoresis <4 g/24 h	
II (intermediate cell mass)	Not stage I or stage III	58 (IIA), 34 (IIB)
III (high cell mass)	Hemoglobin value <8.5 g/dL	45 (IIIA), 24 (IIIB)
	Serum calcium value >12 mg/dL	
	Advanced lytic bone lesions (scale 3)	
	High M-component production rates	
	IgG value >7.0 g/dL	
	IgA value >5.0 g/dL	
	Urine light chain M-component on electrophoresis >12 g/24 h	
	A: relatively normal renal function: serum creatinine < 2.0 mg/dL	
	B: abnormal renal function: serum creatinine >2.0 mg/dL	

Figure 3-17. Durie-Salmon staging system [7]. This staging system has been used for more than two decades and classifies patients into risk groups based on the total body disease burden as identified using a series of laboratory and radiographic tests. Although this was useful for a long period, we have now identified that alternative factors, such as β_2-microglobulin, albumin, and cytogenetics, may be able to provide similar data and are easier to assimilate at the bedside. OS—overall survival.

International Staging System

Stage	Criteria	Median OS, *mo*
I	Serum β_2-microglobulin <3.5 mg/L and albumin >3.5 g/dL	62
II	Not stage I or stage III	44
III	Serum β_2-microglobulin >5.5 mg/L	29

Figure 3-18. International Staging System (ISS) [8]. Recently, large series of patients were combined from myeloma centers around the world in an attempt to simplify the staging criteria for patients with myeloma. The revised ISS was created, and using univariate and multivariate analysis, demonstrated superiority over the Durie-Salmon staging system and was less complicated in terms of the number of tests needed to fully evaluate a patient. This staging system still does not take into account cytogenetics, or emerging data from fluorescence in situ hybridization studies that suggest this may be an important predictor of biologic activity and survival for myeloma patients. OS—overall survival.

Common Cytogenetic Abnormalities in Myeloma
Deletion of chromosome 13
Deletion of chromosome 17p
Translocation (4;14)
Translocation (11;14)
Translocation (14;18)

Figure 3-19. Common cytogenetic abnormalities in myeloma. The identification of cytogenetic abnormalities has allowed for an improved biologic understanding of plasma cell biology. The first to be identified in any large series of patients was deletion of chromosome 13, which was identified as a negative prognostic factor [9]. Unfortunately, only a small percentage of patients with myeloma will have cytogenetically identifiable abnormalities due to the low rate of myeloma cell proliferation. It was not until the widespread use of fluorescence in situ hybridization (FISH) analysis that the higher frequency of cytogenetic abnormalities was further identified. In this setting, the above translocations and deletions were more commonly identified and have now been linked to prognostic information as well. Deletion 13 by cytogenetics has a poor prognostic outcome, likely linked to the fact that cells with cytogenetic abnormalities are proliferating more and thus the disease is not as indolent as most cases of myeloma. Deletion 13 alone as identified by FISH does not carry a negative prognostic effect and, in fact, is noted in close to 50% of patients at the time of diagnosis [10]. Translocation (4;14) is seen in about 10% of patients and is associated with a very poor outcome. Translocation (11;14) is thought to be a positive prognostic finding. Identification of cytogenetic-based staging will likely aid in future risk-adapted therapy approaches [11].

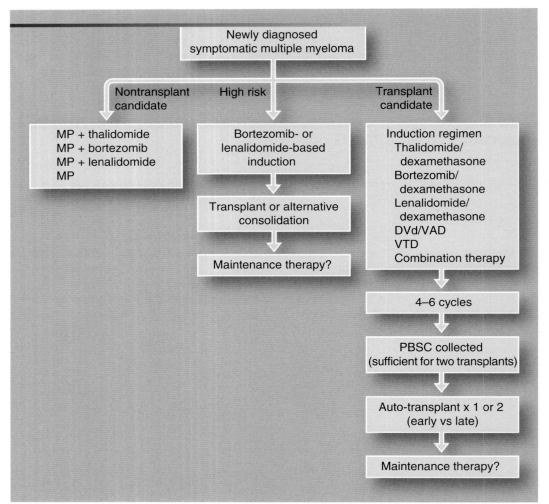

Figure 3-20. Scheme of treatment. Treatment of symptomatic myeloma has been divided into two separate categories. For patients eligible for high-dose therapy and autologous transplantation, alkylate-based induction is avoided. Standard treatment has included the use of dexamethasone, thalidomide, and dexamethasone chemotherapy (VAD [vincristine, doxorubicin, and dexamethasone] or DVd [doxorubicin, vincristine, and dexamethasone]) or, more recently, the use of novel agents such as bortezomib or lenalidomide. The use of novel agents such as bortezomib or lenalidomide with dexamethasone has the ability to induce higher response rates than those of conventional therapy and also induce a higher complete remission rate. Following induction therapy, patients usually move forward with stem cell collection and either early or delayed transplantation.

For patients not eligible for high-dose therapy and transplantation, treatment recently has changed with the observation that melphalan + prednisone + thalidomide is superior to melphalan and prednisone (MP) alone. Newer trials suggest that MP + bortezomib or MP + lenalidomide results in higher response rates, but randomized trials confirming their benefit over MP are currently in progress. PBSC—peripheral blood stem cells; VTD—Velcade (bortezomib), thalidomide, and dexamethasone.

Advantages and Disadvantages of Autologous Peripheral Transplantation for Multiple Myeloma

Advantages
Low mortality
Available for up to 50% of patients
Disadvantages
Contamination by tumor cells
Lack of cure

Figure 3-21. Advantages and disadvantages of autologous peripheral blood stem cell transplantation. Autologous transplantation is applicable for over 50% of patients and should be considered the standard approach for patients deemed suitable candidates for therapy. At this time, there is no upper age limit for consideration of high-dose therapy (HDT). The current mortality for patients in good disease status is less than 2%.

Although transplantation has been demonstrated in at least two large randomized trials to improve survival over conventional therapy [12,13], HDT is not curative [14], with a median duration of remission between 18 and 24 months. Peripheral blood stem cells should be collected before exposure to alkylating agents such as melphalan. To date, the use of HDT in the setting of patients eligible for transplantation represents the sole treatment to have demonstrated a survival benefit over conventional therapy, though the use of novel agents such as bortezomib, thalidomide, and lenalidomide in the induction therapy setting may be able to enhance or supersede the benefits of HDT.

Challenges of Autologous Stem Cell Transplantation

Eradication of multiple myeloma
Removal of myeloma cells and precursors from peripheral blood

Figure 3-22. Challenges of autologous stem cell transplantation. Despite a steep dose-response curve favoring the use of high-dose melphalan, patients continue to relapse. Strategies using combinations of different chemotherapeutic agents or radiation with melphalan have not demonstrated superiority in randomized trials to date, and may be associated with more toxicity than is seen with melphalan alone [15].

Additional efforts to improve response rates and duration of remission by purging the collected bone marrow or stem cell graft using in vitro treatment of the collected graft or CD34+ selection of the graft also have not demonstrated benefit with respect to event-free survival or overall survival [16,17].

Attempts to add novel agents in combination with melphalan are currently being explored. The use of radiolabeled bone-targeted agents with melphalan has been explored in small studies as has the recent combination of melphalan and bortezomib [18].

Current approaches are focusing on improving the response rates and depth of response with the use of more active agents, and determining whether a better pretransplantation response translates into an improved posttransplantation response rate and duration of remission.

Single Versus Double Autologous Stem Cell Transplantation

	EFS at 5 y, %	Survival at 5 y, %
Single	20	40
Double	35	60

Figure 3-23. Survival rates for single versus double autologous stem cell transplantation. It has been suggested that better results may be obtained with double or tandem autologous peripheral stem cell transplants [19]. In a randomized trial of 400 patients reported by the French Myeloma Group, the response rate, event-free survival (EFS), and overall survival were not different for single and double autologous stem cell transplants when evaluated at 2 years. In a subsequent analysis of this study, patients with the double transplant from peripheral stem cells had a better survival than those with a single transplant with stem cells from the bone marrow [20]. Although survival as a whole was improved with double compared with single transplants, there was no benefit for tandem transplants among patients who had already achieved a very good partial response or better following the first transplant. Similar results with the achievement of a very good partial response were reported in preliminary fashion from the Italian MAG group as well.

Advantages and Disadvantages of Allogeneic Bone Marrow or Stem Cell Transplant

Advantages
No tumor cell contamination of the graft
Immunologic graft-versus-myeloma effect
Disadvantages
Few patients have suitable donors or eligibility
High treatment-related mortality
Significant incidence of graft-versus-host disease
Late relapses?/cure?

Figure 3-24. Advantages and disadvantages of allogeneic bone marrow or stem cell transplantation. Major advantages of allogeneic transplantation relate to the absence of tumor cell contamination in the graft and the presence of the graft-versus-myeloma effect [21] that may be useful in the setting of chemotherapy-resistant disease [22].

The recent development of nonmyeloablative transplantation (NMT) has increased the pool of potentially eligible patients, though the long-term results of NMT have yet to demonstrate whether any patients are cured. Additionally, the incidence of graft-versus-host disease seems to occur more commonly with allogeneic transplantation for myeloma, and is even higher with NMT. There was significant enthusiasm with the initial reports from a series of patients treated with tandem autologous/mini-allogeneic transplantation [23]. However, longer follow-up of these patients suggests that relapse and life-limiting graft-versus-host disease continue to be an issue. Final results from a large intergroup US trial comparing tandem autologous transplantation and tandem autologous/mini-allogeneic transplantation are eagerly awaited to address the true utility of mini-allogeneic transplantation for myeloma.

Melphalan and Prednisone Chemotherapy for Multiple Myeloma

Melphalan, 0.15 mg/kg/d, 7 d, + prednisone, 20 mg 3×/d, 7 d
Repeat leukocyte and platelet counts every 3 wk
Repeat cycle every 6 wk
Need modest cytopenia at midcycle

Figure 3-25. Melphalan and prednisone chemotherapy. Chemotherapy with alkylating agents is the preferred initial treatment for patients with symptomatic multiple myeloma who are older than 70 years or for younger patients in whom transplantation is not feasible. The oral administration of melphalan (8 to 10 mg) daily for 7 days and prednisone (20 mg) three times daily for the same 7 days every 6 weeks is a satisfactory regimen. The leukocytes and platelets must be measured every 3 weeks and the dosage of melphalan altered to obtain some reduction of leukocytes or platelets at midcycle (because absorption of melphalan is variable). The patient should receive three courses of melphalan and prednisone before the therapy is discontinued, unless the disease progresses rapidly. The objective response rate is only 50% to 60%.

Single Versus Combination Chemotherapy for Multiple Myeloma

Therapy	Response, %
Melphalan, prednisone	53
Conventional-dose combination therapy	60

Figure 3-26. Melphalan versus combination therapy. Many combinations of chemotherapeutic agents have been used because of the obvious shortcomings of melphalan and prednisone. In a large meta-analysis based on the individual patient data of 4930 patients in 20 prospective trials, the Myeloma Trialists' Collaborative Group found an improved response rate with combination chemotherapy; however, there was no difference in survival and no subset of patients who had a better survival rate than with melphalan and prednisone ($P < 0.00001$) [24].

Novel Combinations for Transplant-Ineligible Patients

Melphalan + prednisone + thalidomide (MPT)
Melphalan + prednisone + bortezomib (MPV)
Melphalan + prednisone + lenalidomide* (MPR)
Melphalan + prednisone + thalidomide + bortezomib* (VMPT)
*Preliminary data from small phase I and II studies only

Figure 3-27. Novel combinations for transplant-ineligible patients. For 30 years, no treatment had been demonstrated to be superior to melphalan + prednisone (MP) as therapy for patients not eligible for high-dose therapy and autologous transplantation. Recent data from the Italian and French groups have demonstrated an improvement in response rate, event-free survival, and overall survival for patients randomly assigned to receive MP + thalidomide over those randomly assigned to receive MP [25,26]. This finding now has effectively replaced the use of MP for patients who are not transplant eligible.

In another phase I/II study, the combination of MP and bortezomib demonstrated impressive activity and is now the subject of a large randomized trial to confirm its activity when compared with MP [27]. The combinations of MP and lenalidomide [28] and MP, thalidomide, and bortezomib [29] have also demonstrated impressive activity, but larger clinical trial data are currently in development. From these trials, it is clear that the addition of novel agents to conventional agents such as MP results in improved responses, and represents a model for future therapy development in this patient population.

Novel and Developing Agents in Multiple Myeloma

Approved agents
Thalidomide
Bortezomib
Lenalidomide
Agents in development
Tanespimycin (KOS-953), heat shock protein-90 inhibitor
Perifosine, AKT inhibitor
CC-4047, immunomodulatory agent
PR-171, second-generation proteasome inhibitor
CCI-779; RAD-001, mammalian target of rapamycin inhibitor

Figure 3-28. Novel and developing agents in multiple myeloma. The development of novel agents has revolutionized myeloma therapy. With the approval of thalidomide, bortezomib, and lenalidomide, patients are achieving better response rates and longer remissions. Lenalidomide and bortezomib both demonstrated improved survival when compared with dexamethasone in large randomized clinical trials [30,31]. Developing agents represent the future of myeloma therapy, with many different targets.

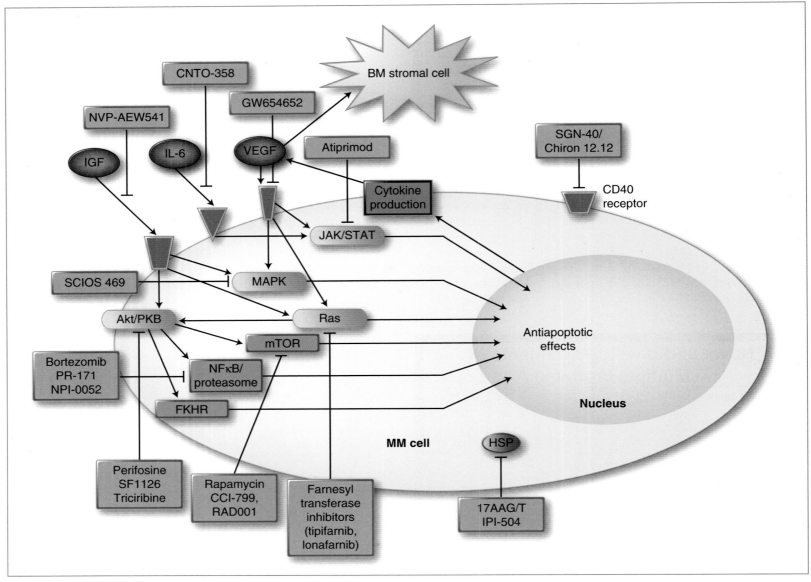

Figure 3-29. Cytokine and target networks in malignant plasma cells. Shown is a pictorial description of multiple potential targets and growth factor receptors on the surface of malignant plasma cells. Many agents for each of these targets are in preclinical and clinical development, demonstrating the challenge in the coming months to further identify suitable agents for future clinical trials. BM—bone marrow; HSP—heat shock protein; IGF—insulin-like growth factor; IL-6—interleukin-6; MM—multiple myeloma; mTOR—mammalian target of rapamycin; NFκB—nuclear factor κB; VEGF—vascular endothelial growth factor.

Complications

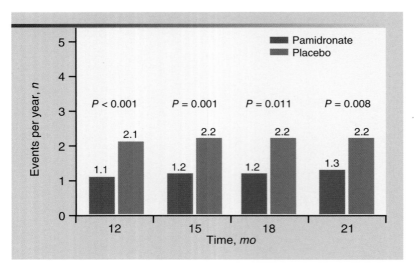

Figure 3-30. Skeletal complications. Skeletal involvement often leads to pain, pathologic fractures, hypercalcemia, or cord compression. Bisphosphonates are specific inhibitors of osteoclastic activity and have been used as adjunctive therapy in multiple myeloma. In a prospective study, 377 patients with myeloma who had bone lesions were randomly assigned to receive pamidronate 90 mg intravenously every 4 weeks or placebo. Patients receiving pamidronate had a significant reduction in skeletal events (pathologic fractures, need for surgery to treat or prevent pathologic fractures, need for radiation to bone, or spinal cord compression). The pamidronate group also had a decreased requirement for analgesic drugs and an improved quality of life [32].

Indications for Bisphosphonate Therapy in Myeloma

Bone disease (radiographic evidence of lytic disease or osteopenia)
Pamidronate 90 mg IV every 3–4 wk over 2–4 h
Zolendronic acid 4 mg IV every 3–4 wk over 30 min
Duration of therapy unknown

Figure 3-31. Indications for bisphosphonate therapy in myeloma. Randomized trials have demonstrated a significant reduction in the incidence of skeletal-related events among patients randomly assigned to bisphosphonate use. The two intravenous (IV) formulations available in the United States are listed in the figure and are both suitable options for patients with myeloma bone disease. Both agents are associated with the potential complication of renal insufficiency, through different mechanisms. For this reason, patients on either agent should undergo regular monitoring of renal function and non–light chain protein excretion in the urine.

Duration of therapy with bisphosphonates remains an unknown issue. Most guidelines have recommended indefinite continuation, though with the recent reporting of the complication of osteonecrosis of the jaw, this is being readdressed. Many groups are advocating either discontinuing therapy after 2 years of treatment [33] or changing from a monthly schedule to every 2 to 3 months for patients who have received 2 years of therapy.

Osteonecrosis of the Jaw: A Summary of Reported Data

Study	Patients, n	ONJ, n (%)*	Risk Factors
Durie et al. [69]	1203	75 (6.2)	Zolendronic acid
	904 MM	62 (6.8)	
Bamias et al. [70]	252	17 (6.7)	Dental extractions
	111 MM	11 (9.9)	
Badros et al. [38]	340	11 (3)	Dental extractions
Dimopoulos et al. [37]	202	15 (7.4)	
Zervas et al. [34]	254	28 (11)	Thalidomide
			Increased duration of BP therapy
Hoff et al. [71]	3994	29 (0.73)	Longer duration of therapy
	548 MM	13 (2.4)	
Tosi et al. [72]	259	9 (3.47; 6.6 at 24 mo)	Duration of exposure
*Includes only proven ONJ cases.			

Figure 3-32. Osteonecrosis of the jaw. The recently reported complication of ONJ is a complication that is associated with painful nonhealing bone destruction in the mouth. It is usually associated with some type of dental procedure or trauma. Risk factors include the use of bisphosphonate (BP) therapy, any oral surgical procedure performed while on BP therapy, and chronic infections of the mouth [34–38]. Because of this complication, it is now recommended that all patients undergo dental evaluation before initiating BP therapy and that any dental procedures be delayed until therapy can be held for a period of time. Finally, the use of prophylactic antibiotics during the period of wound healing may reduce the risk of developing this complication. MM—multiple myeloma.

Deep Venous Thrombosis and Myeloma

Baseline risk at the time of induction therapy between 5% and 10%

Risk increased with the following agents

Thalidomide/lenalidomide in combination with high-dose dexamethasone

Thalidomide/lenalidomide in combination with anthracyclines

Lenalidomide in combination with erythropoietin

Combinations of high-dose dexamethasone and anthracyclines

Figure 3-33. Deep venous thrombosis (DVT) and myeloma. DVT has been a well-recognized complication of myeloma therapy for several years now, but with the increased use of the immunomodulatory agents thalidomide and lenalidomide, mitigating factors contributing to this risk have been identified. Thalidomide or lenalidomide without steroids has a relatively low risk of DVT (<5%), but the addition of dexamethasone may increase this risk to between 15% and 20% [39]. Additionally, the concomitant use of erythropoietin has been identified to increase the risk of DVT among patients treated with lenalidomide + high-dose dexamethasone [40]. Mechanisms for this increased risk are poorly understood but are thought to relate to von Willebrand factor levels, endothelial damage, and perturbations of clotting factor levels and activation.

Prophylaxis for DVT has used numerous strategies, such as aspirin, low-dose warfarin, full-intensity warfarin (international normalized ratio 2 to 3), low molecular weight heparin at full dose, or prophylaxis. Currently, no clear consensus exists on which method to use for each situation.

Peripheral Neuropathy and Myeloma Therapy

Seen with conventional agents such as vincristine and cisplatin

Thalidomide

Incidence is dose related

Incidence is related to duration of therapy

May be motor or sensory

Bortezomib

Incidence may be dose related

Reversible if noted early

Predominantly sensory in nature

Lenalidomide

Predominantly seen as sensory

Mostly grade I or II in nature

Very mild compared with thalidomide or bortezomib

Figure 3-34. Peripheral neuropathy and myeloma therapy. Peripheral neuropathy is a complication of myeloma therapy as a result of the use of a number of different agents. Complications due to historical agents such as vincristine and cisplatin are more commonly noted to be sensory in nature and are essentially irreversible when they occur. Thalidomide-induced neuropathy may be both sensory and motor; it is associated with more chronic administration and appears to be less reversible [41]. Bortezomib causes mainly a sensory neuropathy, but it may be associated with pain [42]. Dose reduction and dose holding as the result of side effects may allow for reversal of bortezomib-induced neuropathy. Lenalidomide-induced neuropathy is generally mild and without significant complications.

Variant Forms of Multiple Myeloma

Key Aspects of Plasma Cell Leukemia

Absolute peripheral blood plasma cell count ≥2.0 × 10⁹/L

Usually >20% plasma cells in differential

Figure 3-35. Plasma cell leukemia. Plasma cell leukemia has been defined by the finding of a peripheral blood absolute plasma cell count of at least 2.0×10^9/L and more than 20% plasma cells in the peripheral blood differential leukocyte count. Plasma cell leukemia should be classified as "primary" when it is diagnosed in the leukemic phase or as "secondary" when there is leukemic transformation of a previously recognized multiple myeloma (40%). Patients with primary plasma cell leukemia are younger and have a higher incidence of hepatosplenomegaly and lymphadenopathy, a higher platelet count, fewer bone lesions, a smaller serum M protein component, and a longer survival (median 6.8 vs 1.3 months) than patients with secondary plasma cell leukemia [43,44].

Circulating plasma cells of any significance represent a significant change in the biology of the disease. Plasma cells are usually stromally dependent for their survival and drug resistance. The presence of circulating cells of any sizable proportion indicates that the malignant plasma cells have become stromally independent, and may represent a more resistant phenotype.

Responses may be seen with conventional agents such as vincristine, doxorubicin, and alkylating agents, as well as the novel agents bortezomib [45,46] and lenalidomide. High-dose therapy and autologous transplantation may have some benefit for these patients, though often remission duration is quite short. Data from allogeneic transplantations, both ablative and nonmyeloablative, have been less than satisfying to date in this poor-risk population.

Key Aspects of Nonsecretory Myeloma

No M protein in serum and urine with immunofixation

Bone marrow clonal plasmacytosis ≥10% or plasmacytoma

Related organ or tissue impairment (end-organ damage)

Figure 3-36. Nonsecretory myeloma. Patients with nonsecretory myeloma have no monoclonal protein in either the serum or urine with immunofixation. This occurs in only 3% of patients with symptomatic multiple myeloma. Renal insufficiency is less common than in patients with secretory myeloma, but the survival is not different [6]. Two thirds of patients with nonsecretory multiple myeloma based on immunofixation have an elevation of free monoclonal light chain of the appropriate isotype in the serum [47]. Because of

the availability of free light assay, most patients who have disease previously defined as nonsecretory can now be followed with an objective marker to assess response. Treatment for nonsecretory myeloma is the same as for that for multiple myeloma. To make the diagnosis, an M protein should be identified in the plasma cells by immunoperoxidase or immunofluorescence methods; in rare instances, no M protein is found in the myeloma cells.

Key Aspects of IgD Myeloma

The λ type is more common than the κ type

Amyloidosis and extramedullary plasmacytomas are more frequent

Figure 3-37. Key aspects of immunoglobulin D (IgD) myeloma. In IgD myeloma, the M protein is smaller than in IgG and IgA myeloma, and λ Bence Jones proteinuria is more common. Amyloidosis and extramedullary plasmacytomas are more frequent

in IgD myeloma. Survival is generally believed to be shorter than with other myeloma types, but often IgD is not diagnosed until later in its course [48–51].

Clinical Features of the POEMS Syndrome

Major features

Chronic inflammatory-demyelinating polyneuropathy with predominantly motor disability and sclerotic skeletal lesions

Possible features

Hyperpigmentation

Hypertrichosis

Gynecomastia

Atropic testes

Other features

Hemoglobin level normal or increased

Thrombocytosis is common

Bone marrow contains <5% plasma cells

Evidence of Castleman's disease

Figure 3-38. The POEMS (polyneuropathy, organomegaly, endocrinopathy, M protein, skin changes) syndrome, or osteosclerotic myeloma. Except for the presence of papilledema, the cranial nerves are not involved and the autonomic nervous system is intact. If the lesions are in a limited area, radiation therapy will produce substantial improvement of the neuropathy in more than one half of patients. If the patient has widespread osteosclerotic lesions, autologous stem cell transplantation or chemotherapy with melphalan and prednisone may be beneficial [52].

Clinical Aspects of Solitary Plasmacytoma of Bone

Single area of bone destruction owing to clonal plasma cells

Bone marrow not consistent with multiple myeloma

Normal skeletal survey (and MRI of spine and pelvis if done)

No related organ or tissue impairment (end-organ damage); small M protein component may be present

Figure 3-39. Solitary plasmacytoma of bone. The diagnosis is based on histologic evidence of a tumor consisting of monoclonal plasma cells identical to those in multiple myeloma. Persistence of the M protein after radiation therapy is associated with an increased risk of progression to multiple myeloma [39]. MRI of the spine and pelvis is helpful for detecting marrow involvement. Almost 50% of patients who have a solitary plasmacytoma are alive at 10 years, and disease-free survival at 10 years ranges from 15% to 25%. Treatment consists of radiation in the range of 40 to 50 Gy. There is no evidence that chemotherapy affects the rate of conversion to multiple myeloma. Progression, when it occurs, usually appears between 3 and 4 years, but the most uncertain criterion for diagnosis is the duration of observation necessary before deciding if the disease will not become generalized. In a group of 23 patients with solitary plasmacytoma of the thoracolumbar spine, multiple myeloma developed in seven of the eight patients with a solitary lesion on roentgenographs alone but in only one of seven patients who also had negative results on MRI [53]. Most patients with solitary plasmacytoma of bone have normal uninvolved immunoglobulin levels [54].

Figure 3-40. Extramedullary plasmacytoma. Extramedullary plasmacytoma is a plasma cell tumor that arises outside the bone marrow. The upper respiratory tract, including the nasal cavity and sinuses, nasopharynx, and larynx, is the most frequent location of lesions. Any organ may be involved. There is a prominence of immunoglobulin A monoclonal protein. The diagnosis is made on the basis of finding a monoclonal plasma cell tumor in an extramedullary site in the absence of multiple myeloma. Treatment consists of tumoricidal irradiation (40 to 50 Gy) and is often curative. In contrast to solitary plasmacytoma of bone, symptomatic multiple myeloma occurs in only 15% of patients [55].

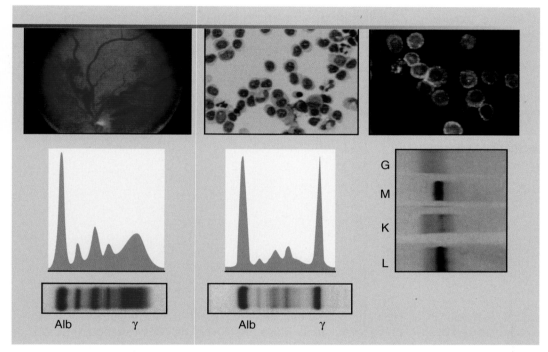

Figure 3-41. Macroglobulinemia. Macroglobulinemia is the result of uncontrolled proliferation of lymphocytes and plasma cells in which a large immunoglobulin M (IgM) protein is produced. The median age is about 65 years, and approximately 60% occur in men. Weakness, fatigue, oronasal bleeding, and blurred vision are common presenting symptoms. Hepatosplenomegaly, lymphadenopathy, retinal hemorrhages and exudates, and sensorimotor neuropathy may be found on examination [56].

Top left, Retinal hemorrhage from hyperviscosity. *Top middle*, Bone marrow showing increased numbers of lymphoid and plasmacytoid cells. *Top right*, Bone marrow showing IgM in cytoplasm of lymphoid cells with immunofluorescence. *Bottom left*, Densitometry tracing showing a broad peak of polyclonal gammopathy, with accompanying agarose gel electrophoresis showing a broad band of γ mobility. *Bottom center*, Densitometry tracing showing a tall, narrow peak with accompanying gel electrophoresis showing a dense band of gamma mobility. *Bottom right*, Immunofixation showing an IgM λ monoclonal protein.

Almost all patients have moderate to severe normocytic, normochromic anemia. The serum protein electrophoretic pattern is characterized by a tall, narrow peak (*bottom center*) or dense band and is usually of γ mobility. A monoclonal light chain, usually small in amount, is present in the urine of 80% of patients. Bone marrow infiltration with lymphoid and plasmacytoid cells expresses CD19, CD20, and CD22 but is usually CD5 and CD10 negative. Alb—albumin.

Therapy for Macroglobulinemia
Rituximab
Fludarabine
Chlorambucil
Cladribine
Autologous stem cell transplantation
Bortezomib

Figure 3-42. Therapy for macroglobulinemia. Patients should not be treated unless they have anemia or constitutional symptoms such as weakness, fatigue, night sweats, weight loss, hyperviscosity, or significant hepatosplenomegaly or lymphadenopathy. Rituximab, a chimeric anti-CD20 monoclonal antibody, produces a response in at least 50% of untreated patients. Fludarabine and cladribine are also effective agents. Chlorambucil produces an objective response in up to 70% of patients. Combinations of alkylating agents, such as the M2 protocol (vincristine, BCNU [carmustine], melphalan, cyclophosphamide, and prednisone) may be beneficial. Autologous stem cell transplantations have been performed in some cases. The use of rituximab either alone or in combination with cytotoxic chemotherapy may be associated with an immunoglobulin M (IgM) flare, or seeming progression of disease with symptomatic hyperviscosity in a previously asymptomatic patient. For this reason, it is suggested that patients receiving rituximab undergo prophylactic plasmapheresis before starting rituximab if there is a high level of disease burden [57].

Recent studies suggest that the proteasome inhibitor bortezomib also has activity in the setting of macroglobulinemia. Studies have been performed in the settings of relapse and newly diagnosed disease, and in combination with rituximab, impressive activity has been demonstrated [58]. The use of bortezomib with rituximab has the added benefit of potentially reducing the IgM flare that occurs with the use of single-agent rituximab in these patients.

Clinical Features of Systemic Amyloidosis
Nephrotic syndrome
Diastolic dysfunction or symptomatic heart failure
Postural hypotension/syncope
Peripheral or central neuropathy
Diarrhea/malabsorption/weight loss

Figure 3-43. Clinical features of systemic amyloidosis. Systemic amyloidosis is a protein conformational disorder characterized by the deposition of aggregated and insoluble amyloid fibrils in tissue. The net result of this deposition is organ dysfunction that may affect nearly every tissue within the body. Diagnosis requires the histologic demonstration of amyloid deposition in tissue, which may be observed in bone marrow aspirates, abdominal fat pad aspirates, lip biopsies, rectal biopsies, or the end organ involved, such as cardiac, renal, or hepatic biopsies. For patients to be categorized as having primary (AL) amyloidosis, there must be demonstration of a clone of plasma cells with the presence of a monoclonal protein by serum or urine protein electrophoresis. More recently, the use of the plasma free light assay has been demonstrated to be a good diagnostic and prognostic marker in AL amyloidosis. Treatment for AL amyloidosis is varied and depends on patient age, extent of organ dysfunction, and performance status [59,60].

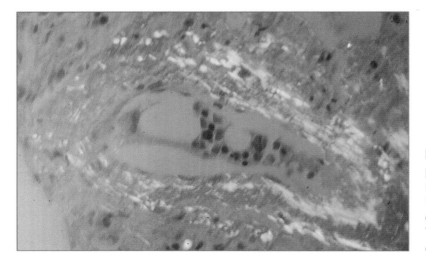

Figure 3-44. Blood vessel from a bone marrow biopsy indicating primary systemic (AL) amyloidosis. Amyloid stained with Congo red produces an apple green birefringence under polarized light. It is a fibrous protein that consists of linear, nonbranching aggregated fibrils of 7.5 to 10.0 nm in width and of indefinite length. The amyloid fibrils in AL amyloidosis consist of a variable portion of a monoclonal light chain. (*From* Kyle and Gertz [61].)

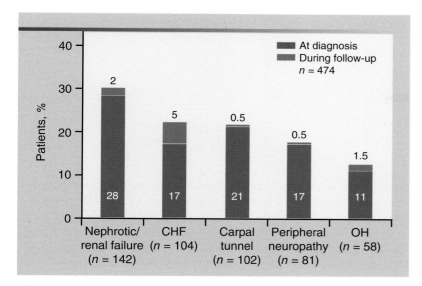

Figure 3-45. Primary systemic (AL) amyloidosis [62]. The median age at diagnosis is 65 years, and only 1% of patients are younger than age 40. Weakness, fatigue, dyspnea, edema, paresthesias, lightheadedness, and syncope are frequently present. Physical findings include a palpable liver in one fourth of patients, but splenomegaly in only 5% and macroglossia in 10%. Nephrotic syndrome, carpal tunnel syndrome, congestive heart failure (CHF), peripheral neuropathy, and orthostatic hypotension (OH) are major presenting syndromes. The presence of one of these syndromes and an M protein in the serum or urine is a strong indication of amyloidosis. A monoclonal protein is found in the serum or urine in almost 90% of patients at diagnosis.

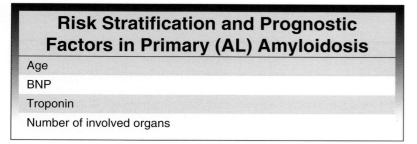

Figure 3-46. Risk stratification and prognostic factors in primary (AL) amyloidosis. AL amyloidosis patients require close scrutiny when deciding on a treatment approach. Mortality for aggressive therapy such as high-dose therapy and autologous transplantation is directly linked to features such as patient age (higher mortality for those >65 years) and the presence of cardiac involvement as defined by an abnormal level of brain natriuretic peptide (BNP) and/or troponin [62]. In a recent publication from the Mayo Clinic group, patients were grouped into three stages of disease by the presence or absence of normal or abnormal BNP and troponin levels within the peripheral blood. Patients with normal values for both were considered stage 1, with a median overall survival (OS) of 26 months, whereas patients with abnormal values for either BNP or troponin were considered stage II, with a median OS of 10.5 months. Patients with abnormal values for both BNP and troponin were considered stage III and had a median OS of 3.5 months. Thus, with easily attainable clinical and laboratory studies, patients can easily be put into risk strata that can be used to define treatment approaches.

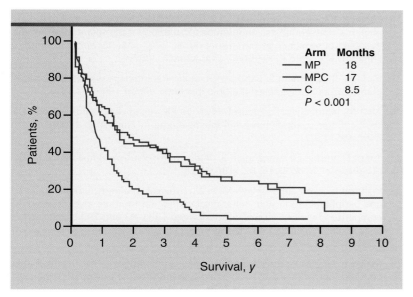

Figure 3-47. Survival of patients with primary systemic (AL) amyloidosis. Therapy for AL amyloidosis is not satisfactory. In a randomized trial, regimens containing melphalan, prednisone, and colchicine (MPC) provided better survival (18 vs 8.5 months) than colchicine (C) alone. Encouraging results have been reported with high-dose intravenous melphalan (140 to 200 mg/m²) followed by autologous peripheral stem cell rescue. However, patients with significant cardiac involvement should not have stem cell transplantation because of the increased mortality [63,64].

Treatment Options for Patients with Primary (AL) Amyloidosis

Oral melphalan-based therapy
High-dose therapy and autologous transplantation
Thalidomide
Lenalidomide
Bortezomib

Figure 3-48. Treatment options for patients with primary (AL) amyloidosis. Treatment options for patients with AL amyloidosis range in intensity and efficacy based on the level of organ dysfunction and patient performance status. For patients ineligible for high-dose therapy and autologous transplantation, standard therapy involves the use of oral melphalan and prednisone or dexamethasone [65]. For patients suitable for high-dose therapy, no induction therapy is needed. Patients may move directly to stem cell mobilization and melphalan-based autologous transplantation. Autologous transplantation in the appropriate setting may result in long-term remissions in certain subsets of patients and may be most suitable for patients with predominantly renal manifestations of their disease [66]. In the setting of relapse, thalidomide may offer some benefit, though the use of thalidomide in amyloidosis is associated with significant toxicity and side effects [67]. Phase II data with lenalidomide suggest that it may have activity in amyloid, and is better tolerated than thalidomide [68]. Bortezomib is being explored in early-phase studies and also shows promise as a single agent.

REFERENCES

1. Annesley TM, Burritt MF, Kyle RA: Artifactual hypercalcemia in multiple myeloma. *Mayo Clin Proc* 1982, 57:572–575.

2. Kyle R: *Classification and Diagnosis of Monoclonal Gammopathies*, vol 152, edn 3. Washington, DC: American Society of Microbiology Press; 1986.

3. Kyle RA, Therneau TM, Rajkumar SV, *et al.*: A long-term study of prognosis in monoclonal gammopathy of undetermined significance. *N Engl J Med* 2002, 346:564–569.

4. Criteria for the classification of monoclonal gammopathies, multiple myeloma and related disorders: a report of the International Myeloma Working Group. *Br J Haematol* 2003, 121:749–757.

5. Rajkumar SV, Kyle RA, Therneau TM, *et al.*: Serum free light chain ratio is an independent risk factor for progression in monoclonal gammopathy of undetermined significance. *Blood* 2005, 106:812–817.

6. Kyle RA, Gertz MA, Witzig TE, *et al.*: Review of 1027 patients with newly diagnosed multiple myeloma. *Mayo Clin Proc* 2003, 78:21–33.

7. Durie BG, Salmon SE: A clinical staging system for multiple myeloma. Correlation of measured myeloma cell mass with presenting clinical features, response to treatment, and survival. *Cancer* 1975, 36:842–854.

8. Greipp PR, San Miguel J, Durie BG, *et al.*: International staging system for multiple myeloma. *J Clin Oncol* 2005, 23:3412–3420.

9. Shaughnessy J, Barlogie B: Chromosome 13 deletion in myeloma. *Curr Top Microbiol Immunol* 1999, 246:199–203.

10. Avet-Loiseau H, Attal M, Moreau P, *et al.*: Genetic abnormalities and survival in multiple myeloma: the experience of the Intergroupe Francophone du Myelome. *Blood* 2007, 109:3489–3495.

11. Stewart AK, Bergsagel PL, Greipp PR, *et al.*: A practical guide to defining high-risk myeloma for clinical trials, patient counseling and choice of therapy. *Leukemia* 2007, 21:529–534.

12. Attal M, Harousseau JL, Stoppa AM, *et al.*: A prospective, randomized trial of autologous bone marrow transplantation and chemotherapy in multiple myeloma. Intergroupe Francais du Myelome. *N Engl J Med* 1996, 335:91–97.

13. Child JA, Morgan GJ, Davies FE, *et al.*: High-dose chemotherapy with hematopoietic stem-cell rescue for multiple myeloma. *N Engl J Med* 2003, 348:1875–1883.

14. Lemoli RM, Martinelli G, Zamagni E, *et al.*: Engraftment, clinical, and molecular follow-up of patients with multiple myeloma who were reinfused with highly purified CD34+ cells to support single or tandem high-dose chemotherapy. *Blood* 2000, 95:2234–2239.

15. Attal M, Harousseau JL: Randomized trial experience of the Intergroupe Francophone du Myelome. *Semin Hematol* 2001, 38:226–230.

16. Vescio R, Schiller G, Stewart AK, *et al.*: Multicenter phase III trial to evaluate CD34(+) selected versus unselected autologous peripheral blood progenitor cell transplantation in multiple myeloma. *Blood* 1999, 93:1858–1868.

17. Stewart AK, Vescio R, Schiller G, *et al.*: Purging of autologous peripheral-blood stem cells using CD34 selection does not improve overall or progression-free survival after high-dose chemotherapy for multiple myeloma: results of a multicenter randomized controlled trial. *J Clin Oncol* 2001, 19:3771–3779.

18. Lonial S, Kaufman J, Langston A, *et al.*: A randomized phase I trial of melphalan + bortezomib as conditioning for autologous transplant for myeloma: the effect of sequence of administration. In: *2007 BMT Tandem Meetings*. Edited by Korngold R. Keystone, CO: ASBMT; 2007:56.

19. Barlogie B, Jagannath S, Desikan KR, *et al.*: Total therapy with tandem transplants for newly diagnosed multiple myeloma. *Blood* 1999, 93:55–65.

20. Attal M, Harousseau JL, Facon T, *et al.*: Single versus double autologous stem-cell transplantation for multiple myeloma. *N Engl J Med* 2003, 349:2495–2502.

21. Tricot G, Vesole DH, Jagannath S, *et al.*: Graft-versus-myeloma effect: proof of principle. *Blood* 1996, 87:1196–1198.

22. Gahrton G, Svensson H, Cavo M, *et al.*: Progress in allogenic bone marrow and peripheral blood stem cell transplantation for multiple myeloma: a comparison between transplants performed 1983–93 and 1994–8 at European Group for Blood and Marrow Transplantation centres. *Br J Haematol* 2001, 113:209–216.

23. Maloney DG, Molina AJ, Sahebi F, *et al.*: Allografting with nonmyeloablative conditioning following cytoreductive autografts for the treatment of patients with multiple myeloma. *Blood* 2003, 102:3447–3454.

24. Combination chemotherapy versus melphalan plus prednisone as treatment for multiple myeloma: an overview of 6633 patients from 27 randomized trials. Myeloma Trialists' Collaborative Group. *J Clin Oncol* 1998, 16:3832–3842.

25. Palumbo A, Bringhen S, Caravita T, *et al.*: Oral melphalan and prednisone chemotherapy plus thalidomide compared with melphalan and prednisone alone in elderly patients with multiple myeloma: randomised controlled trial. *Lancet* 2006, 367:825–831.

26. Facon T, Mary J, Harousseau J, *et al.*: Superiority of melphalan-prednisone (MP) + thalidomide (THAL) over MP and autologous stem cell transplantation in the treatment of newly diagnosed elderly patients with multiple myeloma. *J Clin Oncol (Meeting Abstracts)* 2006, 24:1.

27. Mateos MV, Hernandez JM, Hernandez MT, *et al.*: Bortezomib plus melphalan and prednisone in elderly untreated patients with multiple myeloma: results of a multicenter phase 1/2 study. *Blood* 2006, 108:2165–2172.

28. Palumbo A, Falco P, Falcone A, *et al.*: Oral Revlimid(R) plus melphalan and prednisone (R-MP) for newly diagnosed multiple myeloma: results of a multicenter phase I/II study. *ASH Annual Meeting Abstracts* 2006, 108:800.

29. Palumbo A, Ambrosini MT, Benevolo G, *et al.*: Combination of bortezomib, melphalan, prednisone and thalidomide (VMPT) for relapsed multiple myeloma: results of a phase I/II clinical trial. *ASH Annual Meeting Abstracts*. 2006, 108:407.

30. Richardson PG, Sonneveld P, Schuster MW, *et al.*: Bortezomib or high-dose dexamethasone for relapsed multiple myeloma. *N Engl J Med* 2005, 352:2487–2498.

31. Weber DM, Chen C, Niesvizky R, *et al.*: Lenalidomide plus high-dose dexamethasone provides improved overall survival compared to high-dose dexamethasone alone for relapsed or refractory multiple myeloma (MM): results of a North American phase III study (MM-009). *J Clin Oncol (Meeting Abstracts)* 2006, 24:7521.

32. Berenson JR, Lichtenstein A, Porter L, *et al.*: Long-term pamidronate treatment of advanced multiple myeloma patients reduces skeletal events. Myeloma Aredia Study Group. *J Clin Oncol* 1998, 16:593–602.

33. Lacy MQ, Dispenzieri A, Gertz MA, *et al.*: Mayo clinic consensus statement for the use of bisphosphonates in multiple myeloma. *Mayo Clin Proc* 2006, 81:1047–1053.

34. Zervas K, Verrou E, Teleioudis Z, *et al.*: Incidence, risk factors and management of osteonecrosis of the jaw in patients with multiple myeloma: a single-centre experience in 303 patients. *Br J Haematol* 2006, 134:620–623.

35. Melo MD, Obeid G: Osteonecrosis of the jaws in patients with a history of receiving bisphosphonate therapy: strategies for prevention and early recognition. *J Am Dent Assoc* 2005, 136:1675–1681.

36. Mehrotra B, Ruggiero S: Bisphosphonate complications including osteonecrosis of the jaw. *Hematology Am Soc Hematol Educ Program*. 2006:356–360.

37. Dimopoulos MA, Kastritis E, Anagnostopoulos A, *et al.*: Osteonecrosis of the jaw in patients with multiple myeloma treated with bisphosphonates: evidence of increased risk after treatment with zoledronic acid. *Haematologica* 2006, 91:968–971.

38. Badros A, Weikel D, Salama A, *et al.*: Osteonecrosis of the jaw in multiple myeloma patients: clinical features and risk factors. *J Clin Oncol* 2006, 24:945–952.

39. Zonder JA: Thrombotic complications of myeloma therapy. *Hematology Am Soc Hematol Educ Program*. 2006:348–355.

40. Niesvizky R, Spencer A, Wang M, *et al.*: Increased risk of thrombosis with lenalidomide in combination with dexamethasone and erythropoietin. *J Clin Oncol (Meeting Abstracts)* 2006, 24:7506.

41. Mileshkin L, Stark R, Day B, *et al.*: Development of neuropathy in patients with myeloma treated with thalidomide: patterns of occurrence and the role of electrophysiologic monitoring. *J Clin Oncol* 2006, 24:4507–4514.

42. Richardson PG, Briemberg H, Jagannath S, *et al.*: Frequency, characteristics, and reversibility of peripheral neuropathy during treatment of advanced multiple myeloma with bortezomib. *J Clin Oncol* 2006, 24:3113–3120.

43. Noel P, Kyle RA: Plasma cell leukemia: an evaluation of response to therapy. *Am J Med* 1987, 83:1062–1068.

44. Garcia-Sanz R, Orfao A, Gonzalez M, *et al.*: Primary plasma cell leukemia: clinical, immunophenotypic, DNA ploidy, and cytogenetic characteristics. *Blood* 1999, 93:1032–1037.

45. Gertz MA: Managing plasma cell leukemia. *Leuk Lymphoma* 2007, 48:5–6.

46. Finnegan DP, Kettle P, Drake M, *et al.*: Bortezomib is effective in primary plasma cell leukemia. *Leuk Lymphoma* 2006, 47:1670–1673.

47. Drayson M, Tang LX, Drew R, *et al.*: Serum free light-chain measurements for identifying and monitoring patients with nonsecretory multiple myeloma. *Blood* 2001, 97:2900–2902.

48. Wechalekar A, Amato D, Chen C, *et al.*: IgD multiple myeloma—a clinical profile and outcome with chemotherapy and autologous stem cell transplantation. *Ann Hematol* 2005, 84:115–117.

49. Sinclair D: IgD myeloma: clinical, biological and laboratory features. *Clin Lab* 2002, 48:617–622.

50. Blade J, Kyle RA: Nonsecretory myeloma, immunoglobulin D myeloma, and plasma cell leukemia. *Hematol Oncol Clin North Am* 1999, 13:1259–1272.

51. Blade J, Kyle RA: IgD monoclonal gammopathy with long-term follow-up. *Br J Haematol* 1994, 88:395–396.

52. Dispenzieri A, Kyle RA, Lacy MQ, *et al.*: POEMS syndrome: definitions and long-term outcome. *Blood* 2003, 101:2496–2506.

53. Liebross RH, Ha CS, Cox JD, *et al.*: Solitary bone plasmacytoma: outcome and prognostic factors following radiotherapy. *Int J Radiat Oncol Biol Phys* 1998, 41:1063–1067.

54. Dimopoulos MA, Moulopoulos LA, Maniatis A, Alexanian R: Solitary plasmacytoma of bone and asymptomatic multiple myeloma. *Blood* 2000, 96:2037–2044.

55. Alexiou C, Kau RJ, Dietzfelbinger H, *et al.*: Extramedullary plasmacytoma: tumor occurrence and therapeutic concepts. *Cancer* 1999, 85:2305–2314.

56. Ghobrial IM, Gertz MA, Fonseca R: Waldenstrom macroglobulinaemia. *Lancet Oncol* 2003, 4:679–685.

57. Gertz MA: Waldenstrom macroglobulinemia: a review of therapy. *Am J Hematol* 2005, 79:147–157.

58. Treon SP, Soumerai JD, Patterson CJ, *et al.*: Bortezomib, dexamethasone and rituximab (BDR) is a highly active regimen in the primary therapy of Waldenstrom's macroglobulinemia: planned interim results of WMCTG clinical trial 05-180. *ASH Annual Meeting Abstracts* 2006, 108:2765.

59. Gertz MA, Lacy MQ, Dispenzieri A, Hayman SR: Amyloidosis: diagnosis and management. *Clin Lymphoma Myeloma* 2005, 6:208–219.

60. Gertz MA: Diagnosing primary amyloidosis. *Mayo Clin Proc* 2002, 77:1278–1279.

61. Kyle R, Gertz M: *Amyloidosis*, vol 4. Philadelphia: Current Medicine; 1995.

62. Dispenzieri A, Gertz MA, Kyle RA, *et al.*: Prognostication of survival using cardiac troponins and N-terminal pro-brain natriuretic peptide in patients with primary systemic amyloidosis undergoing peripheral blood stem cell transplantation. *Blood* 2004, 104:1881–1887.

63. Gertz MA, Lacy MQ, Dispenzieri A, *et al.*: Risk-adjusted manipulation of melphalan dose before stem cell transplantation in patients with amyloidosis is associated with a lower response rate. *Bone Marrow Transplant* 2004, 34:1025–1031.

64. Gertz MA, Lacy MQ, Dispenzieri A, *et al.*: Transplantation for amyloidosis. *Curr Opin Oncol* 2007, 19:136–141.

65. Palladini G, Perfetti V, Obici L, *et al*.: Association of melphalan and high-dose dexamethasone is effective and well tolerated in patients with AL (primary) amyloidosis who are ineligible for stem cell transplantation. *Blood* 2004, 103:2936–2938.

66. Dispenzieri A, Kyle RA, Lacy MQ, *et al*.: Superior survival in primary systemic amyloidosis patients undergoing peripheral blood stem cell transplantation: a case-control study. *Blood* 2004, 103:3960–3963.

67. Dispenzieri A, Lacy MQ, Rajkumar SV, *et al*.: Poor tolerance to high doses of thalidomide in patients with primary systemic amyloidosis. *Amyloid* 2003, 10:257–261.

68. Dispenzieri A, Lacy MQ, Zeldenrust SR, *et al*.: The activity of lenalidomide with or without dexamethasone in patients with primary systemic amyloidosis. *Blood* 2007, 109:465–470.

69. Durie BG, Katz M, Crowley J: Osteonecrosis of the jaw and bisphosphonates. *N Engl J Med* 2005, 353:99–102.

70. Bamias A, Kastritis E, Bamia C, *et al*.: Osteonecrosis of the jaw in cancer after treatment with bisphosphonates: incidence and risk factors. *J Clin Oncol* 2005, 23:8580–8587.

71. Hoff AO, Toth B, Altundag K, *et al*.: Osteonecrosis of the jaw in patients receiving intravenous bisphosphonate therapy. *J Bone Miner Res* 2005, 20(Suppl 1):1218.

72. Tosi P, Zamagni E, Cangini D: Osteonecrosis of the jaws in newly diagnosed multiple myeloma patients treated with zoledronic acid and thalidomide-dexamethasone. *Blood* 2006, 108:3951–3952.

CHAPTER 4

Myeloid Disorders

James M. Foran, Karen L. Chang, and Stephen J. Forman

Acute myeloid leukemia (AML, also known as acute myelogenous leukemia) is a result of a somatic mutation in a pluripotent stem cell or, in some cases, a more differentiated cell derived from stem cells. The disease is mostly of unknown etiology except in cases of prior radiation (eg, Hiroshima, Chernobyl, Marshall Islands, or radiation therapy) or chronic exposure to benzene. An increasing number of cases have developed after exposure of the patient to cancer chemotherapeutic agents. Very simplistically, these toxic insults putatively confer upon the cells a growth or survival advantage when compared with normal (unexposed) stem cells. As the mutant cells proliferate and accumulate, normal hematopoiesis is inhibited, resulting in changes in the normal red cell, neutrophil, and platelet levels in the blood and marrow. Patients often present with weakness, exertional fatigue, skin changes (related to thrombocytopenia), and because of neutropenia, infection, poor wound healing, or bleeding. As discussed in this chapter, the diagnosis of AML is made by a measurement of the blood counts and an examination of the bone marrow, as well as numerous ancillary studies. In some cases, the leukemic stem cell is capable of some degree of differentiation that gives the cells a specific morphology or immunophenotype, features that can be exploited for diagnosis, monitoring, and therapy. In addition, cytogenetic analysis of the cells may show specific recurring abnormalities that are used to classify the leukemia, detect minimal residual disease, and provide information regarding the underlying mechanisms of leukemogenesis.

The myelodysplastic syndromes (MDSs) represent a group of dysfunctional neoplastic myeloid disorders that are clonal in origin and have propensity to evolve to acute leukemia over time. Although rare in childhood, the incidence increases after the age of 50 years, with most cases appearing in patients over the age of 60 years. MDS is usually a primary disorder but may also occur as a consequence of marrow injury caused by chemotherapeutic agents (eg, alkylating agents, topoisomerase II inhibitors) or radiation used to treat prior benign or malignant conditions. The diseases show a propensity to cytopenia and dysplastic morphology involving one or more cell lines, giving rise to ineffective hematopoiesis and peripheral cytopenia. In some nonprogressive cases, the hallmark is anemia accompanied by only slight variations in neutrophil and platelet count, whereas in other cases, pancytopenia is noted at diagnosis and represents the major clinical problem. Clonal cytogenetic abnormalities are often detected, and each of the various subtypes has the propensity to evolve into frank acute myelogenous leukemia, depending on their risk factors at the time of diagnosis. Even in the absence of leukemic evolution, most patients with MDS succumb to infection or transfusion-related complications, such as platelet alloimmunization or iron overload.

The myeloproliferative diseases (MPDs) are a group of disorders that are characterized by the slow but relentless progressive expansion of a clone of hematopoietic cells generally limited to a single myeloid lineage. With varying frequencies, these diseases evolve into bone marrow failure (due to myelofibrosis or ineffective hematopoiesis at the late stages) or an acute blastic stage. Similar to the MDSs, the MPDs seem to result from the neoplastic transformation at the level of pluripotent hematopoietic stem cell. In distinct contrast to MDSs, which are characterized by ineffective hematopoiesis from the onset, the proliferation associated with MPDs is initially effective and often of long duration, resulting in increased numbers of red blood cells, granulocytes, or platelets in varying degrees.

The myelodysplastic syndrome/myeloproliferative disorder (MDS/MPD) category includes myeloid disorders that have both dysplastic and proliferative features at the time of initial presentation and that do not meet the criteria for any of the previously defined diseases in the MDS or MPD categories. The three major diseases in the MDS/MPD category are chronic myelomonocytic leukemia, atypical chronic myeloid leukemia, and juvenile myelomonocytic leukemia. The clinician may view each individual patient in the context of whether proliferative or dysplastic manifestations predominate and treat accordingly.

Signs and Symptoms of Acute Myeloid Leukemia
Fatigue, bruising, bleeding
Fever
Bone pain
White blood cell elevation
Pancytopenia
Leukostasis
Hepatosplenomegaly
Visceral involvement
Central nervous system involvement

Figure 4-1. Signs and symptoms of leukemia. Leukemia manifests itself symptomatically by its impact on normal hematopoiesis, resulting in fatigue due to anemia, bruising and bleeding due to thrombocytopenia, and fever due to a decrease in functional neutrophils. Although bone pain is common in children with acute lymphoblastic leukemia, it is less common in adults. A marked elevation in the white blood cell count is typically associated with acute leukemia, but pancytopenia is actually more common, particularly in older patients with acute myeloid leukemia (AML) who may have underlying marrow dysfunction. Only 10% of newly diagnosed patients present with white counts greater than 100 K/μL and actually have a poor prognosis. They are at risk for intravascu-lar clumping of blasts, resulting in marked leukostasis with manifestations of altered mental status and cranial nerve palsies. Some patients may display pleuritic chest pain due to small leukemic emboli in the pulmonary vasculature. Mild hepatosplenomegaly is often present, but massive hepatosplenomegaly should raise the suspicion of a leukemia arising out of a prior hematologic disorder, such as chronic myelogenous leukemia. Visceral involvement in AML occurs in less than 5% of patients. Tumors resulting from a focal collection of blasts, called *chloromas*, may present throughout the body. Central nervous system involvement is uncommon at presentation and is usually restricted to involvement of the leptomeninges, as parenchymal mass lesions are uncommon.

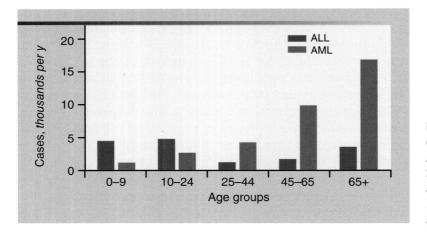

Figure 4-2. Relative incidence of acute lymphoblastic leukemia (ALL) versus acute myeloid leukemia (AML) in different age groups. AML causes approximately 1.2% of all cancer deaths in the United States, with an annual death rate of 2.2 per 100,000 people. There are approximately 9200 new cases of AML each year. As is shown in the figure, AML represents approximately 90% of the cases of all adult acute leukemias [1].

Chemical Exposure and Leukemia

Chemical Exposure and Leukemia
Occupation related
Benzene (chronic exposure)
Toluene
Other industrial solvents?
Pesticides?
Hair dyes?
Cancer chemotherapy related
Alkylating agents
Topoisomerase inhibitors
Epipodophyllotoxins
Anthracyclines
Actinomycin D
Anthracenediones
Recreational
Cigarette smoke

Conditions Predisposing to Acute Myeloid Leukemia, Myelodysplasia, and Myeloproliferative Disorders

Conditions Predisposing to Acute Myeloid Leukemia, Myelodysplasia, and Myeloproliferative Disorders
Older age
Congenital disorders
Down syndrome
Monozygous twinning
Hereditary disorders
Bloom's syndrome
Fanconi's anemia
Other constitutional bone marrow failure syndromes
Systemic mastocytosis
Urticaria pigmentosa
Paroxysmal nocturnal hemoglobinuria
Idiopathic sideroblastic anemia?
Pernicious anemia?
Exposures
Ionizing radiation
Chemicals
Cigarette smoke
Viruses (HTLV-1, EBV?)
Occupation
Farmers
Miners?
Petroleum workers?
Rubber film workers

Figure 4-3. Chemical exposure and leukemia. Certain occupational, iatrogenic, or lifestyle exposures to a number of chemical substances may play a role in the etiology of acute myeloid leukemia (AML) [2]. In these settings, the leukemias are mostly AML, and in some cases, antecedent myelodysplasia is detected. The best-known exposure associated with AML development is benzene. Individual susceptibility to benzene toxicity is related to high CYP2E1 enzyme activity and low or disturbed NQO1 reductase activity (enzymes related to activation and detoxification of benzene metabolites, respectively), as well as to low or reduced glutathione transferase activity in the liver. Many cytostatic drugs are associated with an increased risk of therapy-related myelodysplastic syndrome and therapy-related AML. The first alkylating agents found to be leukemogenic were nitrogen mustard, given in association with radiotherapy in patients with Hodgkin's disease, and melphalan, used for patients with myeloma. In essence, all alkylating agents in clinical use today are leukemogenic [3].

More recently, a variety of topoisomerase II inhibitors have also been shown to be leukemogenic. The leukemogenicity of etoposide (used in combination with other agents) was first demonstrated when it was administered in combination with platinum for patients with non–small cell lung cancer and in patients with acute lymphoblastic leukemia and germ cell cancers. Likewise, the anthracyclines have also been demonstrated to be leukemogenic and, thus, all patients treated with these drugs need to be observed over a long period to ensure that the genetic damage to hematopoietic stem cells that occurred during treatment does not lead to overt evolution to dysplasia in subsequent years.

Figure 4-4. Conditions predisposing to acute myeloid leukemia, myelodysplasia, and myeloproliferative disorders. In the absence of an obvious toxic exposure, most cases of acute leukemia, myelodysplasia, and myeloproliferative disorders develop in humans without an identifiable preexistent cause. Despite this, there are many conditions associated with an increased risk for the development of leukemia and myelodysplasia, including certain clinical and genetic disorders [2]. Congenital disorders (eg, Down syndrome), diseases associated with genomic instability (eg, Bloom's syndrome, Fanconi's anemia, ataxia-telangiectasia, Diamond-Blackfan syndrome), and immunodeficient states (eg, Wiskott-Aldrich syndrome) carry a higher risk for the development of leukemia and myelodysplasia. A significant number of acquired hematologic disorders have a slight to moderate propensity for the development of acute myelogenous leukemia or myelodysplasia, particularly paroxysmal nocturnal hemoglobinuria, which in some series has had a transformation rate of 9%. EBV—Epstein-Barr virus; HTLV-1—human T-lymphotropic virus 1.

Summary of the World Health Organization Classification of Myeloid Neoplasms

Acute myeloid leukemias

  AMLs with recurrent cytogenetic abnormalities

  AML with multilineage dysplasia

  AML and myelodysplastic syndrome, therapy related

  AML not otherwise categorized

  Acute leukemia of ambiguous lineage

Myelodysplastic syndromes

  Refractory anemia

  Refractory anemia with ringed sideroblasts

  Refractory cytopenia with multilineage dysplasia

  Refractory anemia with excess blasts

  Myelodysplastic syndrome associated with isolated del (5q) chromosome abnormality

  Myelodysplastic syndrome, unclassifiable

Chronic myeloproliferative diseases

  Chronic myelogenous leukemia

  Chronic neutrophilic leukemia

  Chronic eosinophilic leukemia/hypereosinophilic syndrome

  Polycythemia vera

  Chronic idiopathic myelofibrosis

  Essential thrombocythemia

  Chronic myeloproliferative disease, unclassifiable

Myelodysplastic/myeloproliferative diseases

  Chronic myelomonocytic leukemia

  Atypical chronic myeloid leukemia

  Juvenile myelomonocytic leukemia

  Myelodysplastic/myeloproliferative diseases, unclassifiable

Figure 4-5. Summary of the World Health Organization (WHO) classification of myeloid neoplasms. The classification of myeloid neoplasms incorporates morphologic, immunophenotypic, genetic, and clinical features to define clinically relevant and biologically homogeneous entities [4,5]. The WHO classification incorporates information obtained from previous classification schemes and symposia, including the French-American-British (FAB) Cooperative Group for acute myeloid leukemias (AML) and myelodysplasia (MDS), the Polycythemia Vera Study Group (PVSG) for chronic myeloproliferative disorders (MPD), and the Year 2000 Mast Cell Disease Symposium [6–9]. The FAB classification, which was a comprehensive, widely accepted, and long-standing scheme, was initially proposed in 1976, and over the ensuing 20 to 25 years, provided a consistent morphologic and cytochemical framework to the majority of cases of AML and MDS. However, information from techniques not widely available at the onset of the FAB group led to observations that FAB classification of certain types of AML and MDS cases was not prognostically useful. For instance, the behavior of cases of AML and MDS associated with recurring genetic abnormalities is more accurately predicted by their genetic change than by their morphologic or cytochemical phenotype. Also, in many cases, either morphology or genetic defects show no correlation or the underlying genetic and molecular defects cannot be identified. The WHO proposed that genetic findings might predict the prognosis and biologic properties of the leukemia more consistently than does morphology. Likewise, the discovery of the molecular basis (*BCR/ABL*) of t(9;22) involving the Philadelphia chromosome led to more definitive understanding of some of the chronic MPDs and further refinement of certain entities, such as chronic myelogenous leukemia. The WHO classification retains the FAB and PVSG reliance on morphologic, cytochemical, and immunophenotypic features of the neoplastic cells to establish their lineage and degree of maturation and furthermore continues to recognize the practical importance of the "blast count" in categorizing myeloid disease and in predicting prognosis. However, the WHO offers some different criteria for blast morphology and a different blast threshold for AML diagnosis, and introduces clonally recurring cytogenetic abnormalities as a basis for diagnosing AML. In addition, the classification and diagnostic criteria for MDS and MPD have been reorganized.

The WHO classification lists the myeloid entities as AML, MDS, chronic MPD, and MDS/MPD. Each of these categories is a heterogeneous collection that contains well-defined diseases as well as diseases for which molecular data are still emerging.

World Health Organization Classification of Acute Myeloid Leukemia

AML with recurrent genetic abnormalities

  AML with t(8;21) (q22;q22), (*AML1/ETO*)

  AML with abnormal bone marrow eosinophils and inv(16)(p13q22) or t(16;16)(p13;q22), (*CBF/MYH11*)

  Acute promyelocytic leukemia with t(15;17)(q22;q12), (*PML/RAR*) and variants

  AML with 11q23 (*MLL*) abnormalities

AML with multilineage dysplasia

  Following MDS or MDS/MPD

  Without antecedent MDS or MDS/MPD, but with dysplasia in at least 50% of cells in two or more cell lineages

AML and myelodysplastic syndromes, therapy related

  Alkylating agent/radiation-related type

  Topoisomerase II inhibitor-related type (some may be lymphoid)

  Others

AML, not otherwise categorized

  AML, minimally differentiated

  AML without maturation

  AML with maturation

  Acute myelomonocytic leukemia

  Acute monoblastic/acute monocytic leukemia

  Acute erythroid leukemia (erythroid/myeloid and pure erythroleukemia)

  Acute megakaryoblastic leukemia

  Acute basophilic leukemia

  Acute panmyelosis with myelofibrosis

  Myeloid sarcoma

Acute leukemia of ambiguous lineage

Figure 4-6. The World Health Organization (WHO) classification of acute myeloid leukemia (AML). The acute leukemias are divided into myeloid or lymphoid based on the lineage of the blast cells. This chapter discusses the myeloid but not the lymphoid leukemias. There are four main categories of AMLs, with the first three being well defined, albeit open-ended for inclusion of more entities as required [10]. The final "category" is not by itself well defined or homogeneous but rather, incorporates all leukemias not fulfilling criteria for the first three categories. The three true categories are AML with recurrent genetic abnormalities, AML with multilineage dysplasia, and AML and myelodysplastic syndromes, therapy related. The final category is AML not otherwise categorized. Another category, acute leukemia of ambiguous lineage, has some features of AML and is also included in this chapter.

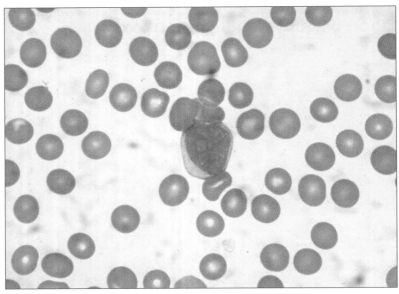

Figure 4-7. Peripheral blood blasts. The World Health Organization (WHO) recommends that morphologic parameters (percentage of blasts, degree of maturation, determination of dysplastic features) should be obtained from a 200-cell leukocyte differential from a peripheral blood smear or a 500-cell differential from an aspirate smear stained with Wright-Giemsa or May-Grünwald-Giemsa. The blast percentage should also be correlated with an estimate of the blast count from a trephine biopsy section. In actual practice, a 200-cell differential will suffice for blast count in both specimen types, with the caveat that a representative and technically optimal area is chosen for enumeration. The aspirate smears should be thoroughly assessed for maturational abnormalities, scanning the entire slide at low power for megakaryocytic abnormalities and at least 40x magnification for assessing myeloid and erythroid abnormalities. At least three aspirate smears should be used for blast count and morphology assessment if the specimen is poorly particulate. The percentage of blasts proposed by the WHO to categorize a specific case comprises the percent blasts as a component of all nucleated marrow cells, with the exception of acute erythroleukemia. If a myeloid neoplasm is found concomitantly with another neoplasm (hematologic or otherwise), the cells of the nonmyeloid neoplasm should be excluded from the denominator when calculating blast percentage. Ancillary studies (cytochemistry and/or immunophenotyping studies) should be used to prove that blasts belong to one of the three cell lines (erythroid, myeloid, megakaryocytic) unless this is obvious from specific morphologic findings, such as Auer rods.

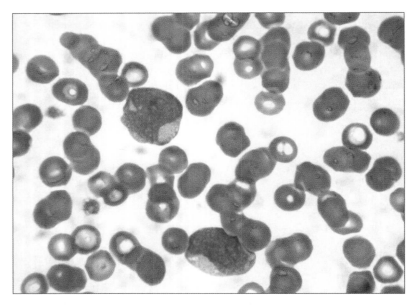

Figure 4-8. Monoblasts and other blast equivalents. Myeloblasts were historically divided into three types, distinction of which is not so important today. In addition to myeloblasts, one may count other cell types as a "blast equivalent" for the purpose of establishing a leukemic diagnosis. Megakaryoblasts are found in acute megakaryoblastic leukemia. The abnormal promyelocytes in acute promyelocytic leukemia have a reniform or bilobed nucleus and cytoplasm with broad cytologic variability, from heavily granulated with bundles of Auer rods to virtually agranular. Monoblasts and promonocytes are seen in acute monoblastic/monocytic leukemia and acute myelomonocytic leukemia. Keep in mind these cells may also be seen in cases of chronic myelomonocytic leukemia, as long as they are less than 20% of marrow cells.

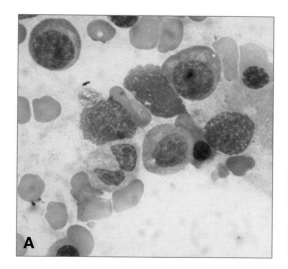

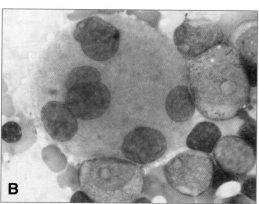

Figure 4-9. Certain cell types that should not be included in a differential count of blasts. **A,** Erythroid precursors (erythroblasts) are included in the blast count only in cases of "pure" erythroleukemia. **B,** Dysplastic micromegakaryocytes are excluded from the blast percentage. The percentage of CD34$^+$ cells is not considered a substitute for a morphologic blast count or estimate from aspiration or trephine biopsy. Not all blasts express CD34. However, evaluating the number of CD34$^+$ cells offers valuable data for diagnostic and prognostic purposes.

Methods to Detect Minimal Residual Disease

Detection Method	Target	Sensitivity, %*
Pathology examination	Cellular morphology	5
Metaphase cytogenetics	Chromosome structure	1–5
Fluorescence in situ hybridization	Chromosome structure	1
Flow cytometry	Surface antigen expression	0.1–1.0
Clonogenic assays	Growth of malignant cells	0.0001–0.1000
Polymerase chain reaction	DNA-RNA sequence	0.0001–0.1000

Sensitivity is defined as the ability to detect a leukemic cell in a background of normal marrow. Thus, an assay that can detect one leukemic cell in a background of 10 normal cells has a sensitivity of 10%.

Figure 4-10. Methods to detect minimal residual disease. The diagnostic approach to patients with acute myeloid leukemia (AML) utilizes a combination of modalities to supplement clinical findings and morphology. Cytochemistry utilizes various chemical reactions to cytoplasmic constituents found in abundance in leukemic blasts. Immunologic testing includes flow cytometry or immunohistochemistry, which detect antigens present on the cell surface or cytoplasm of leukemic cells. Molecular methods, including Southern blot hybridization, polymerase chain reaction, and cytogenetics, help detect changes at the gene level. Some of the molecular targets in AML are highly specific for a disease, such as the t(15;17) of acute promyelocytic leukemia, whereas other targets, such as *MLL*, are indicators of malignancy but not necessarily of a specific AML subtype. Cytochemistry, immunohistochemistry, and flow cytometry require the use of a group of stains/antibodies to observe differential expression of the target constituents, as no single stain or antibody is exclusive and pathognomonic for a particular AML subtype. These techniques have varying sensitivity for detection of malignant cells [11].

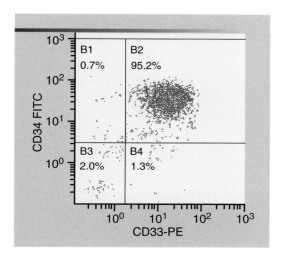

Figure 4-11. Flow cytometry histogram of a group of blasts. The diagnosis of acute myeloid leukemia (AML) can usually be made by morphology alone, and can be confirmed by a positive myeloperoxidase cytochemical stain, which can be easily performed in less than 15 minutes. Immunophenotyping may be helpful in several instances including 1) cases of undifferentiated AML (AML-M0), which is by definition cytochemical myeloperoxidase-negative; 2) cases of biphenotypic AML, which requires knowledge of B-cell or T-cell antigen expression, in addition to a myeloid phenotype; and 3) cases in which a certain phenotype is highly predictive of cytogenetic abnormalities. Most AML cases are positive for CD13 and CD33, using a CD45/side scatter gating strategy. In this histogram, a group of blasts show strong CD34 positivity (y-axis) and CD33 positivity (x-axis), indicative of an immature myeloid population. FITC—fluorescein isothiocyanate. PE—phycoerythrin.

FAB Subtypes, Immunophenotype, and Cytogenetic Abnormalities

Correlation of FAB Subtypes with Monoclonal Antibodies and Cytogenetic Abnormalities of AML

FAB class	Cytochemistry			Monoclonals for Precursor Cells			Myeloid-associated Markers			Monocyte-associated Markers			Cytogenetics
	MPO	PAS	Esterase	TdT	HLA-DR	CD34	CD13	CD33	CD15	CD11	CD14	Other	
M0 (undifferentiated)	< 3%+	-	-	±	+	+	+	±	±	-	-		11q 13
M1 (myeloid)	< 3%+	-	-	±	+	+	+	+	-	±	-		-5, -7, -17, del 3p, +21, +8
M2 (myeloid with differentiation)	> 10%+	-	-	-	+	+	+	+	+	±	-		t(8;21), del 3p, or inv 3,-5, -7, t(6;9), +8
M3 (promyelocytic APL)	++	-	-	-	-	-	+	+	±	-	-		t(15;17)
M4 (myelomonocytic)	+	-	+	-	+		+	+	+	+	+		inv(16) or -16q, t(16;16), occ t(8;21), -5, -7, t(6;9)
M5 (monocytic)	-	+ block	++	-	+		±	+	+	+	+		t(9;11), (p21;p23), +8
M6 (erythroid)	-	++	-	-	±	-	±	±	-	±	-	Glyphorin A	-5q, -5, -7, -3, +8
M7 (megakaryocytic)	-	±	-	-	+	+	-	±	-	-	-	Platelet glycoprotein	inv or del 3, +8, +21

Figure 4-12. FAB subtypes, immunophenotype, and cytogenetic abnormalities (AML). Certain immunophenotypes of acute myeloid leukemia may suggest, but are not diagnostic of, particular cytogenetic abnormalities [12]. CD34, CD117, CD7, and HLA-DR are usually negative or very weak and are present only on a subset of leukemic cells of acute promyelocytic leukemia (APL). Also, CD15 is negative or dim, and CD13 and CD33 expressions are bright and homogeneous. CD19 expression in AML is often present in, but not specific for, t(8;21) abnormality. Approximately 15% of AML cases are also TdT positive. AML—acute myeloid leukemia; FAB—French-American-British; HLA-DR—human leukocyte antigen D–related; MPO—myeloperoxidase; PAS—periodic acid-Schiff; TdT—terminal deoxynucleotidyl transferase.

Turnaround Time for Minimal Residual Disease Detection Methods

Test Method	Target	Turnaround Time
Pathology examination	Morphology	24 h
Flow cytometry	Cell surface antigen	4 h
Southern blot hybridization	DNA or RNA sequences	1–2 wk
Polymerase chain reaction	DNA or RNA sequences	24 h–1 wk
FISH	Chromosome structure	2–5 d
Metaphase cytogenetics	Chromosome structure	3–7 d

Figure 4-13. Turnaround time for minimal residual disease detection methods. Molecular study of the neoplastic cells should be performed initially and at regular intervals throughout the disease course to establish a complete genetic profile and to detect possible genetic evolution. The techniques may include classic karyotyping, reverse transcriptase-polymerase chain reaction (RT-PCR), or fluorescent in situ hybridization (FISH) studies [11]. Because of the turnaround time associated with these tests, the inclusion of genetic information has been criticized as an obstacle to facile use of the World Health Organization classification. However, as technology continuously improves test availability, such data can easily be incorporated for proper diagnosis and treatment.

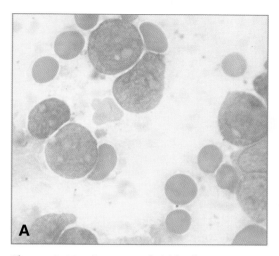

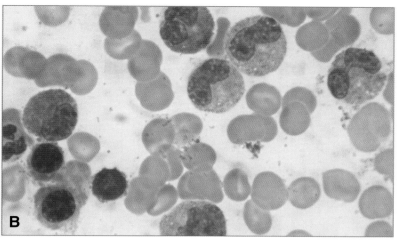

Figure 4-14. Acute myeloid leukemia (AML) with recurrent cytogenetic abnormalities. The new World Health Organization (WHO) classification recognizes the importance of certain cytogenetic translocation as predictors of response to therapy. Patients with certain clonal, recurring cytogenetic abnormalities should be considered to have AML with recurrent genetic abnormalities regardless of the blast percentage. Over one-fourth of patients with de novo AML will have one of these four well-defined recurring genetic abnormalities: t(8;21)(q22;q22), inv(16)(p13q22) or t(16;16)(p13;q22), t(15;17)(q22;q12), or AML with 11q23 [4]. Leukemias with t(8;21), inv(16) or t(16;16), and t(15;17) are considered distinct clinicopathologic-genetic entities. They show a strong correlation between the genetic findings and the morphology, and they have a favorable response to therapy. The t(8;21) blasts (**A**) have characteristic large salmon-pink, waxy-appearing cytoplasmic inclusions. The inv(16) leukemic blasts (**B**) have a mixture of chunky eosinophilic and basophilic cytoplasmic granules and abnormally heavily granulated eosinophils. In contrast, abnormalities of 11q23 have no definitive or consistent morphologic features. The 11q23 abnormalities may be associated with myelomonocytic or monocytic differentiation, and they may be involved in some cases of therapy-related leukemia as well as acute lymphoblastic leukemias and biphenotypic leukemias. The WHO classification also includes some "proposed" (*ie*, not definitive or established) recurring genetic abnormalities, including t(8;16), t(6;9), or t(3;3). Whether these cytogenetic abnormalities define a unique disease or are mainly of prognostic significance within other subgroups remains to be established.

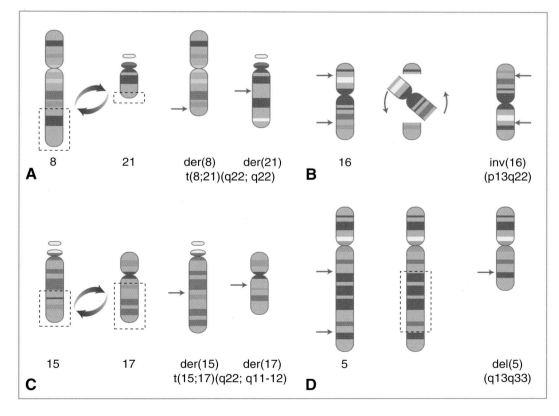

Figure 4-15. Acute myeloid leukemia (AML) with recurrent cytogenetic abnormalities. These are four recurring chromosomal abnormalities characteristic of AML that are detectable by standard cytogenetic evaluation of patient material. Their chromosomal abnormalities are important for the specific characterization of the leukemia, and each has an important prognostic association as well as therapeutic implications in some cases [13]. Patients who have the 8;21 translocation (**A**) or the inv(16) (**B**) have high remission rates and generally do well with postremission therapy. Patients with the 15;17 translocation (**C**) are treated in a completely different manner, built around anthracyclines and all-transretinoic acid (ATRA). Cytogenetic abnormality del(5) (**D**) is commonly observed in patients with myelodysplasia and AML; these patients tend to have a poor prognosis.

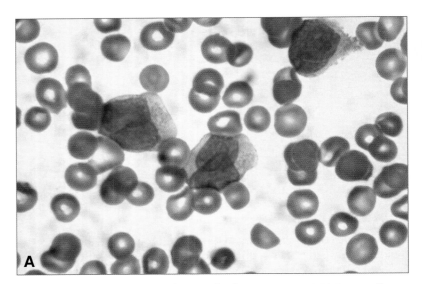

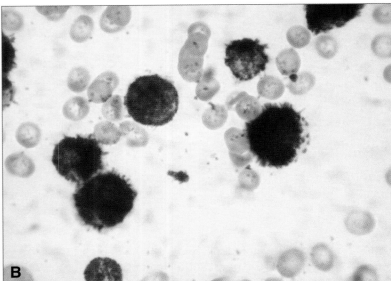

Figure 4-16. Acute promyelocytic leukemia (APL). APL is usually the most easily diagnosed acute myeloid leukemia because the cytoplasm of the malignant cells (**A**) is replete with large eosinophilic granules and Auer rods. The nuclei are often multilobed with indistinguishable nucleoli and are heavily weighted with variably colored granules. A microgranular variant of APL may be recognized by the multilobate nuclei and occasional Auer rods, as well as strong cytochemical myeloperoxidase positivity (**B**), out of proportion to the few number of visible granules. Most patients with APL have evidence of disseminated intravascular coagulation.

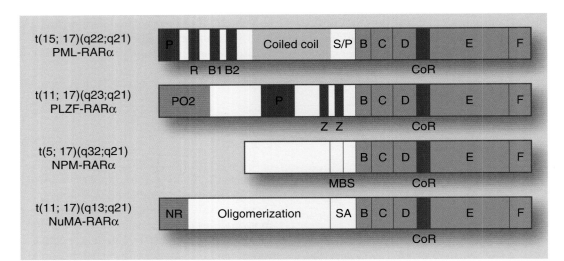

Figure 4-17. Translocations associated with acute promyelocytic leukemia (APL). APL represents a uniquely homogeneous subset of acute myelogenous leukemia defined by its cytogenetic abnormality, t(15;17)(q22;q21), which results in the fusion of retinoic acid receptor *RARα* gene on chromosome 17 with a promyelocyte leukemia (*PML*) gene on chromosome 15. This abnormality yields the PML/ RARα fusion protein that is detectable both by cytogenetics as well as by polymerase chain reaction techniques that are useful both in the diagnosis and evaluation of minimal residual disease. Three other translocations involving the *RARα* gene are associated with APL [5,11,14].

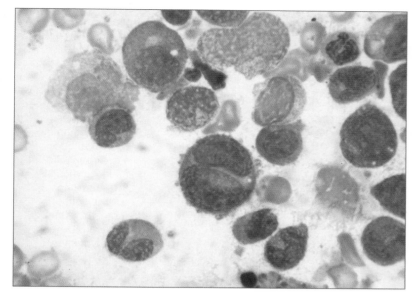

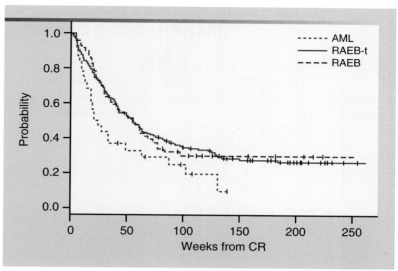

Figure 4-18. Acute myeloid leukemia (AML) with multilineage dysplasia. The French-American-British criteria for myelodysplastic syndrome (MDS) indicated that patients with more than 5% blasts in the peripheral blood and 20% to 29% blasts in the marrow were classified in the MDS subgroup of "refractory anemia with excess of blasts in transformation" and that patients with 30% or more blasts in the marrow were classified as AML. The blast threshold for the diagnosis of AML in the World Health Organization (WHO) classification is lowered to 20% blasts in the blood or marrow. Therefore, most patients with 20% to 29% blasts and myelodysplasia will be classified in the WHO scheme as AML with multilineage dysplasia. The WHO classification also is designed to address the issue that in many older patients, there is evidence of marrow dysfunction that antedates the onset of AML. In these patients, the MDS is characterized by ineffective hematopoiesis and the abnormalities that accompany the disorder or evolve as part of AML development are characterized by the loss of chromosomal material, particularly loss of chromosomes 5 or 5q, 7 or 7q, 3, or 20 [15]. The diagnosis of AML with multilineage dysplasia is easily made in patients who have a well-documented history of MDS or an MDS/myeloproliferative disease (MPD) that has been present for at least 6 months prior to the onset of overt AML. However, this diagnosis is difficult when the leukemia is present in the absence of good clinical documentation. For cases of new-onset AML with morphologic evidence of multilineage dysplasia and no prior history or clinical suspicion of MDS, the WHO classification suggests the term *AML with multilineage dysplasia without antecedent MDS or MDS/MPD*. Multilineage dysplasia is generally defined as 50% or more cells in two or more cell lines showing dysplasia in a pretreatment sample. Some pathologists use a lower threshold (20% dysplastic cells in two or more cell lines). Multilineage dysplasia has been shown to be an independent prognostic factor only in patients who have favorable cytogenetics but has no additional adverse impact in patients with poor-risk cytogenetics.

Figure 4-19. Probability of event-free survival from time of complete remission (CR) in subgroups of acute myeloid leukemia (AML), refractory anemia with excess of blasts in transformation (RAEB-t), and refractory anemia with excess of blasts (RAEB). RAEB patients fared worse than the RAEB-t and AML patients (log rank $P = 0.017$) [16]. The blast threshold for AML diagnosis was lowered because a number of studies observed that patients with 20% to 29% blasts in their bone marrow had similar clinical and biologic features as those with 30% blasts or greater. These similarities included poor-risk cytogenetic abnormalities (including chromosome 7 anomalies and complex abnormalities), increased expression of multidrug-resistance glycoproteins, and poor response to chemotherapy. When matched for similar disease features, such as white blood cell or cytogenetic abnormalities, patients with RAEB-t and AML had similar response to therapy and similar survival times if treated with identical therapy. In addition, myeloid cells from patients with RAEB-t and myelodysplasia (MDS)-related AML had nearly identical proliferation and apoptosis profiles, which differ from those in refractory anemia, refractory anemia with ringed sideroblasts, and RAEB. Data from the International MDS Risk Analysis Workshop indicated that RAEB-t showed a high rate of AML progression within a short time period. With this information, the World Health Organization suggested that patients with 20% to 29% blasts in the blood and/or bone marrow accompanied by multilineage MDS be placed in the same category as those with AML with multilineage dysplasia and 30% or more blasts. Therapeutic decisions for patients with MDS-related AML should be based not only on the percentage of blasts but also on clinical findings, the rate of disease progression, and genetic data.

Contrasting Features of Therapy-related Myeloid Leukemia Secondary to Either Alkylating Agents or Topoisomerase II Inhibitors

	Chromosome Abnormality	Preleukemia Phase	FAB Classification	Age	Latency	Response to Induction Chemotherapy	Long-term Survival	Chemotherapy Drugs
Akylating agents	-5/del(5q), B23 -7/del(7q) syndrome	Myelodysplasia	Not classifiable	Typically older patients	5–7 y	Poor	Poor	Melphalan, mechlorethamine, chlorambucil, cyclophospha-mide, carmustine, lomustine, semustine, procarbazine, dacarbazine, mitolactol
Topoiso-merase II inhibitor	t(11q23)	None	Usually M4, M5; some M1, M2, and ALL	Younger patients	6 mo–5 y	Good	Poor	Etoposide, teniposide, actinomycin D, doxorubicin, 4 epidoxocorubicin, mitroxantrone
	t(21q22)							
Various agents	t(15;17)	None	M3	Younger patients	2–3 y	Good	Good	Bimolane
	inv(16)	None	M4Eo		< 3 y	Good	Good	

Figure 4-20. Contrasting features of therapy-related myeloid leukemia secondary to either alkylating agents or topoisomerase II inhibitors. The increasing use and success of cancer chemotherapy has led to the observation that patients who have been exposed to these agents are at more risk for developing acute myeloid leukemia (AML) and/or myelodysplasia (MDS) in later years [13]. Although morphologically similar, there are a number of features that distinguish therapy-related myeloid leukemia from patients who develop sporadic MDS, including the age at diagnosis and frequency of cytogenetic abnormalities [5]. The most common type typically presents with a latency of approximately 5 years in patients who received alkylating agents. Approximately two thirds of cases present with MDS and the remainder as AML with myelodysplastic features. The morphologic features of therapy-related AML (t-AML) and AML with multilineage dysplasia are identical, and in fact, knowledge of a predisposing etiologic agent is the major difference between these two categories. However, t-AMLs also have a higher incidence of chromosomes 5 and/or 7 anomalies and a worse clinical outcome than AML with multilineage dysplasia. A second type was first observed among patients receiving high cumulative doses of etoposide for lung cancer but has also been seen in patients receiving other drugs known to inhibit topoisomerase II. Clinically, this disease has a shorter latency period of 1 to 2 years and manifests itself with overt leukemia, often with monocytic features. This subtype rarely presents with low-grade MDS. Balanced translocations involving the *MLL* gene at 11q23 and *AML 1* gene at 21q22 are common in this subgroup. A third group of t-AML is therapy-related acute promyelocytic leukemia characterized by typical translocation of gene chromosomes 15 and 17 and prior treatment for psoriasis with bimolane. In general, nearly all therapy-related MDS and AML will have these cytogenetic abnormalities, whereas approximately 40% of patients with primary MDS will have a normal karyotype. ALL—acute lymphoblastic leukemia; FAB—French-American-British.

Subtypes of "Acute Myeloid Leukemia, Not Otherwise Categorized"

Acute myeloid leukemia, minimally differentiated
Acute myeloid leukemia without maturation
Acute myeloid leukemia with maturation
Acute myelomonocytic leukemia
Acute monoblastic leukemia
Acute monocytic leukemia
Acute erythroid leukemia
Acute megakaryoblastic leukemia
Acute basophilic leukemia

Figure 4-21. Subtypes of "acute myeloid leukemia (AML), not otherwise categorized." The majority of cases of AML fall into this fourth subgroup [10]. This entity incorporates the cases that do not satisfy the criteria for any of the other three subgroups, or for which no genetic data can be obtained. Such a large "wastebasket" category may be frustrating for the treating clinician as well as the very ill patient. However, the category provides a framework for disease classification and as more data become available, for shifting to another, hopefully better-defined subgroup. The entities incorporated into this subgroup are defined almost identically to corresponding entities in the French-American-British classification.

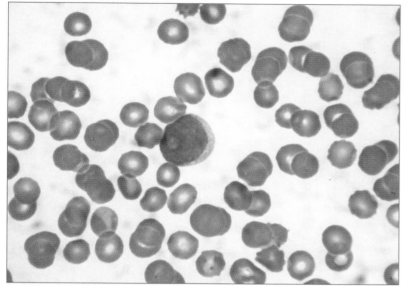

Figure 4-22. Blast of an acute myeloid leukemia (AML), undifferentiated. The blasts have immature nuclear chromatin and no intracytoplasmic granules. Immunophenotyping has helped define a group of patients with undifferentiated myeloid leukemia (AML-M0). These leukemias have a very primitive morphology and lack myeloperoxidase by cytochemistry. In the past, they were likely to be diagnosed and treated as if they had acute lymphoblastic leukemia. Flow cytometry shows expression of at least one early marker of myeloid antigen, usually CD13 or CD33, and there is no expression of T-cell or B-cell markers. Because of these immunophenotypic data, these undifferentiated leukemias are treated in a similar manner to myeloid malignancies.

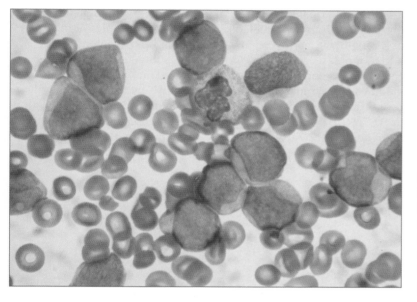

Figure 4-23. Acute myeloid leukemia (AML) without maturation. In AML without maturation, the malignant blasts show great variation in shape, but are homogeneous in staining quality. The blasts contain nuclear chromatin with a characteristic ground-glass texture, pale punched-out nucleoli, and a modest amount of cytoplasm. Myeloperoxidase cytochemistry and the presence of background dysplastic myeloid cells usually distinguish these primitive cells from lymphoblasts.

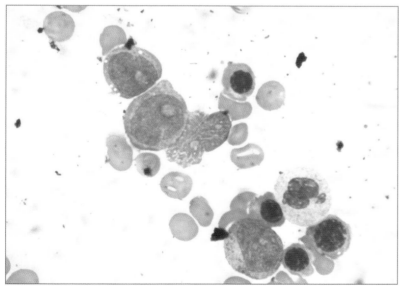

Figure 4-24. The blasts of acute myeloid leukemia (AML) with maturation. These blasts contain primary granules; abundant and basophilic cytoplasm; eccentrically placed nuclei; and delicate, somewhat blotchy chromatin. A small number of Auer rods, which are cylindrical stacks of dysplastic primary granules that fuse into thin needle-like structures, are present in a small to moderate number of blasts in this variant of AML. The primary granules and Auer rods stain strongly with cytochemical myeloperoxidase and α-naphthol AS-D chloracetate esterase.

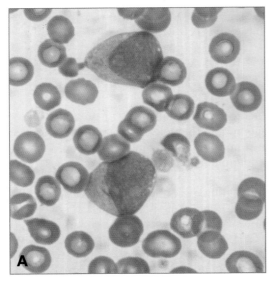
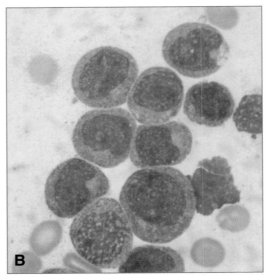

Figure 4-25. Blasts with monocytic differentiation. Acute myelo-monocytic leukemia, acute monoblastic leukemia, and acute monocytic leukemia represent the myeloid leukemias with cytologic and cytochemical features of monocytic differentiation in the World Health Organization classification. They correspond to AML FAB-M4 (**A**), FAB-M5a (**B**), and FAB-M5b, respectively, in the French-American-British (FAB) classification. These three subtypes of acute myeloid leukemias (AMLs) differ solely in the percentage of immature cells showing cytochemical evidence of monocytic differentiation and whether those immature cells are more or less mature. Promonocytes appear immature but retain some features of mature monocytes, such as folded and convoluted nuclear contours with a moderate amount of vacuolated cytoplasm. Monoblasts have an amoeboid quality, with round to oval nuclei with delicate chromatin, prominent nucleoli, and abundant cytoplasm. In assessing bone marrow for AML, we count both promonocytes and monoblasts as "blasts." One distinct subtype of AML, AML-M5b, shows monocytoid blasts with abundant intracytoplasmic granules and prominent erythrophagocytosis by the leukemic cells. This subtype of acute monocytic leukemia is associated with t(8;16)(p11;p13), disseminated intravascular coagulation, and prominent central nervous system and extramedullary involvement [17].

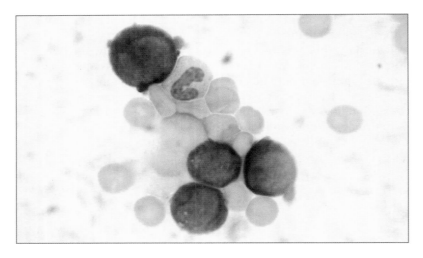

Figure 4-26. α-Naphthyl butyrate esterase cytochemistry in monoblasts. The cytochemical stains most specific for monocytes are α-naphthyl butyrate as substrate and hexa-azotized pararosaniline as coupler (monocyte-specific nonspecific esterase activity). α-Naphthyl acetate and naphthol AS-D acetate are also reactive substrates for monocytes, but specificity for monocytes must be validated by showing fluoride inhibition, which is a unique feature of monocyte esterases.

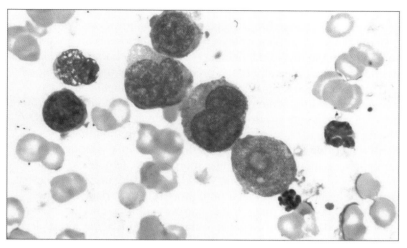

Figure 4-27. Blasts of pure erythroid leukemia. Acute erythroid leukemia has historically encompassed many similar but distinct entities [5]. They are all characterized by a predominant erythroid proliferation in the bone marrow. The World Health Organization (WHO) classification recognizes two subtypes on the basis of having a significant percentage of myeloblasts (acute erythroid/myeloid leukemia) or not (pure erythroid leukemia). In the past, pure erythroid leukemia was also known as diGugliemo disease, acute erythremic myelosis, true erythroleukemia, and minimally differentiated erythroleukemia. Acute erythroid/myeloid leukemia is defined as having erythroid precursors that account for 50% or more of the entire marrow nucleated cell population and myeloblasts that account for 20% or more of the nonerythroid cell population. This entity corresponds to AML FAB-M6. All stages of erythroid matura-

tion are found, and there is usually markedly left-shifted maturation. The distinction between acute erythroid/myeloid leukemia and acute myelogenous leukemia (AML) with multilineage dysplasia is difficult. The WHO classifies such cases as AML with multilineage dysplasia, acute erythroid/myeloid type. In contrast to acute erythroid/myeloid leukemia, pure erythroid leukemia is composed primarily of immature cells showing an erythroid phenotype and there is no significant number of myeloblasts. More than 80% of all marrow cells are immature erythroid precursors with minimal differentiation. The morphology usually suggests erythroid origin with a round nucleus and intense basophilic cytoplasm. The morphologic suspicions must be confirmed by cytoplasmic staining for periodic acid-Schiff (often in a globular pattern) and lack of cytochemical staining for myeloperoxidase or nonspecific esterase.

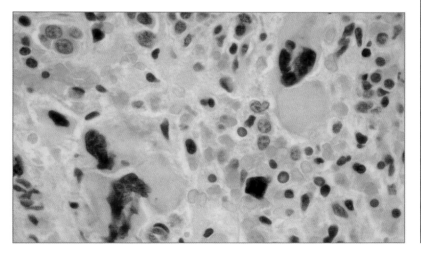

Figure 4-28. Trephine biopsy section, acute megakaryoblastic leukemia. Acute megakaryoblastic leukemia is defined by the presence of 50% or more blasts showing megakaryocytic lineage. This corresponds to AML FAB-7. The blasts are large and have large nuclei with round to slightly irregular nuclear contours, delicate chromatin, and prominent small multiple nucleoli. The cytoplasmic features, including bleb/pseudopod formation and no granules, usually raise the possibility of megakaryocytic lineage. The peripheral blood contains large dysplastic platelets and may show circulating micromegakaryocytes or fragments of mega-karyoblasts. The bone marrow commonly shows trilineage dysplasia and diffuse fibrosis.

Differential Diagnosis of Basophilia
Hematologic malignancies
Acute leukemias, *eg*, myeloid with 12p or t(6;9) abnormalities, rare lymphoblastic types
Chronic myeloproliferative diseases
Myelodysplastic syndromes
Mastocytosis
Acute basophilic leukemia
Hypersensitivity reactions
Hypothyroidism
Ulcerative colitis
Radiation
Infections (varicella, smallpox)
Miscellaneous (renal disease)

Figure 4-29. Differential diagnosis of basophilia. Acute basophilic leukemia is an extremely rare entity and lacks definitive diagnostic criteria. The blasts are morphologically undifferentiated. Recognizing the presence of coarse basophilic granules suggests the possibility of this disease. By cytochemistry, the granules are metachromatic-positive with toluidine blue and negative for myeloperoxidase. Immunophenotyping studies show expression of myeloid markers (usually CD34, CD33, and CD13); CD9 and CD25 expression have also been reported. No consistent cytogenetic abnormalities have been reported. Reports of the presence of Philadelphia chromosome or abnormalities of chromosome 12p, and t(6;9) most likely represent cases of chronic myelogenous leukemia in blast crisis (Philadelphia chromosome) or acute myelogenous leukemia with basophilia: 12p abnormalities, t(6;9) [18].

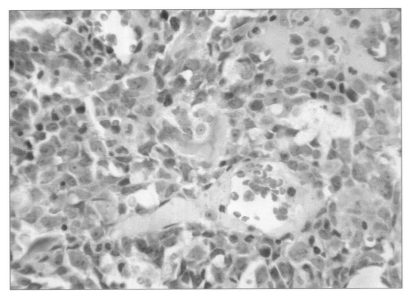

Figure 4-30. Trephine biopsy section, acute panmyelosis with myelofibrosis. Acute panmyelosis with myelofibrosis is an uncommon subtype of acute myeloid leukemia (AML) and is characterized by dysplasia in multiple cell lines, a predominance of megakaryoblasts and megakaryocytes, and extensive fibrosis. Historically, this disease was known as acute myelosclerosis, acute myelofibrosis, acute myelodysplasia with myelofibrosis, and malignant myelosclerosis. The morphologic features overlap with AML with multilineage dysplasia and in fact, may represent different manifestations of the same process. It also shows similar morphologic features to acute megakaryoblastic leukemia. The World Health Organization suggests that these entities be separated until more scientific data become available to delineate them. If the marrow is fibrotic and the leukemic cells are predominantly megakaryoblasts, the term *acute megakaryoblastic leukemia* should be used. If all the cell lines appear immature and dysplastic and the marrow is fibrotic, the term *acute panmyelosis with myelofibrosis* is preferred. This entity represents approximately 1% of all acute leukemias and has a poor prognosis.

Modified Scoring System for Biphenotypic Acute Leukemia*

Points	B Lineage	T Lineage	Myeloid Lineage
2	CD79a	c/sCD3	Myeloperoxidase cytochemistry
	cIgM	Anti-TCRα/β	
	cCD22	Anti-TCRγ/δ	
1	CD19	CD2	CD13
	CD10	CD5	CD33
	CD20	CD8	CD65
		CD10	Anti-MPO
			CD117
0.5	TdT	TdT	CD11c
	CD24	CD7	CD14
		CD1a	CD15

*More than two points each for the myeloid and one of the lymphoid lineages is required for a diagnosis of biphenotypic acute leukemia.

Figure 4-31. Modified scoring system for biphenotypic acute leukemia. A subset of patients with leukemia exhibit features of both myeloid and lymphoid differentiation. Patients with a leukemia clone that expresses two or more acute lymphoblastic leukemia (ALL) antigens and one myeloid antigen comprise about 20% of adult ALL [19]. C—cytoplasmic; s—surface.

Acute Myeloid Leukemia Induction and Consolidation Therapy

Induction		Consolidation
AML induction and consolidation		
Ara-C	200 mg/mg² IV as continuous infusion × 7 d	3 g/m² q12h IV as 2- to 3-h infusion on d 1, 3, 5; repeat q 28d × 4 cycles*
Idarubicin†	12 mg/m² IV on d 1–3	
ALSG regimen		
Ara-C*	3 g/m² IV q12h as 2- to 3-h infusion on days 1, 3, 5, 7 (8 doses)	100 mg/m² IV as continuous infusion × 5 d
Daunorubicin	50 mg/m² IV on days 1–3	50 mg/m² IV × 2 d
VP-16	75 mg/m² IV × 7 d	75 mg/m² IV × 5 d

*For patients < 60 y of age.
†Idarubicin has been substituted for daunorubicin, 45 mg/m², which had been the prevalent anthracycline used in clinical trials prior to 1993. Mitoxantrone, 10 mg/m² × 5 d, has also been used as an alternative.

Figure 4-32. Induction and consolidation therapy for acute myeloid leukemia (AML). The treatment approach for AML can be divided into two phases. Induction therapy is the initial treatment designed to clear the marrow of overt leukemia. Induction therapy usually involves the use of multiple drugs that cause pancytopenia for 2 to 3 weeks. Consolidation therapy is given after a patient is in remission. The regimens noted above are the two most commonly used drug combinations for most types of AML (excluding acute promyelocytic leukemia) [12]. Depending on the cytogenetic analysis of the leukemia, remissions range from 50% to over 80% with induction therapy. ALSG—Australian Leukemia Study Group; Ara-C—cytarabine; VP-16—etoposide.

Complete Remission and Overall Survival by Cytogenetic Risk Status

Risk Status	Total Patients, n	CRs/Pts*	Complete Remission CR rate, %	95% CI	Overall Survival Died, n	RR	95% CI
Favorable	121	98/117	84	77–90	53	1	
Intermediate	278	205/270	76	71–81	168	1.5	1.10–2.05
Unfavorable	184	96/173	55	48–63	162	3.33	2.43–4.55
Unknown	26	13/24	54	33–74	20	2.66	1.59–4.45

*Denominator is the number of patients who were evaluated for response.

Figure 4-33. Complete remission (CR) and overall survival by cytogenetic risk status. An analysis of preinduction therapy cytogenetics of a large group of patients undergoing similar therapy suggests that the cytogenetic characterization predicts not only the postremission outcome but also the ability of a patient to achieve an initial remission. In one large series of 584 patients treated with induction therapy utilizing daunorubicin and cytarabine, 79% of patients achieved a remission [20]. The CR rate varied significantly among the three groups of known cytogenetic risk status, ranging from 84% for "favorable" to 76% for "intermediate risk" to 55% for "unfavorable risk." The major difference in outcome was largely due to the lower CR rate in the unfavorable group compared with the other two combined, as the difference between the intermediate and favorable groups was not significant. RR—relative risk.

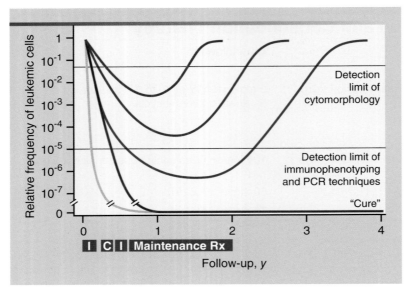

Figure 4-34. The putative relative frequencies of leukemic cells in peripheral blood or bone marrow of acute leukemia patients during and after chemotherapy and during development of relapse [21]. The detection limit of cytologic or morphologic methods is indicated, as well as the detection limit of immunophenotyping and polymerase chain reaction (PCR) techniques.

The induction of remission in itself is not curative for patients with acute myeloid leukemia. This is because initial treatment protocols are not capable of eliminating all clonogenic malignant cells in the patient despite the achievement of a morphologic remission. The detection limit of a cytomorphologic technique is not lower than 1% to 5%, implying that a patient may still have a significant leukemia burden without any morphologic evidence of disease. More sensitive techniques are required for the detection of these malignant cells following treatment, and this is referred to as *detection of minimal residual disease*. Newer techniques are allowing the detection of minimal residual disease, at a sensitivity of at least 10^{-3} (one malignant cell within 1000 normal cells). It is important that these techniques have specificity, ability to discriminate between malignant and normal cells without false-positive results, reproducibility, and feasibility, as well as availability for clinical application. C—consolidation; I—induction; Rx—treatment.

Options for Postremission Therapy for Acute Myeloid Leukemia

Conventional consolidation chemotherapy: a regimen the same as or different from that used to induce CR
Chemotherapy followed by maintenance therapy, which is less myelosuppressive than that administered during remission induction and given for a prolonged period
A high-dose Ara-C—containing regimen
High-dose therapy with autologous hematopoietic progenitor cell support
Allogeneic transplantation

Figure 4-35. Options for postremission therapy for acute myeloid leukemia (AML). Depending on patient age, the cytogenetic evaluation of the diagnostic material and the response to therapy influence the strategy for postremission therapy to address minimal residual disease and cure the patient with leukemia. Historically, all patients with AML were treated as if they had one disease. In many clinical trials, the chemotherapy and autologous and allogeneic transplantation did not distinguish among cytogenetic risk groups. Current practice, as well as the availability of information about the leukemic cells, now helps identify patients at higher and lower risk and provides a basis for choosing the best postremission treatment for patients with AML. Improvements in the supportive care of patients have also allowed the possibility for considering autologous and allogeneic transplantation in patients who are older and whose leukemias are less likely to have good prognosis cytogenetic characteristics. Ara-C—cytarabine; CR—complete remission.

Poor-risk Factors in Patients with Acute Myeloid Leukemia Treated with Chemotherapy Alone

Age > 60 y
Poor-risk cytogenetics
WBC count at diagnosis > 100 K/μL
Absence of CD34 expression
MDR1 expression
Mutation in *FLT3* or lack of mutation in nucleophosmin
FAB M0, M1, M5, M6, M7
Secondary AML (therapy-related or developing after MDS)
Dysplastic morphology at diagnosis
Extramedullary disease at diagnosis
More than one cycle of induction chemotherapy required to achieve complete remission

Figure 4-36. Poor-risk factors in patients with acute myeloid leukemia (AML) treated with chemotherapy alone. There are many characteristics of the leukemic cell that help clinicians determine the best approach for patients who achieve a remission with standard induction therapy for AML. This table lists poor-risk factors that portend the likelihood that the leukemia will relapse. In general, the factors predict which patients will not remain in remission while receiving standard therapy. These patients are candidates for more intensive therapy focused on eliminating the usually larger burden of residual disease, most often by either allogeneic transplantation from a related or unrelated donor. The risk factors are used to determine the most appropriate postremission therapy [22]. FAB—French-American-British (classification); MDS—myelodysplastic syndrome; WBC—white blood cell.

High-dose Ara-C as Postremission Therapy

Study	Patients, n	Median Age, y	Remission Induction Therapy	CR Rate, %	Postremission Therapy	Median Duration of CR, mo	Patients in CR at 5 y, %	Treatment-related Deaths, %
Open phase II	87	38	N/ST	N/ST	HD ara-C	47	49	5
Open phase II studies	56	47	DAT	63	HD ara-C + DNR	23	32 at 4 y	6
CALGB trial	187	43			HD ara-C	19	44	5
	206	49	3 + 7	64	Ara-C:400 mg/m2	19	29	6
	203	48			Ara-c:100 mg/mL	13	24	1
ECOG trial	99	44	DAT	68	HD ara-C + mAMSA	N/ST	28	12
	94	44	DAT	68	Ara-C + 6-TG	N/ST	15	—

Figure 4-37. High-dose cytarabine (ara-C) as postremission therapy. Once remission has been achieved in a patient with acute myeloid leukemia (AML), further intensive therapy is required to prevent relapse. Many trials suggest that exposure to high-dose ara-C consolidation therapy may have a beneficial impact on disease-free survival in patients not undergoing transplantation [23]. The Cancer and Leukemia Group B (CALGB) conducted a study to determine a dose/response effect for ara-C in patients with AML and whether the beneficial effect extended to all subtypes of AML. These studies have influenced the treatment of patients with all AML types, but its most significant impact has been in patients with abnormalities characterized by t(8;21) or inv(16). Patients whose leukemia expressed core binding factor abnormalities, such as t(8;21) or inv(16), showed a 50% likelihood of remaining in remission at 5 years, compared with 32% and 15% with normal karyotype or other cytogenetic abnormalities, respectively. Thus, for most patients with AML, particularly older patients, use of high-dose ara-C has a limited impact on the clinical outcome once a patient has received achieved remission. CR—complete remission; DAT—daunorubicin + ara-C + 6-thioguanine; DNR—daunorubicin; ECOG—Eastern Cooperative Oncology Group; HD—high-dose; mAMSA—amsacrine; N/ST—not stated; 6-TG—6-thioguanine.

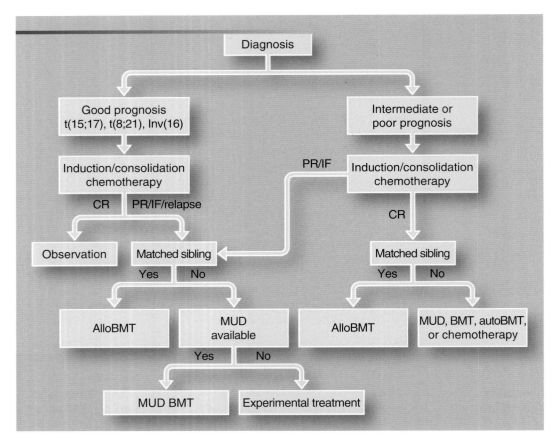

Figure 4-38. This algorithm helps determine postremission (PR) therapy in patients with newly diagnosed acute myeloid leukemia (AML) [24]. All patients and their siblings should undergo human leukocyte antigen (HLA) typing at the time of diagnosis, even if allogeneic transplantation is not considered as initial PR therapy. The initial approach for a patient is determined in large part by cytogenetic risk factors, availability of an HLA-matched sibling donor, and the response to induction therapy. Patients with good prognosis cytogenetics who achieve complete remission (CR) with induction and consolidation therapy are often observed treated with intensive consolidation therapy, with delay until the patient relapses. Patients with intermediate or poor-risk cytogenetics who achieve a CR with induction and consolidation therapy should proceed to allogeneic transplantation if a donor is available. For some patients, an autologous transplant in first remission is also considered, particularly if there is not a family donor. For patients who do not enter CR or who relapse after standard therapy, allogeneic transplantation from a sibling or unrelated donor is the only potential curative therapy for AML. Obviously, this approach needs to be individualized for each patient based on performance status, patient preference, age, and co-existing medical problems. alloBMT—allogeneic bone marrow transplantation; autoBMT—autologous bone marrow transplantation; BMT—bone marrow transplantation; IF—interferon; MUD—matched-unrelated donor.

Acute Myeloid Leukemia: Relapse Therapy

Drug	Dosage	Paired Drugs	Dosage
Ara-C	2-3 g/m² IV q 12h as 3-h infusion × 8 doses	+ Mitoxantrone	12 mg/m² IV on days 1-3 or
		Daunorubicin	60 mg/m² IV on days 5, 6, or
		VP-16	100 mg/m² IV daily × 5 d
Topotecan	1.25 mg/m² q24h continuous infusion × 5 d	+ Ara-C	1 g/m² over 2 h on days 1-5 and
		Amifostine	200 mg/m² qod on days 6-7
			until ANC > 1500/µL
Ara-C	2 g/m²/d IV × 5 d	+ FdURD	300 mg/m²/d × 5 d + G=CSF +/- idarubicin 10 mg/m²/d on days 1-3
Mitoxantrone	10 mg/m² IV daily × 5 d	+ VP-16	100 mg/m² IV as 2 h infusion daily × 5 d

Figure 4-39. Acute myeloid leukemia (AML) relapse therapy. Patients who do not respond to initial therapy or who relapse within 6 months of attaining complete remission are considered to have relatively resistant disease. Efforts to achieve a second remission and overcome drug resistance are focused on high-dose cytarabine (ara-C)-containing regimens, new agents, targeted therapy using leukemia-specific monoclonal antibodies conjugated with either radionuclides or toxins, and the use of nonchemotherapeutic agents to block the drug efflux pump associated with *MDR1* gene expression [10]. High-dose ara-C paired with mitoxantrone, etoposide (VP-16), methotrexate, and fludarabine (FdURD) have produced short-lived complete remissions in 40% to 60% of relapsed AML patients. Combinations of mitoxantrone and etoposide produced 40% to 50% complete remission rates. Cyclosporine, a potent inhibitor of P-glycoprotein–mediated drug efflux, although not improving the overall response rate, appears to prolong the remission in patients who actually achieve a remission.

Although none of the above options offer more than a 10% to 50% chance of long-term disease-free survival, they do provide temporary cytoreduction sufficient to permit further high-dose treatment strategies, such as marrow transplantation from a sibling or unrelated donor. Allogeneic transplantation achieves a 30% to 40% disease-free survival at 5 years when performed after a first relapse or in second remission. Reduced-intensity conditioning regimens are being explored as treatment options in older patients and in those who have other medical problems that would otherwise preclude full-dose allogeneic transplantation. ANC—absolute neutrophil count; G-CSF—granulocyte colony-stimulating factor.

Gemtuzumab Ozogamicin (CMA-676, Mylotarg)

Anti-CD33 antibody conjugated to calicheamicin, a potent anthracycline
Phase I-II study as single agent given twice 2 w apart
Dose of up to 9 mg/m²
30% complete remission in patients in first relapse (older and younger)
Mild infusional toxicity, pancytopenia but no gastrointestinal toxicity

Figure 4-40. Gemtuzumab ozogamicin. This anti-CD33 antibody conjugated to calicheamicin has recently been approved by the US Food and Drug Administration for treatment of relapsed acute myeloid leukemia (AML) in older patients [25]. In phase I and phase II trials, between 25% and 35% of patients with AML who relapsed after a complete remission of more than 6 months achieved clearance of marrow and peripheral blood blasts. Treatment-related toxicity is very low, with infusional side effects of fever and chills and a slow platelet and granulocyte recovery. No cardiac or cerebellar toxicities were noted nor was there any significant mucositis, although liver function abnormalities were reported in 20% to 30% of patients. The drug gives a potential therapeutic option to patients who have AML but may not be in adequate condition to undergo a standard induction therapy. Currently, phase II trials are exploring the addition of gemtuzumab to daunomycin and cytarabine as induction therapy while other groups are studying its potential for preventing disease recurrence by its use in consolidation therapy after achievement of a remission.

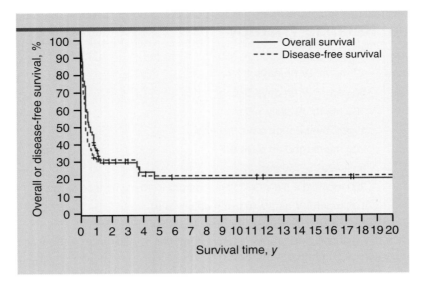

Figure 4-41. Overall survival versus disease-free survival with standard induction chemotherapy. Although the majority of patients with acute myeloid leukemia will achieve a remission, approximately 20% to 30% will not go into remission with induction chemotherapy. This represents a poor prognostic factor and, in general, multiple courses of chemotherapy are not effective in achieving remission and achieving cure of the disease. Under these circumstances, allogeneic transplantation can sometimes be curative and is the treatment of choice before pursuing additional courses of chemotherapy that are unlikely to be effective and will make transplantation more difficult. The figure shows that approximately 30% of patients can become long-term disease-free survivors despite failing to achieve remission with initial chemotherapy (Unpublished data, Dr. Henry Fung, Duarte, CA).

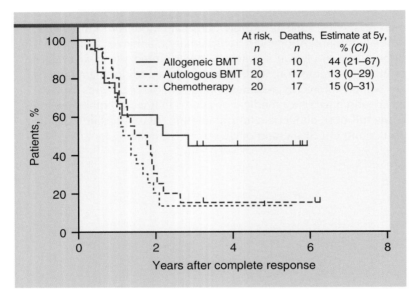

Figure 4-42. Curative impact of transplantation for patients with poor-risk cytogenetics. Allogeneic transplantation is a particularly important therapeutic consideration for patients with acute myeloid leukemia who have poor-risk cytogenetics and have achieved a remission. In general, autologous transplantation or continued chemotherapy has not been effective in providing long-term disease-free survival for the majority of these patients. An intergroup trial conducted in the United States comparing autologous and allogeneic transplantation to chemotherapy was particularly demonstrative in showing the potential curative impact of transplantation on this group of patients [20]. BMT—bone marrow transplantation.

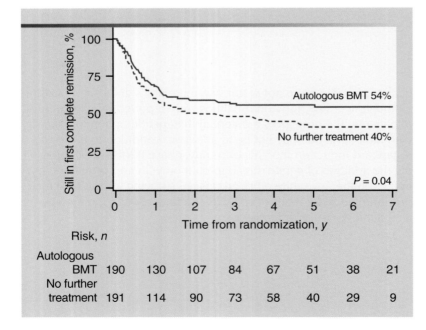

Figure 4-43. Disease-free survival of patients randomly assigned either autologous transplantation or intensive chemotherapy in the British Medical Research Council's AML 10 trial [26]. Many studies have reported the use of unpurged or purged autologous marrow for the treatment of patients with acute myeloid leukemia (AML), usually after consolidation therapy. Disease-free survival rates for patients transplanted in first remission vary between 34% and 80%. The Medical Research Council Leukemia Working Parties conducted a clinical trial to determine whether the addition of autologous stem cell transplantation to intensive consolidation chemotherapy improved the disease-free survival in patients with AML in first remission. After three courses of consolidation, bone marrow was harvested from patients who lacked a donor. The patients then were randomized to receive either one additional cyclotherapy or autologous transplant. On an intent-to-treat analysis, the number of relapses was lower in the group assigned to autologous transplant (37% vs 58%, P = 0.0007), which resulted in a superior disease-free survival rate at 7 years (53% vs 40%). This benefit of the transplant in preventing relapse was seen in all cytogenetic risk groups. BMT—bone marrow transplantation.

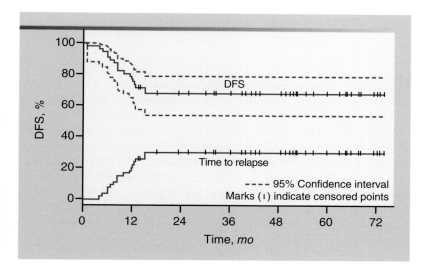

Figure 4-44. Disease-free survival (DFS) versus time to relapse. Several groups have attempted to determine whether the addition of an immunotherapeutic treatment after achievement of minimal residual disease following autologous stem cell transplant might improve DFS [27]. Interleukin-2 (IL-2), a cytokine with a broad range of antitumor effects, has been used in some patients undergoing autologous stem cell transplant to augment indigenous immune functions. One phase II study, which tested high-dose IL-2 following autologous stem cell transplant, showed a 2-year probability of DFS of 73% for a group of patients who actually underwent transplantation in this study. The probability of DFS was 86% for patients with favorable cytogenetics, 70% for patients with intermediate cytogenetics, and 70% for patients with poor-risk cytogenetics.

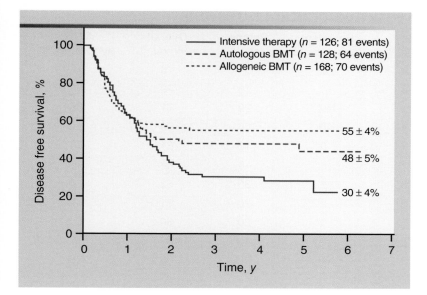

Figure 4-45. Disease-free survival (DFS) with allogeneic bone marrow transplantation (BMT) versus intensive chemotherapy versus autologous BMT. BMT from a human leukocyte antigen (HLA)-matched sibling has been established as a highly effective therapy for achievement of long-term disease control in acute myeloid leukemia (AML) in first remission, with cure rates in the range of 50% to 60% of recipients. The therapeutic effect is dependent on both the intensive preparative regimen and, importantly, on the graft-versus-tumor effect resulting from the alloreactivity of the bone marrow graft. Worldwide, the most common regimens used for allogeneic transplantation have been either busulfan and cyclophosphamide, total-body irradiation and cyclophosphamide, or total-body irradiation and etoposide. The results are dependent on the age of the patient and the cytogenetic risk group. This figure shows the DFS for 422 patients randomly assigned either intensive chemotherapy and autologous transplantation, versus patients who had an HLA-matched sibling donor and underwent allogeneic transplantation, showing the relative efficacy of each of these modalities in controlling leukemia [24]. Based on this and many other studies, with the exception of patients who have AML in first remission with good-risk cytogenetics, allogeneic stem cell transplant is generally recommended when there is an HLA-matched sibling, particularly for patients who have either intermediate- or poor-risk cytogenetics. For patients with poor-risk cytogenetics without a sibling donor, who thus have limited options with chemotherapy or possibly autologous stem cell transplant, an unrelated donor transplant is becoming an increasingly viable option. Although these transplants are associated with enhanced risks of transplant-related complications, the poor prognosis with other modalities would favor this approach as the best means for achieving long-term control.

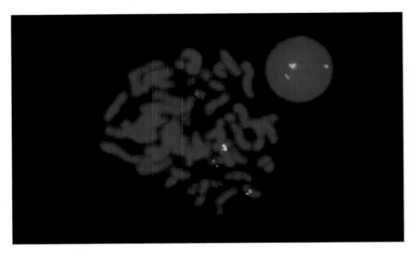

Figure 4-46. Fluorescence in situ hybridization study of t(15;17) in acute promyelocytic leukemia (APL). Involvement of the *RARα* gene in the pathogenesis of APL suggested the use of retinoids as therapy [13]. The HL60 line can be induced to differentiate in cultures with all-*trans*-retinoic acid (ATRA), and in 1988, a study from Shanghai showed a complete remission rate of 85% with this retinoid. When compared with induction chemotherapy, ATRA offers the advantage of a shorter neutropenic period and slightly faster resolution of disseminated intravascular coagulation. Normalization of marrow morphology and cytogenetics requires 30 to 60 days. (*Courtesy of Dr. Marilyn L. Slovak, Duarte, CA.*)

Main Clinical Trials in Acute Promyelocytic Leukemia

Study	Treatment	Complete remission, %	Early death, %	Resistant leukemia, %	Relapse rate, %	Overall survival, %	ATRA syndrome, %
APL 91	ATRA before CT	91	9	0	31	76	5
	CT	81	8	10	78	49	NA
ECOG (0129)	ATRA before CT	76	11	NR	29	71	26
	CT	69	14	NR	58	50	NA
APL 93	ATRA before CD	95	7	0	16	81	20
	ATRA and CT	94	7	0	6	84	11
MRC	Short ATRA before CT	70	23	7	36	52	4
	Extended ATRA and CT	87	12	2	20	71	1
AIDA (0493)	ATRA and CT	95	5	0	20	80	2.5
PETHEMA (LPA96)	ATRA and CT	89	10	2	10	82	6
CALGB	Arsenic trioxide consolidation	89	8	NR	NR	86	NR

Figure 4-47. Main clinical trials in acute promyelocytic leukemia (APL). Initial treatment of APL was addressed in three large studies that showed that all-*trans*-retinoic acid (ATRA), in combination with anthracycline-based chemotherapy (CT), results in improved long-term disease-free survival [13]. When ATRA is used at the time of diagnosis, some patients develop a retinoic acid syndrome characterized by fever, respiratory distress, pulmonary infiltrates, and cardiovascular collapse. This syndrome often correlates with leukocytosis greater than 10,000/mm³, and treatment of the syndrome usually involves temporary discontinuation of ATRA and the use of high-dose steroids or chemotherapy to control leukocytosis. In addition, some patients develop a transient pseudotumor cerebri when treated with ATRA. One of the most noteworthy observations is that when ATRA is combined with idarubicin for induction, the complete remission rate can be as high as 95%, indicating that cytarabine, the mainstay of most other induction regimens for acute myeloid leukemia, is not required to achieve a remission of APL. In APL, reverse-transcriptase polymerase chain reaction for the promyelocytic leukemia RARα fusion protein can be used to follow a response to therapy [27]. The marker clears slowly, with many patients still positive following induction; however, patients with persistence of the gene at the end of consolidation are at high risk for relapse as are those with re-emergence of the marker following a period without detectable protein. The CALGB (Cancer and Leukemia Group B) has shown a survival advantage for consolidation with arsenic trioxide (unpublished data). AIDA—ATRA plus idarubicin; ECOG—Eastern Cooperative Oncology Group; MRC—Medical Research Council; NA—not available; NR—not reported; PETHEMA—Spanish Cooperative Group for Hematological Malignancies Treatment.

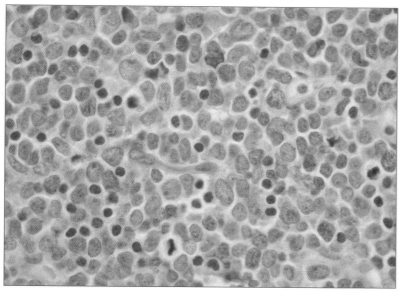

Figure 4-48. Extramedullary myeloid tumors. Myeloid leukemias involving extramedullary sites are known as *myeloid sarcomas* (World Health Organization classification), *extramedullary myeloid tumors* (our preferred term), *granulocytic sarcomas*, or *chloromas*. There are several modes of clinical presentation. Patients with known acute myeloid leukemia may develop leukemic involvement of lymph nodes or soft tissues. Extramedullary myeloid leukemia may be the first sign of blastic transformation in a patient with known chronic myeloid leukemia, other myeloproliferative diseases, or myelodysplasia. Finally, extramedullary involvement by myeloid leukemia may occur in a patient with no known history of leukemia.

The cells of extramedullary myeloid tumor include blasts and eosinophilic myelocytes. The tumor usually has a high mitotic rate, and interspersed tangible body macrophages may lend a starry-sky appearance. Touch imprints or frozen sections, if available, can be examined cytochemically for myeloperoxidase or Sudan black B. Immunohistochemistry is extremely useful, with CD68, antimyeloperoxidase, CD117 (c-kit), CD43, CD15, and antilysozyme each positive in a high percentage of cases. Flow cytometric expression of CD34, CD33, CD13, and CD117 is also seen.

MYELODYSPLASTIC DISORDERS

Crude and Age-specific Incidences of Myelodysplastic Syndrome*					
Study	Aul *et al.*	Radlund *et al.*	Williamson *et al.*	Ma *et al.*	Epling-Burnette *et al.*
Geographic area	Dusseldorf (Germany)	Jönköping (Sweden)	East Dorset (England)	SEER (US)	
Study period	1986–1990	1988–1992	1981–1990	2001–2003	2001–2003
Age group, *y*					
≤ 49	0.2	0.7	0.5		
50–59	4.9	1.6	5.3	2.8	
60–69			15	10	7.4
≥ 80			89	36.2	36.3
All ages	4.1	3.5	12.6	3.4	4.5†

Incidence figures per 100,000 per year.
†*Males.*

Figure 4-49. Crude and age-specific incidences of primary myelodysplastic syndrome (MDS) [28]. Primary MDS has a bimodal age incidence, with the caveat that it has been described in all age groups [28–33]. It appears to primarily be a disease of later life, with approximately 80% of patients with MDS older than age 60 at the time of diagnosis. In one series, 91% of a large number of cases were older than 50 years at the time. Less commonly, primary MDS occurs in the pediatric population and includes specific pediatric syndromes, such as juvenile chronic myeloid leukemia and infantile monosomy 7 syndrome [34,35]. The male-to-female ratio is approximately 1:2. Some studies suggest that the number of MDS cases, independent of chemotherapy, is increasing; this may relate to the increased risk of the aging process itself as well as increased recognition of the causes of anemia in older people.

Signs and Symptoms of Myelodysplastic Syndrome

Symptoms related to anemia
Infection
Bleeding manifestations
Organomegaly and lymphadenopathy

Figure 4-50. Signs and symptoms of myelodysplastic syndrome. Nearly half of patients with myelodysplasia are not symptomatic at the time of initial diagnosis. Symptomatology is related to the effect of the disease on hematopoietic cell production leading to anemia, thrombocytopenia, and leukopenia or combinations of abnormalities. Because the disease is more common in the elderly, symptoms of anemia may range from fatigue to exertional dyspnea that may exacerbate heart disease. Independent of cell number, the functional white cells are often functionally abnormal, and thus about one third of patients have recurrent localized or systemic infections. Similar to disordered granulocytic or monocytic function, patients may have manifestations of bleeding, such as petechiae or gross hemorrhage. Splenomegaly or hepatomegaly is found in up to 20% of patients. Patients with an extremely large spleen and a marrow suggestive of myelodysplasia with increased monocytes should raise the diagnosis of chronic myelomonocytic leukemia.

Primary Diseases with a Verified Increased Risk of Therapy-related Myelodysplastic Syndrome and Therapy-related Acute Myeloid Leukemia After Chemotherapy

Hematologic neoplasms
Hodgkin disease
Non-Hodgkin lymphomas
Multiple myeloma
Polycythemia vera
Essential thrombocythemia
Acute lymphoblastic leukemia
Solid tumors
Breast cancer
Ovarian cancer
Lung cancer
Testicular cancer
Childhood solid tumors
Gastointestinal cancer
Nonmalignant diseases
Rheumatoid arthritis
Psoriasis
Wegener's granulomatosis

Figure 4-51. Primary diseases with a verified increased risk of therapy-related myelodysplastic syndrome (MDS) and therapy-related acute myeloid leukemia (AML) after chemotherapy. Well-defined cohort studies revealed the diseases carrying the highest increased risk of development of therapy-related MDS or therapy-related AML [3]. Complicating these studies was the observation that AML may develop as a part of the natural history of a number of diseases, including polycythemia rubra vera, essential thrombocythemia, and germ cell tumors of mediastinal location. Nevertheless, using chemotherapy in these diseases increases the risk further beyond the baseline. For nonmalignant disorders treated with chemotherapy and for many solid tumors, including breast, ovarian, and lung cancer, the risk of subsequent leukemic development is related to the treatment regimen, which ironically results in the longevity that allows the hematopoietic disorder to evolve.

Comparative Categorization of Myelodysplastic Syndromes with the French-American-British and World Health Organization Classification Systems

FAB	WHO
RA	RA with unilineage dysplasia*
	RCMD
	5q- syndrome[†]
RARS	RARS with unilineage dysplasia*
	RCMD with ringed sideroblasts
RAEB	RAEB-I (5%–9% bone marrow blasts)
	RAEB-II (10%–19% bone marrow blasts)
RA with excess blasts in transformation	Acute myelogenous leukemia (≥ 20% bone marrow blasts)
Chronic myelomonocytic leukemia	Myelodysplastic syndrome/myeloproliferative disorders[‡]
	MDS unclassified

*Requires 6 months of persisting anemia without other cause to establish the diagnosis.
[†]< 5% Marrow blasts, micromegakaryocytes, and thrombocytosis.
[‡]MDS if WBC ≤ 13,000/µL, MPD if WBC > 13,000 µL.

Figure 4-52. Comparative categorization of myelodysplastic syndromes (MDSs) with the French-American-British (FAB) and World Health Organization (WHO) classification systems. A morphologic classification of MDS known as the FAB classification was introduced in 1983 and was based on the number of blasts in blood and bone marrow and on the specific cell lineages affected by the neoplastic process [7]. The classification system for MDS consisted of five subgroups based on the percentage of blasts in the peripheral blood and bone marrow, presence of ringed sideroblasts in the bone marrow, and monocyte count in peripheral blood. The ability of the FAB classification to accurately predict prognosis and progression to acute leukemia was well validated over nearly two decades of widespread use.

The WHO classification for MDS builds on the FAB classification by incorporating new cytogenetic, molecular, and clinical data obtained over the years [5,36,37]. Refractory anemia (RA) with excess blasts (RAEB) in transformation was eliminated because of its similar behavior to acute myeloid leukemia (AML); thus the blast percentage that defines AML is now greater than 20%. Refractory cytopenia with multilineage dysplasia (RCMD) and the 5q- syndrome are regarded as separate entities of MDS within the categories of refractory anemia and refractory anemia with ringed sideroblasts (RARS). Also, the criteria for the lower-grade lesions (RA and RARS) are slightly different between the two classifications. A category is added to include an MDS that is not otherwise classifiable. Chronic myelomonocytic leukemia is included in a separate category of MDS/myeloproliferative disorders because of the overlap of findings between dysplasia and myeloproliferation in this disorder.

World Health Organization Classification of Myelodysplastic Syndromes

Disease	Blood Findings	Bone Marrow Findings
RA	Anemia	Erythroid dysplasia only
	No or rare blasts	< 5% blasts
		< 15% ringed sideroblasts
RARS	Anemia	Erythroid dysplasia only
	No blasts	15% ringed sideroblasts
		< 5% blasts
RCMD	Cytopenias (bicytopenia or pancytopenia)	Dysplasia in ≥10% of cells in 2 or more cell lines
	No or rare blasts	> 5% in marrow
	No Auer rods	No Auer rods
	< 1 K/µL monocytes	< 15% ringed sideroblasts
RCMD-RS	Cytopenias (bicytopenia or pancytopenia)	Dysplasia in ≥ 10% of cells in 2 or more cell lines
	No or rare blasts	> 5% in marrow
	No Auer rods	No Auer rods
	< 1 K/µL monocytes	< 15% ringed sideroblasts
RAEB-1	Cytopenias (bicytopenia or pancytopenia)	Unilineage or multilineage dysplasia
	< 5% blasts	5%–9% blasts
	No Auer rods	No Auer rods
	< 1 K/µL monocytes	
RAEB-2	Cytopenias (bicytopenia or pancytopenia)	Unilineage or multilineage dysplasia
	5%–19% blasts	10%–19% blasts
	Auer rods ±	Auer rods ±
	< 1 K/µL monocytes	
MDS-U	Cytopenias	Unilineage dysplasia in granulocytes or megakaryocytes
	No or rare blasts	< 5% blasts
	No Auer rods	No Auer rods
MDS associated with isolated del (5q)	Anemia	Normal to increased megakaryocytes with hypolobated nuclei
	< 5% blasts	< 5% blasts
	Platelets normal or increased	No Auer rods
		Isolated del(5q)

Figure 4-53. World Health Organization classification of myelodysplastic syndromes (MDSs). The criteria for MDS are well delineated [5,38]. As with acute myeloid leukemia, it is anticipated that additional MDSs with a characteristic constellation of clinical, genetic, and pathologic findings will be identified. MDS-U—MDS, unclassified; RA—refractory anemia; RARS—refractory anemia with ringed sideroblasts; RCMD—refractory cytopenia with multilineage dysplasia; RCMD-RS—RCMD and ringed sideroblasts; RAEB—refractory anemia with excess blasts.

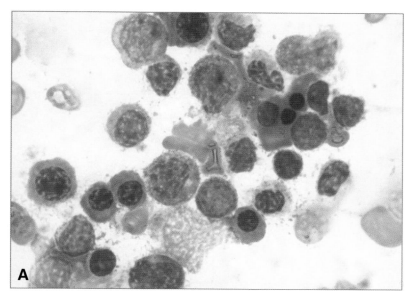
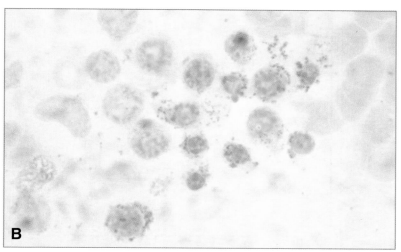

Figure 4-54. Refractory anemia (RA) with multilineage dysplasia. The lower-grade myelodysplastic syndrome (MDS) categories of RA and refractory anemia with ringed sideroblasts (RARS) are to be distinguished from a new World Health Organization (WHO) category of refractory cytopenia with multilineage dysplasia (RCMD) with or without ringed sideroblasts. RA and RARS are defined as diseases in which the dysplasia is morphologically restricted to the erythroid lineage. **A,** The diagnosis of RCMD is made in the presence of multilineage dysplasia, defined as 10% or more dysplastic cells in two or more of the cell lineages, 5% blasts, no Auer rods, and no monocytosis. **B,** Cases that meet those criteria and have at least 15% ringed sideroblasts are considered RCMD with ringed sideroblasts (RCMD-RS). Many investigators consider RCMD and RCMD-RS to represent different manifestations of the same disease, with similar clinical courses and response to therapy. In contrast to patients with RCMD, those with RA or RARS are reported to have longer survival times and a lower rate of transformation to acute myeloid leukemia (AML). Also, the risk of AML transformation may not increase significantly throughout the course of the disease. Compared to patients with RA or RARS, patients with RCMD or RCMD-RS have a higher incidence of cytogenetic abnormalities, more frequent progression to AML, and shorter survival.

One must stringently apply the diagnostic and clinical criteria for RA or RCMD, with or without ringed sideroblasts, to avoid overinterpretation of dyspoiesis secondary to a nonclonal disorder. Erythroid dysplasia is not defined precisely in the French-American-British or WHO classifications, thus the threshold for its recognition shows great interobserver variation. In cases in which patients present with cytopenia affecting more than one cell lineage, multilineage dysplasia affecting less than 10% of cells (*ie,* less than the level required for RCMD diagnosis), and less than 5% blasts in the bone marrow, the pathologist may offer only a descriptive diagnosis with the suggestion of RCMD. Also, in such cases and for cases suspected to be RA, if there is no evidence of clonality by genetic studies, the WHO recommends observation for 6 months prior to making a diagnosis of MDS.

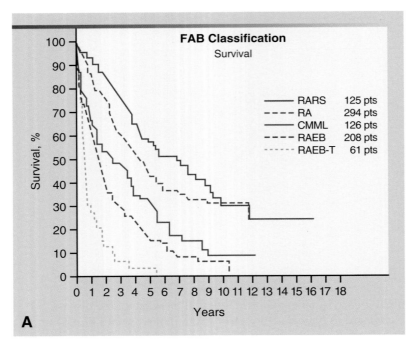

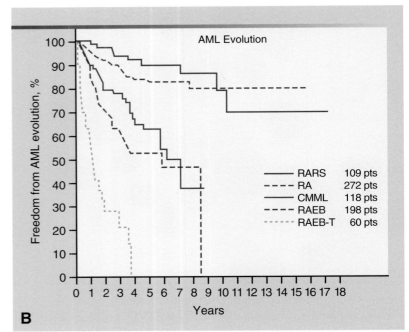

Figure 4-55. Survival (**A**) and freedom from acute myeloid leukemia (AML) evolution (**B**) of patients with myelodysplastic syndromes (MDSs) related to their French-American-British (FAB) classification. The World Health Organization classification indicates that the category of refractory anemia (RA) with excess blasts (RAEB) is further divided into two subgroups, depending on the number of blasts in the blood and bone marrow and the presence or absence of Auer rods. The two subtypes of RAEB are RAEB-1, with 5% to 9% marrow blasts, and RAEB-2, with 10% to 19% marrow blasts.

Creation of these subtypes is based on data published by the International MDS Risk Analysis Workshop that patients with 10% or more blasts in the bone marrow have a worse clinical outcome than do those with fewer blasts [39]. Patients with 10% or more blasts in the bone marrow have a shorter median survival and a higher rate of transformation to acute leukemia than do those with less than 10% blasts. CMML—chronic myelomonocytic leukemia; RAEB-T—RAEB in transformation; RARS—refractory anemia with ringed sideroblasts.

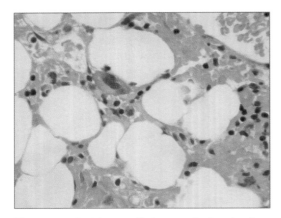

Figure 4-56. Hypocellular myelodysplastic syndrome (MDS). Hypocellular MDS is not a category of MDS in the French-American-British or World Health Organization classification [40]. Nonetheless, it deserves specific mention because of its overlap with aplastic anemia (AA) and paroxysmal nocturnal hemoglobinuria (PNH). It accounts for less than 25% of cases of MDS and is usually defined as having a bone marrow cellularity of less than 30%, or less than the corrected marrow cellularity by age. Cases of hypocellular MDS may be difficult to distinguish from aplastic anemia, but the presence of marrow dysplasia (in the absence of treatment) and a clonal cytogenetic disorder favor MDS. The inter-relationship of hypocellular MDS, AA, and PNH is the source of intense interest and study. Patients diagnosed with hypocellular

MDS may have cells characteristic of PNH, an acquired clonal stem cell disorder characterized by intravascular hemolysis, hyper-coagulability, and relative bone marrow failure. Cells of PNH show exquisite sensitivity to the complement lysis sensitivity test; this abnormal sensitivity is caused by the absence from the erythrocyte membrane of two proteins (CD55 and CD59) that regulate the activation of complement. Many patients with PNH present with marrow aplasia, and it is now apparent that a large number of patients with AA (estimates range from 15% to 50%) also have PNH cells at diagnosis [36,41,42]. PNH cells are not found in patients with constitutional bone marrow failure or bone marrow failure resulting from chemotherapy.

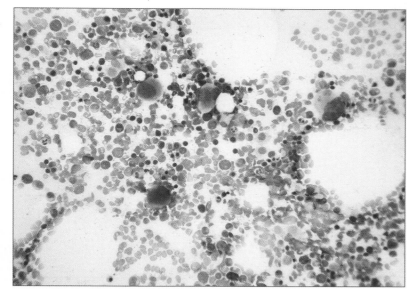

Figure 4-57. The 5q- syndrome. The 5q- syndrome is narrowly defined as de novo myelodysplasia with an isolated cytogenetic abnormality involving deletions between bands q21 and q32 of chromosome 5 [43]. The gene(s) involved in this syndrome is different from that affected in de novo and therapy-related acute myeloid leukemias and myelodysplastic processes associated with del(5q). Patients with the 5q-syndrome usually present with refractory macrocytic anemia, normal to increased platelet count, and increased numbers of megakaryocytes many of which have hypolobate nuclei. The number of blasts in the bone marrow and blood is less than 5%. These findings are associated with long survival. Additional cytogenetic abnormalities or 5% or more blasts in the blood or marrow are exclusionary for the diagnosis.

International Prognostic Scoring System for Myelodysplastic Syndrome

Characteristic	Value	Score
Bone marrow blasts, %	< 5	0
	5–10	0.5
	11–20	1.5
	21–30	2
Karyotype*	Good	0
	Intermediate	0.5
	Poor	1
Cytopenias	0–1	0
	2–3	0.5

Risk Group	Sum of Score
Low	0
Intermediate 1	0.5–1.0
Intermediate 2	1.5–2.0
High	> 2.5

*Good = diploid, -y, del(5q), del(20q); Poor = chromosome 7 abnormalities or complex (≥ 3) abnormalities; intermediate = all others.

Figure 4-58. International prognostic scoring system (IPSS) for myelodysplastic syndrome (MDS). An international MDS risk analysis workshop proposed a system that combines the clinical, morphologic, and cytogenetic data to generate a prognostic system that can be used by physicians to determine therapy and advise patients about prognosis. The IPSS for MDS was first described in 1997 [39]. Its prognostic score includes five variables considered important in predicting the rate of acute myeloid leukemia transformation: bone marrow blast percentage, number of cytopenias, cytogenetic subgroup, age, and gender. The analysis that was performed showed that the most significant independent variables for predicting overall survival were percentage of bone marrow blasts, number of cytopenias, and cytogenetics.

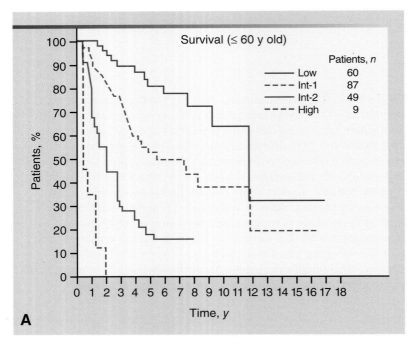

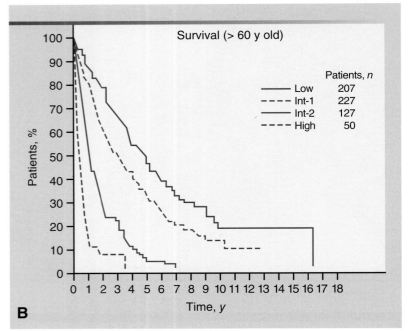

Figure 4-59. Survival for patients with low International Prognostic Scoring System (IPSS) scores. In the IPSS, patients are divided into four risk groups regarding survival as well as evolution into acute myeloid leukemia. When stratified by age (< 60 years [**A**] and > 60 years [**B**]), the analysis showed the four risk groups were also useful in predicting outcome. The figures show survival for patients with low IPSS scores having longer survival than those other groups [39].

Survival and Leukemic Evolution of Myelodysplasia According to the French-American-British Group

	RA	RARS	RAEB	RAEB-T	CMML
Median survival, *mo*	43	73	12	5	20
Transformation to AML, %	15	5	40	50	35
Proportion of patients, %	25	15	35	15	10

Figure 4-60. Survival and leukemic evolution of myelodysplasia according to the French-American-British Morphologic Group. The median on survival relates to the consequences of bone marrow failure, which exposes the patient to life-threatening bleeding and/or infection or evolution to acute myeloid leukemia (AML). Evolution to AML was the basis for the different morphologic groups of patients [36]. Patients with refractory anemia (RA) have an approximately 15% chance of transformation to AML, whereas patients with refractory anemia with excess blasts (RAEB) have an approximately 40% to 50% chance of developing AML. CMML—chronic myelomonocytic leukemia; RAEB-T—RAEB in transformation; RARS—refractory anemia with ringed sideroblasts.

Therapeutic Options for Myelodysplastic Syndrome

Supportive care: antibiotics, transfusions, iron chelation as needed (parenteral or oral)

HGFs: eythropoietin, G-CSF, GM-CSF

BRMs: amifostine, pentoxyfylline, lisofylline, interferon alfa, ATG, cyclosporine, retinoids, vitamin D analogues

Low-intensity chemotherapy: low doses of cytarabine, topotecan, decitabine, azacytidine, hydroxyurea

Immunomodulatory drugs (lenalidomide [Revlemid*]) or thalidomide

High-intensity therapy: AML induction chemotherapy ± MDR modulator (ie, refractory AML therapy); bone marrow or PBSC transplantation; allogenic matched sibling or matched unrelated donor transplantation; autologous

Combinations

*Celgene; Summit, NJ.

Figure 4-61. Therapeutic options for myelodysplastic syndrome (MDS). Options for patients with MDS depend on the degree of cytopenia, risk of acute myeloid leukemia (AML), age of the patient, and any comorbid conditions. Therapy for MDS needs to be individualized. Many patients can be treated with supportive care including antibiotics, transfusion, and iron chelation therapy, with or without hematopoietic growth factor (HGF) support. Other patients, however, require low-intensity chemotherapy as a means of reestablishing more ordered hematopoiesis. The only curative therapy for MDS is allogeneic bone marrow transplantation from a related or unrelated donor. This therapy is often used for younger patients with disease; patients who have therapy-related MDS; or patients whose disease at diagnosis, based on International Prognostic Scoring System (IPSS) score, predicts a shortened survival. In general, the IPSS score at the time of diagnosis and the age of the patient influence the timing and use of transplantation. The major goals of therapy are to improve hematopoietic function and in some cases, replace defective hematopoiesis by transplantation. Newer approaches that focus on differentiation therapy such as 5-azacytidine and decitabine are also being explored for patients with this disorder. ATG—antithymocyte globulin; BRM—biologic response modifier; G-CSF—granulocyte colony-stimulating factor; GM-CSF—granulocyte-macrophage colony-stimulating factor; MDR—multidrug resistance; PBSC—peripheral blood stem cell.

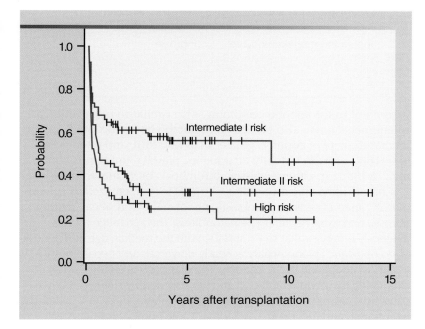

Figure 4-62. Disease-free survival by International Prognostic Scoring System (IPSS) score. Allogeneic transplantation is the only curative therapy available for patients with myelodysplastic syndrome (MDS), and there is a large experience with patients (particularly those under the age of 60) who have been treated with this approach. Approximately 40% to 50% of patients with MDS can become long-term, disease-free survivors after allogeneic transplantation. In the same way that the IPSS score has been applied to patients at diagnosis to determine prognosis, it also has been applied to patients undergoing transplantation to determine the impact of IPSS score on the results of transplantation. The figure shows the impact of those scores on patients in the three different risk groups of newly diagnosed MDS [44]. The IPSS was not designed to evaluate prognosis after a delayed time after diagnosis, as it does with the transplant analysis. Nonetheless, the long-term disease-free survival in the intermediate I, intermediate II, and high-risk groups appears to be better in the transplanted group than the nontransplanted group, thus supporting the decision of early hematopoietic cell transplantation for patients within these risk groups. Consistent with IPSS scores, however, there were significant differences in relapses, with a 2% rate for patients in the lower-risk group and 38% for those in the high-risk group. This risk of relapse was the major factor in long-term disease-free survival for all three groups.

World Health Organization Classification of Chronic Myeloproliferative Diseases

Chronic myelogenous leukemia: Ph chromosome, t(9;22)(q34;q11), BCR/ABL-positive

Chronic neutrophilic leukemia

Chronic eosinophilic leukemia (and the hypereosinophilic syndrome)

Polycythemia vera

Chronic idiopathic myelofibrosis (with extramedullary hematopoiesis)

Essential thrombocythemia

Chronic myeloproliferative disease, unclassifiable

Figure 4-63. The World Health Organization classification of chronic myeloproliferative diseases (CMPDs). This classification comprises seven entities. Only one of the entities, chronic myelogenous leukemia, has a specific genetic abnormality with which it is always associated, namely, the Philadelphia (Ph) chromosome (a reciprocal translocation between chromosomes 9 and 22) or BCR/ABL fusion gene [44]. The other six CMPDs do not have any known specific genetic abnormalities, except for the definitional absence of the Ph chromosome.

Clinical Characteristics of Myeloproliferative Diseases

Characteristic	CML	PV	ET	PMF
Hematocrit	Decreased	Increased	±	Decreased
White cell count	Dramatically increased	Normal or increased	Normal, increased or decreased	Normal, increased or decreased
Differential	All stages, from promyelocytes to PMNs	WNL	WNL	Leukoerythroblastic smear
Platelets	Normal or increased	Normal or increased	Dramatically increased	Normal, increased, or decreased
Bone marrow	Myeloid hyperplasia	Myeloid and erythroid	Increased megakaryocytes	Fibrosis
Special studies	Ph chromosome	Increased RBC mass	___	___
JAK2 mutation	___	++	±	±

Figure 4-64. Clinical characteristics of myeloproliferative diseases. The various myeloproliferative disorders can generally be distinguished by their clinical presentation and by which cell line predominates [45,46]. Chronic myelogenous leukemia (CML) affects mostly adults in their sixth or older decade and is characterized by an increase in granulocytes and their precursor cells in the peripheral blood, splenomegaly, and the presence of the Philadelphia chromosome in the marrow myeloid cells.

Polycythemia vera (PV) is characterized by an expansion of the total red cell mass, often accompanied by splenomegaly and an increase in granulopoiesis and thrombopoiesis. Cytogenetic abnormalities occur in 10% to 15% of patients at diagnosis and commonly include trisomy 8, trisomy 9, and 20q-. In addition to an elevated red cell mass, patients with PV have a low serum erythropoietin level and typically show autonomous growth of erythroid colonies.

Essential thrombocythemia (ET) is characterized by the isolated expansion of the megakaryocytic lineage. Similar to PV, ET occurs at a median age of 60 years. The criteria for diagnosis require exclusion of the other myeloproliferative and myelodysplastic disorders. Most patients present without symptoms or may show vasomotor or thrombotic symptoms. Also similar to polycythemia, splenomegaly may also be detected, but the hallmarks of ET are the increased platelet count to greater than 600 K/µL and often greater than 1000 K/µL. In virtually all patients, platelet function is abnormal, resulting in either excessive thrombosis or increased bleeding.

Chronic idiopathic myelofibrosis (CIMF) is characterized by splenomegaly, anemia, leukoerythroblastic peripheral blood smear, marrow fibrosis, and extramedullary hematopoiesis. The age range for this diagnosis is very similar to ET and PV, with the median age at diagnosis 60 to 65 years. Splenomegaly is nearly universal, and hepatomegaly occurs in about half of the patients. The diagnosis is established by examining the peripheral blood and marrow and by ruling out other causes of marrow fibrosis, such as myelodysplasia, hairy cell leukemia, lymphoma, and metastatic carcinoma. Large numbers of blasts are usually not seen and if present, suggest the diagnosis of acute megakaryoblastic leukemia. Cytogenetic abnormalities occur in about 40% of the patients and frequently involve deletion of the long arm of chromosomes 13 and 20. PMN—polymorphonuclear neutrophil; WNL—within normal limit.

Criteria for Different Phases of Chronic Myelogenous Leukemia

CML, chronic phase
No significant symptoms
None of the features of accelerated or blast phases
CML, accelerated phase
Diagnose if one or more of the following is present:
Blasts 10%–19% of peripheral blood white cells or bone marrow cells
Peripheral blood basophils at least 20%
Persistent thrombocytopenia (< 100 K/μL) unrelated to therapy, or persistent thrombocytosis (> 1000 K/μL) unresponsive to therapy
Increasing spleen size and increasing WBC count unresponsive to therapy
Cytogenetic evidence of clonal evolution (*ie*, the appearance of an additional genetic abnormality that was not present in the initial specimen at the time of diagnosis of chronic phase CML)
CML, blast phase
Diagnose if one or more of following is present:
Blasts 20% or more of peripheral blood white cells or bone marrow cells
Extramedullary blast proliferation
Large foci or clusters of blasts in bone marrow biopsy

Figure 4-65. Criteria for different phases of chronic myelogenous leukemia (CML). CML affects mostly adults 50 years and older and is divided into three phases: chronic, accelerated, and blast [45]. The chronic (or stable) phase is characterized by granulocytosis and few blasts. Accelerated- or advanced-phase CML is characterized by progressive myeloid maturation arrests, increasing resistance to therapy, an increase in bone marrow and peripheral blood blasts, and possibly the development of extramedullary disease. Transformation into the accelerated or blast phases is usually accompanied by acquisition of secondary mutations and in many cases, additional cytogenetic changes (eg, duplication of the Ph chromosome, trisomy 8, and isochromosome 17). Megakaryocytic proliferation in sizable sheets and clusters, associated with marked reticulum or collagen fibrosis and/or severe granulocytic dysplasia, should be considered suggestive of the accelerated phase of CML. These findings have not yet been analyzed in large clinical studies, however, so it is not clear if they are independent criteria for accelerated phase. They often occur simultaneously with one or more of the other features listed.

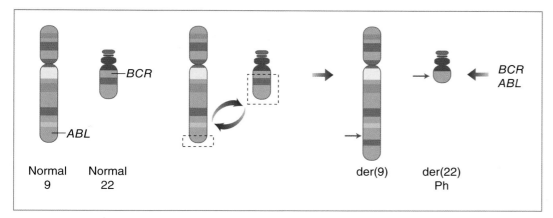

Figure 4-66. The Philadelphia (Ph) chromosome was identified in 1960 as a shortened chromosome 22 [47]. The introduction of banding techniques in the 1970s allowed the observation that the Ph chromosome resulted from a reciprocal translocation between chromosomes 9 and 22 [48]. The application of molecular biology techniques in 1980 revealed that the Ph chromosome involved a rearrangement of the *ABL* gene on chromosome 9 and the *BCR* (breakpoint cluster region) gene on chromosome 22, leading to the creation of a *BCR/ABL* fusion gene [49]. It was then recognized that the *BCR/ABL* gene encodes an abnormal abl-related protein (p210) with deregulated tyrosine kinase activity. This pointed to a potential molecular mechanism whereby hematopoietic cells that contain this abnormal gene gain a proliferative advantage over their normal counterparts. Ultimately, it was demonstrated that hematopoietic cells transduced with *BCR/ABL* could induce a chronic myelogenous leukemia (CML)-like illness in mice, thus providing the first direct evidence that the product of this gene is the important factor in the development of CML and also providing the information that led to directed or targeted therapy for the disease designed to inhibit the kinase function of the bcr-abl protein.

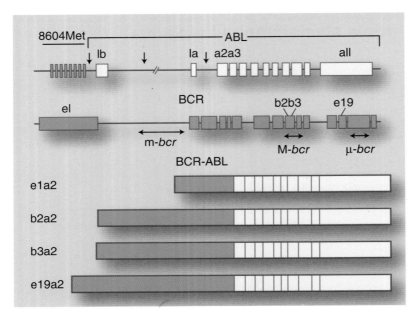

Figure 4-67. *BCR/ABL* gene rearrangements. In chronic myelogenous leukemia (CML), the fusion protein product of *BCR/ABL* varies in size depending on the site of the BCR breakpoint [50]. Three breakpoints are described: M-bcr, m-bcr, and μ-bcr. The breakpoint is usually with a 5.8-kb segment, the major breakpoint cluster region (M-bcr) either between bcr exons b2 and b3 or between exons b3 and b4. As a result, the bcr/abl translocation leads to the production of two different fusion gene transcripts (p210). In 40% of CML patients, the mRNA transcript has a b2a2 junction, and in 40%, the mRNA transcript has a b3a2 junction (with the a2 exons representing ABL breakpoints). When the breakpoint is within the minor breakpoint cluster region (m-bcr), a p190bcr/abl is produced. This 190-kb variant bcr/abl protein usually is associated with Philadelphia (Ph) chromosome–positive acute lymphoblastic leukemia and is present in low amounts in 90% of CML patients. A rare third breakpoint cluster region known as the mu (μ) region (μ-bcr), downstream of M-bcr, has also been described and results in a protein of 230 kb. Strong evidence suggests that the position of the breakpoint in the bcr region influences the disease phenotype in CML. In rare cases of CML, p190 is a predominant gene product and these patients have a prominent monocytic component, are older, and generally do not have splenomegaly. The clinical significance of chromosomal abnormalities in addition to the Ph chromosome that are present at diagnosis is not known. However, evidence of clonal evolution after diagnosis is usually associated with transformation to more aggressive disease.

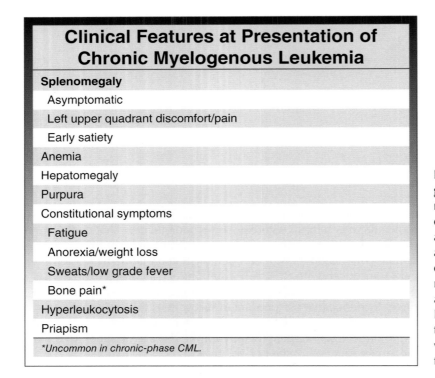

Clinical Features at Presentation of Chronic Myelogenous Leukemia
Splenomegaly
Asymptomatic
Left upper quadrant discomfort/pain
Early satiety
Anemia
Hepatomegaly
Purpura
Constitutional symptoms
Fatigue
Anorexia/weight loss
Sweats/low grade fever
Bone pain*
Hyperleukocytosis
Priapism
*Uncommon in chronic-phase CML.

Figure 4-68. Clinical features at presentation of chronic myelogenous leukemia (CML). The presenting clinical features of CML may be as indolent as the asymptomatic patient in whom the diagnosis is discovered on complete blood count as part of an annual examination or for an unrelated disorder or may be as severe as significant fatigue, weight loss, sweats, abdominal discomfort, or the discovery of an abdominal mass that is found to be splenomegaly. Splenomegaly is the most common physical finding of CML and may in fact be the only abnormality on physical examination. Lymphadenopathy is very uncommon and when found, suggests that there has been transformation of the disease. Patients who present with central nervous system syndromes or priapism require urgent treatment with leukapheresis to relieve the problems.

Laboratory Features at Presentation of Chronic Myelogenous Leukemia	
Peripheral Blood	**Bone Marrow**
Neutrophil leukocytosis with "left shift"	Myeloid hyperplasia
Basophilia/eosinophilia	Blasts < 10% in chronic phase
Thrombocytosis	Minimal/no dysplasia
Anemia	Increased megakaryocytes
Blasts < 10% in chronic phase	Myelofibrosis (mild/moderate)
↓LAP score	Monocytes usually < 3%
↑Lactic dehydrogenase	
↑Uric acid	
↑Vitamin B12/transcobalamin	
Cytogenetic analysis-Ph chromosome positive (90%–95%)	
Molecular analysis-*bcr/abl* positive (> 95%)	

Figure 4-69. Laboratory features at presentation of chronic myelogenous leukemia (CML). Patients with CML have a characteristic peripheral blood smear that shows large numbers of early precursors of granulocytic development. This peripheral blood leukocytosis, combined with the presence of the Philadelphia (Ph) chromosome, establishes the diagnosis of CML. On some occasions, it may be necessary to rely on molecular studies to reveal the presence of the *BCR/ABL* fusion gene if the Ph chromosome is not seen by classic cytogenetic analysis. Absolute numbers of basophils and eosinophils are often elevated, and the patient may also have an elevated platelet count. A number of conditions bear a morphologic resemblance to CML, including other myeloproliferative disorders, such as polycythemia vera in its proliferative phase, as well as chronic myelomonocytic leukemia. In this latter condition, which represents an overlap between myelodysplastic and myeloproliferative disorders, the Ph chromosome is not found, but other cytogenetic abnormalities can be detected. Leukemoid reactions—in which a reactive leukocytosis occurs in response to malignancy, infection, or hemolysis—may be confused with CML. Patients with leukemoid reactions usually have a high leukocyte alkaline phosphatase (LAP) level, which is low in CML or chronic myelomonocytic leukemia.

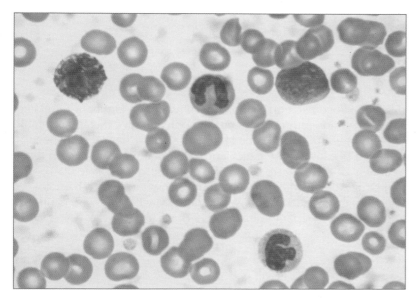

Figure 4-70. Peripheral blood smear, chronic myelogenous leukemia (CML). The peripheral blood smear shows a characteristic leukocytosis, with a WBC count in the range of 100 to 400 K/μL. There is marked neutrophil and myelocyte predominance. Basophils and eosinophils are also elevated in number, usually less than 5% of the total WBC count. Basophils and eosinophils are always present and rarely decreased in number. One should guard against making the diagnosis of CML in the absence of basophils (even one will suffice!). Absolute monocyte counts are also elevated but comprise less than 4% to 5% of the total WBC count. Patients usually also have moderate normochromic, normocytic anemia and a slightly elevated platelet count.

The bone marrow is hypercellular with trilineage hematopoiesis and marked myeloid and megakaryocytic hyperplasia. Gaucher-like histiocytes are often plentiful because of the high cell turnover. Early in the disease course, fibrosis is not common, but later, myelofibrosis may be quite prominent. As the patient enters the accelerated phase, the mature blood cells transition from "leukemic and functional" to accumulation of nonfunctional blast cells. Most commonly, the blasts have a myeloid phenotype, but lymphoid, mixed or undifferentiated phenotypes have also been described. Only rarely has transformation shown erythroblastic, megakaryoblastic, or T-lymphoblastic differentiation.

Definition of Response in Chronic Myelogenous Leukemia

Response*	Category	Criteria
Hematologic remission	Complete	Normalization of WBC counts to < 9 K/µL with normal differential; normalization of platelet counts to < 450 K/µL; disappearance of all signs and symptoms of disease
Cytogenetic response	Complete†	No evidence of Ph chromosome–positive cells
	Partial	5%–34% of metaphases Ph chromosome–positive cells
	Minor	35%–95% of metaphases Ph chromosome–positive cells
	None	Persistence of Ph chromosome in all analyzable cells

*Response assessed on routine cytogenic analysis with at least 20 metaphases counted.
†Major cytogenetic response includes complete and partial cytogenetic responses.

Figure 4-71. Response definitions in chronic myelogenous leukemia (CML). Most patients will respond well to initial treatment for CML, with normalization of blood counts and disappearance of splenomegaly and systemic symptoms.

Response in CML can be divided between hematologic remission, in which the blood counts normalize with therapy, and a cytogenetic response. Historically, better patient survival has depended on achieving either a major or complete cytogenetic response to therapy; thus it is an important component in the evaluation of any therapy for CML.

Presently, molecular analysis of residual disease has not been a criterion for treatment response, as evidence of disease can be detected in nearly all patients treated with therapies other than allogeneic transplantation. In fact, allogeneic transplantation remains the only therapy that has been proven to be effective in achieving a long-term, durable molecular remission of the disease [51].

Therapy for Chronic Myelogenous Leukemia

Busulfan
Hydroxyurea
Interferon alfa
Imatinib mesylate
Dasatinib
Interferon and cytosine arabinoside
Allogeneic transplantation (sibling)
Allogeneic transplantation (unrelated)
Autologous transplantation

Figure 4-72. Therapy for chronic myelogenous leukemia (CML). CML therapy has evolved over many years and has gone from a point where control of the blood counts was the major and only therapeutic potential to one where the disease can be cured by allogeneic transplantation. The introduction of imatinib mesylate recently has revolutionized the therapeutic approach and has provided a reliable medication for achieving both hematologic control and in many patients, a cytogenetic remission of the disease

[52,53]. Allogeneic transplantation from either a family or unrelated matched donor currently remains the only curative therapy available to patients with CML, but the treatment strategy has recently been modified because of the major impact of imatinib mesylate on the treatment of the disease. Dasatinib, now approved by the US Food and Drug Administration, was recently shown to induce hematologic and cytogenetic responses in patients with CML who cannot tolerate or are resistant to imatinib [54].

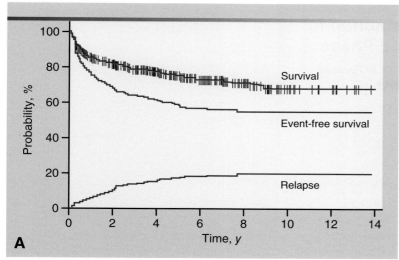

A

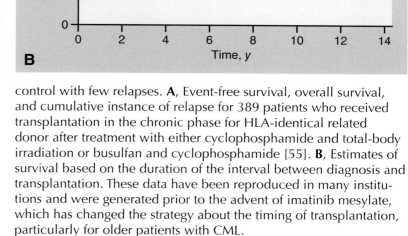

B

Figure 4-73. Long-term disease-free survival (DFS). Long-term DFS can be anticipated in 45% to 80% of patients with chronic myelogenous leukemia (CML) undergoing related-donor transplantation during the chronic phase. The beneficial effects are most evident in younger patients transplanted early in the course of disease, optimally within 1 year of diagnosis. In this group of patients, more than 70% experience long-term DFS. The most common effective transplant regimens for patients in the chronic phase involve the use of total-body irradiation with cyclophosphamide, or high-dose busulfan and cyclophosphamide. Both of these result in good disease control with few relapses. **A**, Event-free survival, overall survival, and cumulative instance of relapse for 389 patients who received transplantation in the chronic phase for HLA-identical related donor after treatment with either cyclophosphamide and total-body irradiation or busulfan and cyclophosphamide [55]. **B**, Estimates of survival based on the duration of the interval between diagnosis and transplantation. These data have been reproduced in many institutions and were generated prior to the advent of imatinib mesylate, which has changed the strategy about the timing of transplantation, particularly for older patients with CML.

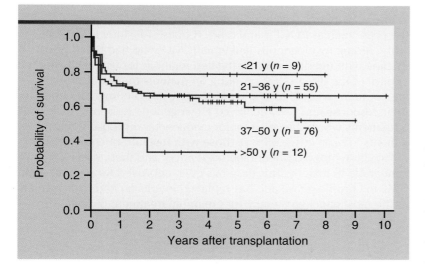

Figure 4-74. Overall survival of patients with chronic myelogenous leukemia (CML) undergoing matched unrelated donor transplantation, stratified by age [55]. For CML patients who do not have a family donor, an HLA-matched unrelated donor can be considered, particularly for younger patients [24]. The chance for good outcome of CML and overall survival following transplantation approach those obtained with a family donor. The same good-risk factors for related donors also apply to patients undergoing transplantation from an unrelated donor, including younger age, HLA matching, and a short interval from diagnosis to transplantation.

Risk of Relapse after Bone Marrow Transplantation for Chronic Myelogenous Leukemia in Chronic Phase

	Patients, *n*	Relative Risk of Relapse
Allogeneic		
No GVHD	115	1
Acute GVHD only	267	1.15
Chronic GVHD only	45	0.28
Acute and chronic GVHD	164	0.24
Syngeneic	24	2.95
Allogeneic, T-cell depleted	154	5.14

Figure 4-75. Risk of relapse after bone marrow transplantation for chronic myelogenous leukemia (CML) in the chronic phase [56]. The cure achieved by allogeneic stem cell transplantation is mediated in large part by the allogeneic stem cell graft itself. Although the preparative regimen achieves significant cytoreduction, the actual cure of the disease, namely, the elimination of minimal residual disease, is probably mediated by T cells present in the donor hematopoietic cell graft. Patients who receive T-cell–depleted transplants have a higher incidence of relapse after transplantation. Patients who manifest graft-versus-host reaction after transplantation have a decreased risk of relapse compared with patients who had no graft-versus-host disease (GVHD). This has led to the exploration of transplantation regimens that focus on engraftment and the initiation of a graft-versus-tumor effect, particularly in older patients who may not be able to tolerate the high-dose regimens used in a traditional transplantation. Among this patient group, there are disorders for which a graft-versus-tumor effect has been demonstrated, and CML appears to be the most susceptible to this immunologic, allogeneic effect.

Tyrosine Kinase Inhibitors

Imatinib mesylate (STI-571, Gleevec)

Specific inhibitor of bcr-abl

Inhibitor of tyrosine kinase activity mediated by bcr-abl

High degree of specificity

Competitive inhibitor of ATP binding site of the bcr-abl-encoded kinase

Prevents phosphorylation of substrates involved in bcr-abl signal transduction

Initial treatment 400 mg/d, but may be more effective at 600 mg/d

Dasatinib (Sprycel)

Dual kinase inhibitor (ABL and Src)

Initial treatment 70 mg PO bid (lower-dose or once daily dosing regimens may also be effective)

Figure 4-76. Imatinib mesylate is a potent inhibitor of the tyrosine kinase activity of bcr-abl and a few other tyrosine kinases found in the cells, such as PDGF-r and c-Kit. A phase I-II study in patients with chronic myelogenous leukemia (CML) who had failed prior therapy with interferon-α investigated imatinib for its toxicity and control of the disease [52]. Among 54 patients treated at doses greater than or equal to 300 mg/day, 98% had a complete hematologic response and 54% achieved a cytogenetic response, including 17 patients who achieved a major cytogenetic response. Among patients in blast crisis, 55% of those with myeloid phenotype and 75% with lymphoid phenotype responded, and there was no significant grade III toxicity. This drug has been approved for patients with CML in chronic phase and has replaced interferon and hydroxyurea as the most effective therapy for the initial treatment of CML.

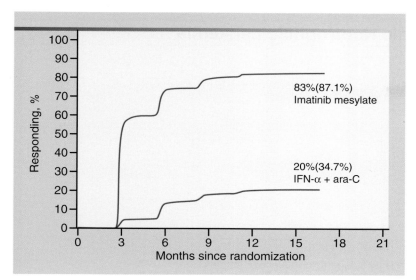

Figure 4-77. Results of a trial to determine the efficacy of interferon alfa (IFN-α) and cytarabine (ara-C) versus imatinib mesylate. Between June 2000 and January 2001, an international study of 1106 patients newly diagnosed with chronic myelogenous leukemia participated in a randomized trial to determine the relative efficacy of IFN-α and ara-C compared with imatinib mesylate [57]. A crossover was built into the study that allowed patients to receive the alternative drug if they had an increase in white blood cell count, loss of hematologic control, intolerance, and failure to achieve a major cytogenetic response at 12 months. As shown here, major cytogenetic responses with imatinib mesylate occurred rapidly within the first 3 months and most patients showed the maximum response by 12 months.

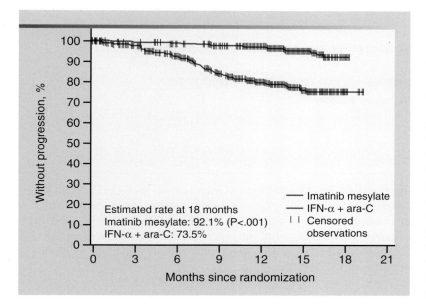

Figure 4-78. Results showing superior efficacy of imatinib mesylate. In this study, imatinib mesylate was superior to interferon alfa (IFN-α)/cytarabine (ara-C) in preventing disease progression at 18 months [57]. Seventy-three percent of patients receiving IFN-α/ara-C were stable, whereas 92% of patients receiving imatinib as initial therapy were stable, suggesting better disease control with imatinib. Of note was that 58% of the patients receiving IFN-α/ara-C crossed over to receive imatinib sometime during the study, with the major indication being the intolerance of therapy, or lack or loss of hematologic control of the disease. In this study, imatinib was superior to IFN-α/ara-C in achieving complete immunologic response, major cytogenetic response, progression to accelerated phase and blast crisis, or tolerance of the drug itself. Studies are now ongoing to determine whether a higher dose, namely, 800 mg, would be more effective in achieving a deeper cytogenetic response in patients with newly diagnosed chronic myelogenous leukemia.

Comparison of Hydroxyurea, Interferon Alfa, and Imatinib Mesylate for the Treatment of Chronic Myelogenous Leukemia

Variable	Hydroxyurea	Interferon alfa	Imatinib mesylate
Mechanism of action	Ribonucleotide reductase inhibitor	Not known	Selective inhibitor of bcr-abl
Oral administration	Yes	No	Yes
High cost of drug	No	Yes	Yes
Induces rapid hematologic responses	Yes	No	Yes
Induces cytogenetic responses	No	Yes	Yes
Commonly toxic	No	Yes	No
Active against blast phase	No	No	Somewhat
Improves survival	No	Yes	Unknown
May worsen results of allogeneic stem-cell transplantation	No	Perhaps*	Unknown

*Prolonged therapy with interferon alfa appears to worsen the outcome, but not if treatment with the drug is stopped at least 3 months before transplantation.

Figure 4-79. Comparison of hydroxyurea, interferon alfa, and imatinib mesylate for the treatment of chronic myelogenous leukemia (CML). The introduction of imatinib mesylate has modified the treatment approach to patients with CML, including the timing of transplantation. The table compares the three most commonly used nontransplant drugs—namely, hydroxyurea, interferon, and imatinib mesylate—for treatment of CML, emphasizing the superiority of imatinib in treating this disease [58].

Diagnostic Criteria for Chronic Neutrophilic Leukemia

Peripheral blood leukocytosis ≥ 25 K/μL

  Segmented neutrophils and bands > 80% of WBCs

  Immature granulocytes (promyelocytes, myelocytes, metamyelocytes) < 10% of WBCs

  Myeloblasts < 1% of WBCs

Hypercellular bone marrow biopsy

  Neutrophilic granulocytes increased in percentage and number

  Myeloblasts < 5% of nucleated marrow cells

  Neutrophilic maturation pattern normal

Hepatosplenomegaly

No identifiable cause for physiologic neutrophilia

  No infectious or inflammatory process

  No underlying tumor, or if present, demonstration of clonality of myeloid cells by cytogenic or molecular studies

No Ph chromosome or *BCR-ABL* fusion gene

No evidence of another myeloproliferative disease

  No evidence of polycythemia vera, *ie*, normal red cell mass

  No evidence of chronic idiopathic myelofibrosis, ie, no abnormal megakaryocytic proliferation, no reticulin or collagen fibrosis, no marked red blood cell poikilocytosis

  No evidence of essential thrombocythemia, *ie*, platelets < 600 K/μL, no proliferation of mature, enlarged megakaryocytes

No evidence of a myelodysplastic syndrome or a myelodysplastic/myeloproliferative disorder

  No granulocytic dysplasia

  No myelodysplastic changes in other myeloid lineages

Monocytes < 1 K/μL

Figure 4-80. Diagnostic criteria for chronic neutrophilic leukemia (CNL). CNL is an extremely rare disease of dubious existence; less than 100 reported cases exist. The criteria for CNL are nonspecific and include sustained peripheral blood neutrophilia, bone marrow hypercellularity due to neutrophilic granulocytic proliferation, and hepatosplenomegaly. The diagnosis is essentially that of exclusion of all causes of reactive neutrophilia and all other myeloprolifera-tive diseases. The World Health Organization included CNL in the category of chronic myeloproliferative diseases, with the recommendation that the possibility of an underlying disease be carefully excluded. If another neoplasm, such as myeloma, is present, the diagnosis of CNL should be made only if there is genetic evidence of a myeloid neoplasm.

Diagnosis of Chronic Eosinophilic Leukemia and Hypereosinophilic Syndrome

Required: persistent eosinophilia ≥ K/µL in blood, increased numbers of bone marrow eosinophils, and myeloblasts < 20% in blood or marrow
Exclude all causes of reactive eosinophilia secondary to:
Allergy
Parasitic disease
Infectious disease
Pulmonary diseases (*eg*, hypersensitivity pneumonitis, Loeffler's)
Collagen vascular diseases
Exclude all neoplastic disorders with secondary, reactive eosinophilia:
T-cell lymphomas, including mycosis fungoides, Sézary syndrome
Hodgkin lymphoma
Acute lymphoblastic leukemia/lymphoma
Mastocytosis
Exclude other neoplastic disorders in which eosinophils are part of the neoplastic clone:
Chronic myelogenous leukemia (Ph chromosome or *BCR/ABL* fusion gene positive)
Acute myeloid leukemia, including those with inv(16), t(16;16) (p13;q22)
Other myeloproliferative diseases (PV, ET, CIMF)
Myelodysplastic syndromes
Exclude T-cell population with aberrant phenotype and abnormal cytokine production
If there is no demonstrable disease that could cause the eosinophilia, not abnormal T-cell population, and no evidence of a clonal myeloid disorder, diagnose HES
If all of the requirements, including first four conditions, have been met, and if the myeloid cells demonstrate a clonal chromosomal abnormality or are shown to be clonal by other means, or if blast cells are present in the peripheral blood (> 2%) or are increased in the bone marrow (> 5% but less than 19% of nucleated bone marrow cells), diagnose CEL

Figure 4-81. Diagnosis of chronic eosinophilic leukemia (CEL) and hypereosinophilic syndrome (HES). HES is a rare hematologic disorder manifested by the sustained overproduction of eosinophils in the bone marrow, eosinophilia in blood, tissue infiltration, and organ damage [45]. Diagnostic criteria that have been established are sustained eosinophilia for more than 6 months; the absence of other causes of eosinophilia, including parasitic infections and allergies; and signs of organ involvement, most frequently of the heart, central and peripheral nervous system, lungs, and skin. The differential diagnosis includes specific subtypes of leukemia in which eosinophilic proliferation is common [59]. The most clearly defined entities are chronic myelomonocytic leukemia with eosinophilia associated with the translocation t(5;12)(9q33;p13) and chronic leukemia with evolution to acute myeloid leukemia and T-lymphoblastic lymphoma associated with t(8;13)(p11;q12) or other cytogenetic aberrations with an 8p11-12 breakpoint. The syndrome is more common in men than in women and occurs predominantly between the ages of 20 and 50 years. Total leukocyte counts are usually less than 25 K/µL but include 30% to 75% eosinophils. Bone marrow eosinophils are increased, but myeloblasts are not. In some cases, the syndrome has been proven to be clonally derived, as demonstrated by clonal karyotypic abnormalities and X-inactivation assays. A large number of diseases, syndromes, and inflammatory processes are associated with peripheral blood and/or tissue eosinophilia. The most common associations are infections with parasitic helminths and allergic disorders and their related inflammatory reactions. Effective clinical assessment of the patient with eosinophilia requires the physician to take a detailed history that includes travel information, where the patient lives, medication use, vitamin supplements, and allergic symptomatology. Because many of these disorders are systemic, patients may present with fever, weight loss, arthralgias, rashes, and lymphadenopathy. Only after exclusion of these disorders by history, physical examination, and laboratory evaluation, should one consider a disorder such as idiopathic hypereosinophilic syndrome or chronic eosinophilic leukemia. CIMF—chronic idiopathic myelofibrosis; ET—essential thrombocythemia; PV—polycythemia vera.

Major Organ Involvement and Prominent Clinical Features in Patients with the Hypereosinophilic Syndrome

Primary Organ Involvement	Clinical Manifestations
Cardiovascular	Eosinophilic endomyocardial disease
	Pericarditis
	Arrhythmias
Cutaneous	Skin lesions, eg, angioedema, urticaria
	Thromboembolic disease
Hematologic/splenic	Lymph node and/or spleen enlargement
	Splenic infarction
Ocular	Ophthalmologic complications
Gastrointestinal/hepatic	Gastrointestinal involvement, including diarrhea
	Diarrhea alone
Pulmonary	Pulmonary involvement
Neurologic	Central nervous system disease
	Psychiatric disturbance
Renal	Renal impairment
Systemic	Anorexia and weight loss
	Myalgia
	Arthralgia
	Fever, excessive sweating.

Figure 4-82. Organ involvement and prominent features in patients with the hypereosinophilic syndrome (HES) [60]. Patients with the HES may present with a variety of clinical manifestations. Cardiac manifestations may be considerable, occurring in 50% to 60% of the patients and can lead to eosinophilic endomyocardial fibrosis. Fifty percent of patients may show pulmonary involvement with a chronic, persistent nonproductive cough, which is the most common respiratory syndrome. Neurologic syndromes are also quite common and are related to thromboemboli that may result from cardiac thrombi. Some patients may present with primary diffuse central nervous system dysfunction of unknown etiology, including changes in behavior, confusion, ataxia, and loss of memory. Other patients, however, present with peripheral neuropathies; these occur in 50% of patients. Skin manifestations are also very common and include angioedema, urticaria, pleuritic papules and nodules, and in some cases, mucosal ulcerations.

Treatment for Hypereosinophilia Syndrome

Corticosteroids
Hydroxyurea
Vincristine
Alkylating agents
Interferon
Cardiac surgery
Anticoagulation
Imatinib mesylate
Allogeneic stem cell transplantation

Figure 4-83. Treatment for chronic eosinophilic leukemia/hypereosinophilic syndrome. The indications for initial treatment are evidence of progressive organ involvement and symptoms. Given the frequency and potential severity of cardiac involvement, echocardiographic follow-up is important. Prednisone is considered the first-line agent for patients with organ involvement. The presence of angioedema and urticaria, elevated serum IgE levels, and a rapid drop in eosinophil counts in response to the initiation of steroids are good prognostic signs. Patients with splenomegaly, established cardiac dysfunction, or neurologic symptoms at the time of presentation respond poorly to steroids. Over time, many patients become steroid refractory and require other agents, such as chemotherapy. Although there is limited experience for bone marrow transplantation, several reports have shown that this may be a successful approach, particularly for patients with advanced disease who have not done well with alternative therapies. Given the improvements in transplantation care, a patient with this syndrome who is poorly responsive to initial agents or who has complications that would predict shorter survival should be considered for transplantation. Recently, several groups have reported that some cases of hypereosinophilic syndrome respond to imatinib mesylate [61]. In one series, 10 of 11 patients treated with the medication entered a complete remission. All of them had life-threatening manifestations of the syndrome. Studies were performed that showed that a deletion of chromosomal material from 4q12 had left fragments of two genes, FIP1L1 and PDGFRA, which fused to form a novel gene, FIP1L1-PDGFRA, resulting in a tyrosine kinase that remains consistently active by virtue of the fusion. This is analogous to imatinib-sensitive bcr-abl enzyme in chronic myelogenous leukemia (CML). Thus, as for CML, imatinib will likely become the mainstay of therapy for patients with hypereosinophilic syndrome, particularly those who do not respond initially to steroids.

Stages of Polycythemia Vera

Stage	Clinical Findings
Asymptomatic	Splenomegaly
	Isolated erythrocytosis
	Isolated thrombocytosis
Erythrocytotic phase (polycythemic)	Erythrocytosis
	Thrombocytosis
	Leukocytosis
	Splenomegaly
	Thrombosis
	Hemorrhage
	Pruritus
Inactive phase	No longer requires phlebotomy or chemotherapy
	Possibly iron deficient
Postpolycythemic myeloid metaplasia	Anemia
	Leukoerythroblastosis
	Thrombocytopenia or thrombocytosis
	Enlarging splenomegaly
	Systemic symptoms (fever, weight loss)
Acute myeloid leukemia	

Figure 4-84. Stages of polycythemia vera. Polycythemia vera is a clonal stem cell disorder characterized by increased red blood cell production and escape of normal erythropoiesis [62]. The disease manifests in two stages: the initial proliferative phase and the end stage, or "spent" phase. A small percentage of cases also progress to acute leukemia. Polycythemia vera differs from many other hematologic malignancies in that patients often have a prolonged course manifested solely by the excess production of red blood cells and platelets. This stage can be controlled by either phlebotomy or medication. However, over the course of time, the disease can evolve into several other syndromes, such as myelofibrosis and acute leukemia. In the initial *polycythemic stage*, the patient has splenomegaly and the peripheral blood is characterized by increased red blood cell mass with normochromic normocytic red blood cells; thrombocytosis; and normal leukocyte count. One may see a superimposed iron deficiency anemia with hypochromic microcytic red blood cells due to excessive bleeding. There may also be neutrophilia or basophilia or left shift, but generally, there are no blasts. The bone marrow is typically hypercellular. After some time, the *erythrocytotic phase* of the disease frequently becomes less active and the patient may no longer suffer from sequelae of excessive red blood cell production nor require any treatment. Subsequently, these patients may develop what is called the *spent-phase* or *postpolycythemic myeloid metaplasia*, which is very similar to chronic idiopathic myelofibrosis. A significant proportion of these patients will eventually go on to develop acute myelogenous leukemia.

World Health Organization Criteria for Polycythemia Vera

Present criteria

A1: Elevated RBC mass > 25% above mean normal predicted value, or Hb > 18.5 g/dL in men, 16.5 g/dL in women*

A2: No cause of secondary erythrocytosis, including

Absence of familial erythrocytosis due to

No elevation of EPO due to

  hypoxia (arterial $PO_2 \leq 92\%$)

  high oxygen affinity hemoglobin

  truncated EPO receptor

  inappropriate EPO production by tumor

A3: splenomegaly

A4: clonal genetic abnormality other than Ph chromosome or *BCR/ABL* fusion gene in marrow cells

A5: endogenous erythroid colony formation in vitro

B1: Thrombocytosis > 400 K/μL

B2: WBC > 12 K/μL

B3: Bone marrow biopsy showing panmyelosis with prominent erythroid and megakaryocytic proliferation

B4: Low serum erythropoietin levels

Diagnose PV when A1 + A2 and any other category A are present, or when A1 + A2 and any two of category B are present

Proposed revised criteria†

Major criteria

  Hemoglobin > 18.5 g/dL in men, 16.5 g/dL in women, or other evidence of increased red cell volume‡

  Presence of *JAK*2617V>F or other functionally similar mutation such as *JAK*2 exon 12 mutation

Minor criteria

  Bone marrow biopsy showing hypercullularity for age with trilineage growth (panmyelosis) with prominent erythroid, granulocytic, and megakaryocytic proliferation

  Serum erythropoietin level below the reference range for normal

  Endogenous erythroid colony formation in vitro

Or > 99th percentile of method-specific reference range for age, sex, altitude of residence.
†*Diagnosis would require the presence of both major criteria and 1 minor criterion or the presence of the first major criterion together with 2 minor criteria.*
‡*Hemoglobin or hematocrit > 99th percentile of method-specific reference range for age, sex, altitude of residence or hemoglobin > 17 g/dL in men, 15 g/dL in women if associated with a documented and sustained increase of at least 2 g/dL from an individual's baseline value that cannot be attributed to correction of iron deficiency, or elevated red call mass > 25% above mean normal predicted value.*

Figure 4-85. World Health Organization criteria for polycythemia vera (present and proposed revised). In most patients, the diagnosis of polycythemia vera is easy to make because the patient will have erythrocytosis, leukocytosis, and thrombocytosis, reflecting the myeloproliferative nature of the disease, with the bone marrow showing trilineage hyperplasia [45,46]. Splenomegaly is also common. Initially, it is important to discriminate polycythemia vera from the large number of other causes of secondary erythrocytosis.

Not all patients with an elevated hemoglobin or hematocrit have true polycythemia [63,64]. In some cases, the red cell value is relative or spurious secondary to dehydration. Polycythemia may be caused by a number of clinical situations, including chronic hypoxemia, renal disease, and selected tumors, as well as various syndromes. In some cases, the diagnosis may be difficult to make, particularly in the absence of leukocytosis, thrombocytosis, or splenomegaly. Other findings, such as arterial blood gas values, serum vitamin B12 levels, leukocyte alkaline phosphatase scores, and a careful examination of the marrow cellularity along with erythropoietin (EPO) levels, can help establish the diagnosis. Hb—hemoglobin.

Treatment of Polycythemia Vera

Treatment	Advantages	Disadvantages
Phlebotomy	Low risk, simple to perform	Does not control thrombocytosis or leukocytosis
Hydroxyurea	Controls leukocytosis and thrombocytosis; low leukemogenic risk	Continuous therapy required
Busulfan	Easy to administer; prolonged remissions; risk of leukemogenesis probably not high	Overdose produces prolonged marrow suppression; risks of leukemogenesis, long-term pulmonary and cutaneous toxicity
32P	Patient compliance not required; prolonged control of thrombocytosis and leukocytosis	Expensive and relatively inconvenient; moderate leukemogenic risk
Chlorambucil	Easy to administer; good control of thrombocytosis and leukocytosis	High risk of leukemogenesis
Interferon	Low leukemogenic potential; effect on pruritus	Inconvenient, costly, frequent side effects
Anagrelide	Selective effect on platelets	Selective effect on platelets

Figure 4-86. Treatment of polycythemia vera. A number of treatments have evolved for the treatment of polycythemia vera. The simplest is phlebotomy, which does not expose the patient to potentially leukemogenic therapies, such as hydroxyurea or 32P [64]. In some cases, combinations of therapies are required, particularly if a patient develops thrombocytosis while undergoing phlebotomy. Nevertheless, in most patients during the proliferative phase of disease, blood counts can be controlled and the patient can maintain a relatively asymptomatic life. In general, it is desirable to maintain a hematocrit between 42% and 45%. Hyperuricemia should be treated with allopurinol. Elective surgery or dental procedures should be delayed until the red cell mass and platelet counts have been normalized for a few months.

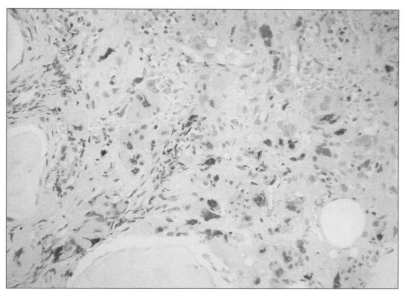

Figure 4-87. Chronic idiopathic myelofibrosis (CIMF), fibrotic stage. CIMF is a clonal myeloproliferative disease characterized by marked myeloid and megakaryocytic hyperplasia and associated with extramedullary hematopoiesis and reticulin or collagen fibrosis [65]. CIMF is synonymous with agnogenic myeloid metaplasia and myeloid metaplasia with myelofibrosis. Approximately 0.5 to 1.5 per 100,000 individuals per year are diagnosed, with a male-to-female ratio of 1:1. Patients are usually in their 60s; the disease rarely occurs in children. Nearly one-third of patients are asymptomatic, with a diagnosis suspected only when routine physical examination reveals splenomegaly or routine laboratory tests show anemia or thrombocytopenia. Symptoms, if present, may include fatigue, dyspnea, weight loss, night sweats, low-grade fever, and bleeding. Splenomegaly is present in approximately 90% of patients and may be accompanied by hepatomegaly in approximately half of those cases. The disease course is characterized by progressive fibrosis and is characteristically divided into two stages: prefibrotic and fibrotic. CIMF has a worse survival than essential thrombocythemia or polycythemia vera.

Median survival times vary from 3 to 5 years, although there is great individual variation in survival lengths [65]. Bone marrow failure may lead to infection and hemorrhage, and patients may also have portal hypertension, cardiac failure, and thromboembolic events. Leukemia transformation may occur in approximately 5% to 20% of cases. Risk factors for poor prognosis include age greater than 70 years, severe anemia (hemoglobin < 10 g/dL), thrombocytopenia (< 100 K/µL), marked peripheral blood granulocytic immaturity, and abnormal karyotype.

Chronic Idiopathic Myelofibrosis: Prefibrotic Stage

Clinical Findings	Morphologic Findings
Spleen and liver	Blood
No or mild splenomegaly or hepatomegaly	No or mild leukoerythroblastosis
Hematologic parameters	No or minimal red blood cell poikilocytosis; few if any dacrocytes
Mild anemia	Bone marrow
Mild to moderate leukocytosis	Hypercellularity
Mild to marked thrombocytosis	Neutrophilic proliferation
	Megakaryocytic proliferation and atypia (clustering of megakaryocytes, abnormally lobulated megakaryocytic nuclei, naked megakaryocytic nuclei)
	Minimal or absent reticulin fibrosis

Figure 4-88. Chronic idiopathic myelofibrosis (CIMF): prefibrotic stage. The diagnosis of CIMF is usually made by noting the presence of a leukoerythroblastic blood smear, organomegaly due to extramedullary hematopoiesis, and myelofibrosis of the bone marrow [45]. An early, prefibrotic stage of CIMF may not show these classic findings. Instead, one may see nonspecific myeloid hyperplasia without diffuse marrow fibrosis, anemia, mild leukocytosis, and mild thrombocytosis. The presence of clusters of bizarre megakaryocytes is a clue to the prefibrotic stage of CIMF. Although megakaryocytic hyperplasia is present in all of the myeloproliferative disorders, only CIMF usually has pleomorphic megakaryocytes.

Chronic Idiopathic Myelofibrosis: Fibrotic Stage

Clinical Findings	Morphologic Findings
Spleen and liver	Blood
Moderate to marked splenomegaly and hepatomegaly	Leukoerythroblastosis
Hematology	Prominent red blood cell poikilocytosis with dacrocytes
Moderate to marked anemia	Bone marrow
Low, normal, or elevated WBC	Reticulin and/or collagen fibrosis
Platelet count decreased, normal, or elevated	Decreased cellularity
	Dilated marrow sinuses with intraluminal hematopoiesis
	Prominent megakaryocytic proliferation and atypia (clustering of megakaryocytes, abnormally lobulated megakaryocytic nuclei, naked nuclei)
	New bone formation (osteosclerosis)

Figure 4-89. Chronic idiopathic myelofibrosis (CIMF): fibrotic stage [45]. Most patients with CIMF are diagnosed in the fibrotic stage, during which organomegaly is common because of extramedullary hematopoiesis. Anemia, leukoerythroblastosis with numerous teardrop cells, and a hypercellular fibrotic marrow are typical of this disease stage. The presence of more than 10% blasts suggests the possibility of an accelerated or blast phase of CIMF. Platelets show marked variation in size and granularity, and circulating megakaryocytic fragments or nuclei may be observed.

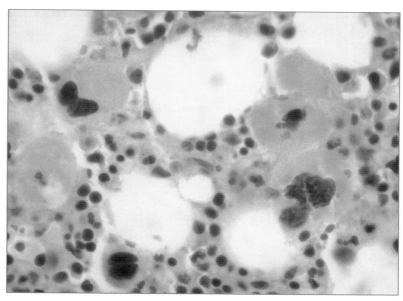

Figure 4-90. Primary thrombocythemia. Essential thrombocythemia is a clonal disorder of multipotential hematopoietic stem cells [66]. The disease is characterized by persistent thrombocytosis in the blood and an increased number of large, mature megakaryocytes in the bone marrow. The underlying mechanism for its predominant phenotype, namely, elevated platelet count, is not yet known, but may be related to preferential responsiveness of the clone to regulatory factors that favor differentiation along the megakaryocytic plate-let pathway. A significant number of patients with this disorder are asymptomatic at presentation. Because platelet counts are included in complete blood counts performed during routine physical examinations, patients may have an incidental finding of thrombocytosis, which may lead to the diagnosis of essential thrombocythemia. Thus constitutional symptoms are rare and physical findings are often limited to mild splenomegaly (present in 40% of patients). The clinical course is punctuated by either hemorrhagic or thrombotic episodes.

Diagnostic Criteria for Essential Thrombocythemia

Present criteria

Positive criteria

 Sustained platelet count > 600 K/μL

 Bone marrow biopsy specimen showing proliferation mainly of the megakaryocytic lineage with increased numbers of enlarged, mature megakaryocytes

Criteria of exclusion

 No evidence of polycythemia vera (PV)

  Normal red cell mass or Hb < 18.5 g/dL in men, 16.5 g/dL in women

  Stainable iron in marrow, normal serum ferritin or normal MCV

  If the first condition is not met, failure of iron trial to increase red cell mass or hemoglobin levels to the PV range

 No evidence of CML

  No Ph chromosome and no *BCR/ABL* fusion gene

 No evidence of chronic idiopathic myelofibrosis

  Collagen fibrosis absent

  Reticulin fibrosis minimal or absent

 No evidence of myelodysplastic syndrome

  No del(5q), t(3;3)(q21;q26), inv(3)(q21q26)

  No significant granulocytic dysplasia, few if any micromegakaryocytes

 No evidence that thrombocytosis is reactive due to:

  Underlying inflammation or infection

  Underlying neoplasm

  Prior splenectomy

Proposed revised criteria

 Sustained platelet count ≥ 450 x 10^9/L*

 Bone marrow biopsy specimen showing proliferation mainly of the megakaryocytic lineage with increased numbers of enlarged, mature megakaryocytes; no significant increase or left-shift of neutrophil granulopoiesis or erythropoiesis

 Not meeting WHO criteria for PV[†], PMF[‡], CML[§], MDS[¶], or other myeloid neoplasm

 Demonstration of *JAK*2617V>F or other clonal marker, or in the absence of a clonal marker, no evidence for reactive thrombocytosis**

Diagnosis requires meeting all four criteria.
During the work-up period.
[†]*Requires the failure of iron replacement therapy to increase hemoglobin level to the PV range in the presence of decreased serum ferritin. Exclusion of PV is based on hemoglobin and hematocrit levels, and red cell mass measurement is not required.*
[‡]*Requires the absence of relevant reticulin fibrosis, collagen fibrosis, peripheral blood leukoerythroblastosis, or markedly hypercellular marrow for age accompanied by megakaryocyte morphology that is typical for PMF—small to large with an aberrant nuclearl-cytoplasmic ratio and hyperchromatic, bulbous or irregularly folded nuclei and dense clustering.*
[§]*Requires the absence of BCR-ABL.*
[¶]*Requires absence of dyserythropoiesis and dysgranulopoiesis.*
**Causes of reactive thrombocytosis include iron deficiency, splenectomy, surgery, infection, inflammation, connective tissue disease, metastatic cancer, and lymphoproliferative disorders. However, the presence of a condition associated with reactive thrombocytosis does not exclude the possibility of ET if the first 3 criteria are met.*

Figure 4-91. Diagnostic criteria for essential thrombocythemia (present and proposed revised). There are no known genetic or biologic markers specific for essential thrombocythemia, thus the diagnosis is one of exclusion [45]. CML—chronic myelogenous leukemia; MCV—mean corpuscular volume.

Major Causes of Thrombocytosis

Clonal thrombocytosis

  Essential (primary) thrombocythemia

  Other myeloproliferative disorders (polycythemia vera, chronic myelogenous leukemia, chronic idiopathic myelofibrosis)

Familial thrombocytosis

Reactive (secondary) thrombocytosis

  Acute blood loss

  Iron deficiency

  Postsplenectomy, asplenic states

  Recovery from thrombocytopenia ("rebound")

  Malignancies

  Chronic inflammatory and infectious diseases (inflammatory bowel disease, connective tissue disorders, temporal arteritis, tuberculosis, chronic pneumonitis)

  Acute inflammatory and infectious diseases

  Response to exercise

  Response to drugs (vincristine, epinephrine, all-trans-retinoic acid, cytokines, and growth factors)

  Hemolytic anemia

Figure 4-92. Major causes of thrombocytosis. Primary thrombocythemia should be distinguished from reactive or secondary forms as well as from other myeloproliferative disorders, such as polycythemia vera, chronic idiopathic myelofibrosis, and chronic myelogenous leukemia (CML), which may also be characterized by thrombocytosis and other hematologic abnormalities. Bone marrow karyotypic analysis is imperative in every patient to exclude an unusual presentation of CML because the disorders are treated differently and CML is potentially curable with marrow trans-plantation. Some patients are not recognized to have CML until the disease actually enters a blast transformation, thus alerting everyone to the correct diagnosis. Occasionally, patients with myelodysplastic syndromes may also present with moderate to marked thrombocytosis, particularly patients with 5q- syndrome or those with acquired sideroblastic anemia. There are many causes of secondary forms of thrombocytosis. Most commonly, patients with iron deficiency anemia may show reactive thrombocytosis, although the platelet count in this situation rarely goes above 700 K/µL.

Treatment of Thrombocytosis

Platelet pheresis in patients with hemorrhagic or thrombotic complications

Anagrelide

Interferon

Hydroxyurea (in patients over age 60)

Discontinue smoking

Figure 4-93. Treatment of thrombocytosis. The major therapeutic decision for the physician in the case of thrombocytosis is whether or not treatment is required to reduce the platelet count. The issue is related to the lack of prospective trials to determine the impact of platelet reduction on the morbidity and mortality in this disorder. Young asymptomatic patients with a platelet count less than 1 million may not need treatment. Some studies have identified high-risk patients as those over 60 years of age with a previous history of thrombosis. A therapeutic goal is to maintain platelet counts, which has been shown to reduce the incidence of subsequent thrombotic episodes. Also, there is a consensus that lowering the platelet count in some patients—those with active or recurrent bleeding or thrombosis—results in symptomatic improvement. In fact, prompt cytoreduction is particularly necessary in patients who have microvascular digital or cerebellar ischemia syndromes. Platelet apheresis is the most effective way of achieving an acute reduction but is also an effective means of long-term control of thrombocytopenia. Hydroxyurea has proven to be a very effective agent for the control of thrombocythemia, although some hesitate to use it because of its potential—although statistically insignificant—trend toward development of acute leukemia. Although the leukemogenic potential of hydroxyurea is substantially less than that of radiophosphorus or alkylating agents, one should consider this effect in the long-term control of platelet counts in younger essential thrombocythemia patients. Anagrelide is very effective in platelet cytoreduction and is probably the best first-line therapy. Unlike hydroxyurea, anagrelide reduces the platelet count without affecting the white blood cell count. In some situations, interferon is used and is also very effective, although the response rate is slower and side effects are more profound than with other agents.

Diagnostic Criteria for Chronic Myelomonocytic Leukemia

Persistent peripheral blood monocytosis > 1 K/µL
No Ph chromosome or *BCR/ABL* fusion gene
< 20% blasts (myeloblasts, monoblasts, and promonocytes) in the blood or bone marrow
Dysplasia in one or more cell lines
If dysplasia is absent or minimal, the diagnosis of CMML may still be made if the other requirements are present, and
An acquired, clonal cytogenetic abnormality is present in the marrow cells, or
The monocytosis has been persistent for at least 3 months, and
All other causes of monocytosis have been excluded

Figure 4-94. Diagnostic criteria for chronic myelomonocytic leukemia (CMML). CMML is a clonal stem cell disorder and shares features of both myeloproliferative disorders (MPDs) (leukocytosis and hepatosplenomegaly) and myelodysplasia (MDS) (trilineage dysplasia) [66]. Because of these mixed features, the classification and recognition of this disease has been somewhat tortuous, with new "criteria" emerging seemingly annually. Under the World Health Organization (WHO) classification, the disease is placed in a separate category that recognizes its overlap between the MPDs and MDSs. However, the WHO classification does not offer the two traditional, separate subtypes of "proliferative" and "nonproliferative" CMML because there appear to be no specific clinical, cytogenetic, or molecular differences based on the magnitude of the white blood cell count. In fact, some patients who initially have low white blood cell counts and minimal if any splenomegaly may eventually develop markedly elevated white blood cell counts and splenomegaly.

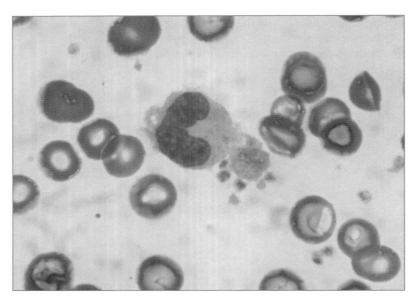

Figure 4-95. Patients with chronic myelomonocytic leukemia (CMML) usually present with splenomegaly, abnormal white blood cell counts, and trilineage dysplasia. Patients usually have at least 10% monocytes in the peripheral blood WBC differential, and always have less than 20% blasts. The peripheral blood monocytosis is also mature but is not reliable by itself for the diagnosis of CMML because mature monocytes may also be seen in the peripheral blood of patients with acute myelomonocytic leukemia or acute monocytic leukemia. The bone marrow of CMML patients is usually hypercellular and contains a proliferation of mature monocytes, which are often dysplastic.

A higher blast count indicates a more unfavorable prognosis, thus CMML is subdivided into two prognostic categories, depending on the percentage of blasts in the peripheral blood and bone marrow. The diagnosis of CMML-1 is made when one sees less than 5% blasts in blood and less than 10% blasts in bone marrow. The diagnosis of CMML-2 is made when the peripheral blood contains between 5% and 19% blasts, the marrow contains between 10% and 19% blasts, or if Auer rods are present and blasts comprise less than 20% of blood or marrow. Twenty percent or more blasts indicate an acute myeloid leukemia rather than CMML. The suffix "with eosinophilia" should be used for CMML-1 or CMML-2 when the above criteria are present and when the eosinophil count in the peripheral blood is greater than 1.5 K/µL.

Flow cytometry studies usually show expression of CD33, CD13, CD4, and CD14. CD34 expression is usually an indicator of increased numbers of blasts. Approximately one-third of CMML patients have clonal cytogenetic abnormalities, such as +8, 7/del(7q), and structural abnormalities of 12p. None of these are specific. 11q23 abnormalities are unusual and suggest the diagnosis instead of acute myelogenous leukemia.

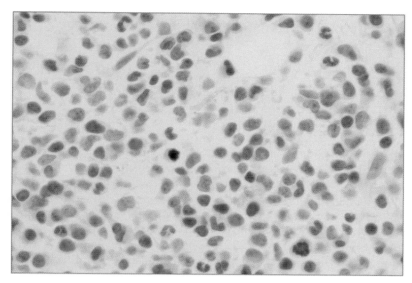

Figure 4-96. Atypical chronic myeloid leukemia (aCML), trephine biopsy section. aCML is a rare and clinically aggressive disease that also displays features of myelodysplastic syndromes and myeloproliferative disorders [4,67]. It is characterized by leukocytosis with dysplastic neutrophils and may be associated with multilineage dysplasia. The disease affects older patients (median age of diagnosis in seventh or eighth decade of life), with reported median survival times of only 11 to 18 months. Despite unfortunate similarities in names, aCML and chronic myelogenous leukemia (CML) have in common only the following superficial features: peripheral blood leukocytosis, hypercellular bone marrow, and more than 20% blasts in the peripheral blood or bone marrow. The diseases are significantly different in many ways; aCML shows absence of Philadelphia chromosome and *BCR/ABL* fusion gene, presence of marked granulocytic dysplasia (not observed during the chronic phase of CML), presence of leukocytosis composed predominantly of neutrophils, no to minimal basophils, no or minimal absolute monocytosis, and presence of dysplasia in the erythroid and megakaryocytic lineages.

No specific immunophenotypic or cytogenetic abnormality has been identified. Over three-fourths of patients have cytogenetic abnormalities, including +8, +13, del(20), i(17q), and del(12p).

Patients with aCML do poorly, with a median survival time of less than 20 months. Poor prognostic factors include thrombocytopenia and marked anemia. Approximately one-third of patients develop acute leukemia, whereas others die of marrow failure.

Helpful Features in the Differential Diagnosis of Chronic Phase of CML, Atypical CML, and CMML in Adults

Feature	CML	Atypical CML	CMML
Ph chromosome and *BCR/ABL*	+	—	—
Peripheral blood white cell count	+++	++	+
Peripheral blood basophils	≥ 2%	< 2%	< 2%
Peripheral blood monocytes	< 3%	3%–10%	Usually > 10%
Peripheral blood promyelocytes, myelocytes, and metamyelocytes	> 20%	10%–20%	≤ 10%
Peripheral blood blasts	< 2%	> 2%	< 2%
Granulocyte dysplasia	—	++	+
Bone marrow erythroid hyperplasia	—	—	+

Figure 4-97. Helpful features in the differential diagnosis of chronic phase of chronic myelogenous leukemia (CML), atypical chronic myeloid leukemia (aCML), and chronic myelomonocytic leukemia (CMML) in adults. Distinguishing aCML from CMML may be difficult. Cases of aCML tend to have more blasts and eosinophils.

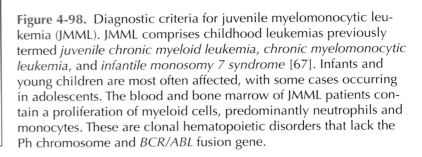

Diagnostic Criteria for Juvenile Myelomonocytic Leukemia
Diagnostic criteria
Peripheral blood monocytosis > 1 K/μL
Blasts, including promonocytes are < 20% of the WBCs in the blood and bone marrow
Absence of Ph chromosome or *BCR/ABL* fusion gene
Plus two or more of the following:
Hemoglobin F increased for age
Immature granulocytes in the peripheral blood
WBC count > 10 K/μL
Clonal chromosomal abnormality (*eg*, may be monosomy 7)
GM-CSF hypersensitivity of myeloid progenitors in vitro

Figure 4-98. Diagnostic criteria for juvenile myelomonocytic leukemia (JMML). JMML comprises childhood leukemias previously termed *juvenile chronic myeloid leukemia, chronic myelomonocytic leukemia,* and *infantile monosomy 7 syndrome* [67]. Infants and young children are most often affected, with some cases occurring in adolescents. The blood and bone marrow of JMML patients contain a proliferation of myeloid cells, predominantly neutrophils and monocytes. These are clonal hematopoietic disorders that lack the Ph chromosome and *BCR/ABL* fusion gene.

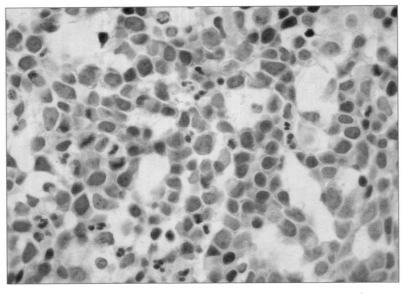

Figure 4-99. Juvenile myelomonocytic leukemia (JMML), trephine biopsy. The incidence of JMML is approximately 1.3 million children less than 14 years old. Although it accounts for less than 3% of leukemias in children, it is the most common myelodysplastic syndrome or myeloproliferative disorder in children. Approximately 10% of cases occur in children with the clinical diagnosis of neurofibromatosis type 1. Blood, bone marrow, liver, and spleen virtually always show a myelomonocytic proliferation, and the lymph nodes, skin, and respiratory tract are also commonly involved. The blood shows leukocytosis, anemia, and often thrombocytopenia. The median WBC is approximately 30 K/μL, but is greater than 100 K/μL in 5% to 10% of children. Neutrophils predominate, and blasts and promonocytes are usually more than 5% of the white cells and by definition, always less than 20%. Eosinophilia and basophilia are rare. The bone marrow is hypercellular and contains a mono-cytic proliferation. Blasts and promonocytes by definition are less than 20%, and Auer rods are never seen. Dysplastic features of the hematopoietic cells are rare. No specific immunophenotypic or cytochemical features have been described. Cytogenetic abnormalities, including monosomy 7, are found in 30% to 50% of children.

In contrast to adult chronic myelomonocytic leukemia, JMML has an aggressive clinical course and poor prognosis. Poor prognostic factors include age greater than 2 years at the time of diagnosis, platelet counts less than 33 K/μL, and hemoglobin F levels greater than 15%. Most patients die from organ failure, such as respiratory failure due to leukemic infiltration. Approximately 10% of patients evolve to acute leukemia. Response to chemotherapy is poor, and currently, bone marrow transplantation is the only therapy that has been shown to clearly improve survival time.

REFERENCES

1. Miller K, Daoust P: Clinical manifestations of acute myeloid leukemia. In *Hematology Basic Principles and Practice*, edn 3. Edited by Hoffman R, Benz EJ Jr, Shattil SJ, *et al*. Philadelphia: Churchill Livingstone Press; 2000:999–1024.

2. Henderson E, McArthur J: Diagnosis, classification, and assessment of response to treatment. In *Leukemia*, edn 7. Edited by Henderson ES, Lister TA, Greaves MF. Philadelphia: WB Saunders Co.; 2002:227–248.

3. Pedersen-Bjergaard J: Chemicals and leukemia. In *Leukemia*, edn 7. Edited by Henderson ES, Lister TA, Greaves MF. Philadelphia: WB Saunders Co.; 2002:171–199.

4. Jaffe ES, Harris NL, Stein H, Vardiman JW: *World Health Organization Classification of Tumours: Pathology and Genetics of Tumours of Haematopoietic and Lymphoid Tissues*. Lyon, France: IARC Press, 2001.

5. Vardiman JW, Harris NL, Brunning RD: The World Health Organization (WHO) classification of the myeloid neoplasms. *Blood* 2002, 100:2292–2302.

6. Bennett JM, Catovsky D, Daniel MT, *et al*.: Proposals for the classification of the acute leukaemias: French-American-British Cooperative Group. *Br J Haematol* 1976, 33:451–458.

7. Bennett JM, Catovsky D, Daniel M, *et al*.: The French-American-British (FAB) Co-operative Group. Proposals for the classification of the myelodysplastic syndromes. *Br J Haematol* 1982, 51:189–199.

8. Murphy S, Peterson P, Iland H, *et al*.: Experience of the Polycythemia Vera Study Group with essential thrombocythemia: a final report on diagnostic criteria, survival and leukemia transition by treatment. *Semin Hematol* 1997, 34:29–39.

9. Valent P, Horny HP, Escribano L, *et al*.: Diagnostic criteria and classification of mastocytosis: a consensus proposal. *Leuk Res* 2001, 25:603–625.

10. Brunning R, Matutes E, Harris N, *et al*.: Acute myeloid leukaemias. In *Pathology and Genetics of Tumours of Haematopoietic and Lymphoid Tissues*. Edited by Jaffe ES, Harris NL, Stein H, Vardiman JW. Lyon, France: IARC Press; 2001:75–107.

11. Radich JP, Slovak ML: The laboratory evaluation of minimal residual disease. In *Hematopoietic Cell Transplantation*, edn 2. Edited by Thomas ED, Blume KG, Forman SJ. Malden, MA: Blackwell Science, Inc.; 1999:235–247.

12. O'Donnell MR: Acute leukemias. In *Cancer Management: A Multidisciplinary Approach*. Edited by Pazdur R, Coia LR, Hoskins WJ, Wagman LD. New York: PRR; 2002:685–707.

13. Rambaldi A, Biondi A: Acute promyelocytic leukemia. In *Leukemia*, edn 7. Edited by Henderson ES, Lister TA, Greaves MF. Philadelphia: WB Saunders Co.; 2002:529–543.

14. Sainty D, Liso V, Cantu-Rajnoldi A, *et al*.: A new morphologic classification system for acute promyelocytic leukemia distinguishes cases with underlying PLZF/RARA gene rearrangements. *Blood* 2000, 96:1287–1296.

15. LeBeau M, Larson R: Cytogenetics and Neoplasia. In *Hematology Basic Principles and Practice*, edn 3. Edited by Hoffman R, Benz EJ Jr, Shattil SJ, *et al*.: Philadelphia: Churchill Livingstone Press; 2000:848–870.

16. Estey E, Thall P, Beran M, *et al*.: Effect of diagnosis (refractory anemia with excess blasts, refractory anemia with excess blasts in transformation, or acute myeloid leukemia [AML]) on outcome of AML-type chemotherapy. *Blood* 1997, 90:2969–2077.

17. Hanslip J, Swansbury G, Pinkerton R, *et al*.: The translocation t(8;16)(p11;p13) defines an AML subtype with distinct cytology and clinical features. *Leuk Lymphoma* 1992, 6:479–486.

18. Hanson CA: Peripheral blood and bone marrow: morphology, counts and differentials, and reactive disorders. In *Clinical Laboratory Medicine*, edn 2. Edited by McClatchey KD. Philadelphia: Lippincott Williams & Wilkins; 2002:797–829.

19. Arber D: Bone marrow. In *Modern Surgical Pathology*, vol 2. Edited by Weidner N, Cote R, Suster S, Weiss L. New York: WB Saunders Co.; 2003:1597–1657.

20. Slovak M, Kopecky K, Cassileth P, *et al*.: Karyotypic analysis predicts outcome of pre-remission and post-remission therapy in adult acute myeloid leukemia: a Southwest Oncology Group/Eastern Cooperative Oncology Group study. *Blood* 2000, 96:4075–4083.

21. Szczepanski T, vanDongen J: Detection of minimal residual disease. In *Leukemia*, edn 7. Edited by Henderson ES, Lister TA, Greaves MF. Philadelphia: WB Saunders Co.; 2002:249–283.

22. Schlenk RF, Corbacioglu A, Krauter J, *et al*.: Gene mutations as predictive markers for postremission therapy in younger adults with normal karyotype AML [abstract]. *Blood* (ASH Annual Meeting Abstracts) 2006, 108:abstract 4.

23. Rohatiner A, Lister T: Acute myelogenous leukemia. In *Leukemia*, edn 7. Edited by Henderson ES, Lister TA, Greaves MF. Philadelphia: WB Saunders Co.; 2002:485–517.

24. Negrin R, Blume K: Hematopoietic cell transplantation in the leukemias. In *Leukemia*, edn 7. Edited by Henderson ES, Lister TA, Greaves MF. Philadelphia: WB Saunders Co.; 2002:459–484.

25. Bross PF, Beitz J, Chen G, *et al*.: Approval summary: gemtuzumab ozogamicin in relapsed acute myeloid leukemia. *Clin Cancer Res* 2001, 7:1490–1496.

26. Burnett AK, Goldstone AH, Stevens RM, *et al*.: Randomized comparison of addition of autologous bone marrow transplantation to intensive chemotherapy for acute myeloid leukemia in first remission: results of MRC AML 10 trial. UK Medical Research Council Adult and Children's Leukaemia Working Parties. *Lancet* 1998, 351:700–708.

27. Stein AS, O'Donnell MR, Slovak ML, *et al*.: Interleukin-2 after autologous stem-cell transplantation for adult patients with acute myeloid leukemia in first complete remission. *J Clin Oncol* 2003, 21:615–623.

28. Aul C, Bowen DT, Yoshida Y: Pathogenesis, etiology, and epidemiology of myelodysplastic syndromes. *Haematologica* 1988, 83:71–86.

29. Chang KL, O'Donnell MR, Slovak ML, *et al*.: Primary myelodyplasia occurring in adults under 50 years old: a clinicopathologic study of 52 patients. *Leukemia* 2002, 16:623–631.

30. Foucar K, Langdon RMI, Armitage JO, *et al*.: Myelodysplastic syndromes. a clinical and pathologic analysis of 109 cases. *Cancer* 1985, 56:553–561.

31. Fenaux P, Preudhomme C, Estienne M, *et al*.: De novo myelodysplastic syndromes in adult aged 50 or less. A report on 37 cases. *Leuk Res* 1990, 14:1053–1059.

32. Ma X, Does M, Raza A, Mayne ST: Myelodysplastic syndromes: incidence and survival in the United States. *Cancer* 2007, 109:1536–1542.

33. Epling-Burnette PK, Bai F, Painter JS, *et al*.: Reduced natural killer (NK) function associated with high-risk myelodysplastic syndrome (MDS) and reduced expression of activating NK receptors. *Blood* 2007, 109:4816–4824.

34. Barnard D, Kalousek D, Wiersma S, *et al*.: Morphologic, immunologic, and cytogenetic classification of acute myeloid leukemia and myelodysplastic syndrome in childhood: a report from the Children's Cancer Group. *Leukemia* 1996, 10:5–12.

35. Passmore SJ, Hann IM, Stiller CA, *et al*.: Pediatric myelodysplasia: a study of 68 children and a new prognostic scoring system. *Blood* 1995, 85:1742–1750.

36. Gotlib J, Greenberg P: Myelodysplastic syndromes. In *Leukemia*, edn 7. Edited by Henderson ES, Lister TA, Greaves MF. Philadelphia: WB Saunders Co.; 2002:545–582.

37. Third MIC Cooperative Study Group: Recommendations for a morphologic, immunologic and cytogenetic (MIC) working classification of the primary and therapy related myelodysplastic disorders. *Cancer Genet Cytogenet* 1988, 32:1–10.

38. Brunning R, Bennett J, Flandrin G, *et al*.: Myelodysplastic syndromes. In *Pathology and Genetics of Tumours of Haematopoietic and Lymphoid Tissues*. Edited by Jaffe ES, Harris NL, Stein H, Vardiman JW. Lyon, France: IARC Press; 2001:61–73.

39. Greenberg P, Cox C, LeBeau M, *et al.*: International scoring system for evaluating prognosis in myelodysplastic syndromes. *Blood* 1997, 2079–2088.

40. Tuzuner N, Cox C, Rowe JM, *et al.*: Hypocellular myelodysplastic syndromes (MDS): new proposals. *Br J Haematol* 1995, 91:612–617.

41. Mathew P, Tefferi A, Dewald GW, *et al.*: The 5q-syndrome: a single-institution study of 43 consecutive patients. *Blood* 1993, 81:1040–1045.

42. Barrett J, Saunthararajah Y, Molldrem J: Myelodysplastic syndrome and aplastic anemia: distinct entities or diseases linked by a common pathophysiology? *Semin Hematol* 2000, 37:15–29.

43. Tooze JA, Marsh JCW, Gordon-Smith EC: Clonal evolution of aplastic anemia to myelodysplasia, acute myeloid leukaemia and paroxysmal nocturnal haemoglobinuria. *Leuk Lymphoma* 1999, 33:231–241.

44. Anderson J: Allogeneic hematopoietic cell transplantation for myelodysplastic and myeloproliferative disorders. In *Hematopoietic Cell Transplantation*, edn 2. Edited by Thomas E, Blume K, Forman S. Malden, MA: Blackwell Science, Inc.; 1999:872–886.

45. Vardiman J, Brunning, R, Harris N: Chronic myeloproliferative diseases. In *Pathology and Genetics of Tumours of Haematopoietic and Lymphoid Tissues*. Edited by Jaffe ES, Harris NL, Stein H, Vardiman JW. Lyon, France: IARC Press; 2001:15–44.

46. Tefferi A, Thiele J, Orazi A, *et al.*: Proposals and rationale for revision of the World Health Organization diagnostic criteria for polycythemia vera, essential thrombocythemia, and primary myelofibrosis: recommendations from an ad hoc international expert panel. Blood 2007, 110:1092–1097.

47. Nowell PC, Hungerford DA: A minute chromosome in human chronic granulocytic leukemia. *Science* 1960, 132:1497–1500.

48. Rowley JD: A new consistent chromosomal abnormality in chronic myelogenous leukaemia identified by quinacrine fluorescence and Giemsa staining [letter]. *Nature* 1973, 243:290–293.

49. Bartram CR, deKlein A, Hagemeijer A, *et al.*: Translocation of c-ab1 oncogene correlates with the presence of a Philadelphia chromosome in chronic myelocytic leukaemia. *Nature* 1983, 306:277–280.

50. Melo JV: The diversity of BCR-ABL fusion proteins and their relationship to leukemia phenotype. *Blood* 1996, 88:2375–2384.

51. Cortes JE, Silver RT, Kantarjian H, Aguayo A: Chronic myelogenous leukemia. In *Cancer Management: A Multidisciplinary Approach*. Edited by Pazdur R, Coia LR, Hoskins WJ, Wagman LD. New York: PRR; 2002:709–720.

52. Druker BJ, Talpaz M, Resta DJ, *et al.*: Efficacy and safety of a specific inhibitor of the BCR-ABL tyrosine kinase in chronic myeloid leukemia. *N Engl J Med* 2001, 344:1031–1037.

53. Druker BJ, Tamura S, Buchdunger E, *et al.*: Effects of a selective inhibitor of the abl tyrosine kinase on the growth of bcr-abl positive cells. *Nat Med* 1996, 2:561–566.

54. Talpaz M, Shah MP, Kantarjian H, *et al.*: Dasatinib in imatinib-resistant Philadelphia chromosome–positive leukemias. *N Engl J Med* 2006, 354:2531–2541.

55. Thomas ED, Clift R: Allogeneic transplantation for chronic myeloid leukemia. In *Hematopoietic Cell Transplantation*, edn 2. Edited by Thomas ED, Blume KG, Forman SJ. Malden, MA: Blackwell Science, Inc.; 1999:807–816.

56. Horowitz MM, Gale RP, Sondel PM, *et al.*: Graft-versus leukemia reactions after bone marrow transplantation. Data from the International Bone Marrow Transplant Registry. *Blood* 1990, 75:555–562.

57. Forman S: ASH Update: Lymphoma/Leukemia Innovations in Treatment. *Southern California Academy of Clinical Oncology 102nd Cancer Seminar*; 2003.

58. Savage D, Antman K: Drug therapy: imatinib mesylate: a new oral targeted therapy. *N Engl J Med* 2002, 346:683–693.

59. Bain BJ: Hypereosinophilia. *Curr Opin Hematol* 2000, 7:21–25.

60. Ackerman S, Butterfield J: Eosinophilia, eosinophil-associated diseases and the hypereosinophilic syndrome. In *Hematology Basic Principles and Practice*, edn 3. Edited by Hoffman R, Benz EJ Jr, Shattil SJ, *et al.* Philadelphia: Churchill Livingstone Press; 2000:702–720.

61. Cools J, DeAngelo DV, Gotlib J, *et al.*: A tyrosine kinase created by fusion of the PDGFRA and FIP1L1 genes as a therapeutic target of imatinib in idiopathic hypereosinophilic syndrome. *N Engl J Med* 2003, 348:1201–1214.

62. Hoffman R: Polycythemia vera. In *Hematology Basic Principles and Practice*, edn 3. Edited by Hoffman R, Benz EJ Jr, Shattil SJ, *et al.* Philadelphia: Churchill Livingstone Press; 2000:1130–1155.

63. Spivak J: Erythrocytosis. In *Hematology Basic Principles and Practice*, edn 3. Edited by Hoffman R, Benz EJ Jr, Shattil SJ, *et al.* Philadelphia: Churchill Livingstone Press; 2000:388–396.

64. Beutler E: Polycythemia. In *Williams Hematology*, edn 6. Edited by Beutler E, Lichtman M, Coller B, *et al.* New York: McGraw Hill; 2001:689–701.

65. Hoffman R: Agnogenic myeloid metaplasia. In *Hematology Basic Principles and Practice*, edn 3. Edited by Hoffman R, Benz EJ Jr, Shattil SJ, *et al.* Philadelphia: Churchill Livingstone Press; 2000:1172–1188.

66. Hoffman R: Primary thrombocythemia. In *Hematology Basic Principles and Practice*, edn 3. Edited by Hoffman R, Benz EJ Jr, Shattil SJ, *et al.*: Philadelphia: Churchill Livingstone Press; 2000:1188–1204.

67. Vardiman J: Myelodysplastic/myeloproliferative diseases. In *Pathology and Genetics of Tumours of Haematopoietic and Lymphoid Tissues*. Edited by Jaffe ES, Harris NL, Stein H, Vardiman JW. Lyon, France: IARC Press; 2001:45–59.

Disorders of Hemostasis and Thrombosis

Steven R. Deitcher

The human hemostatic system consists of multiple independent yet integrally related cellular and protein components that maintain blood fluidity under normal conditions and promote localized, temporary thrombus formation at sites of vascular injury. A normal hemostatic system is the human physiologic defense against exsanguination. An abnormal hemostatic system may result in pathologic bleeding, vascular thrombosis, or both.

Alterations in the quantitative and qualitative status of any hemostatic cellular or protein element may have a significant biologic effect. Platelet deficiency (thrombocytopenia), platelet adhesion defects, and platelet aggregation disorders are associated with an inability to form an adequate primary hemostatic platelet plug and may lead to significant mucocutaneous bleeding and post-traumatic, life-threatening hemorrhage. In contrast, a marked increase in platelet count (thrombocytosis) and accentuated platelet aggregation ("sticky platelet syndrome") have been associated with thromboembolic events. Deficiency of a procoagulant factor integral to the intrinsic (factors XI, IX, VIII), extrinsic (factor VII), or common (factors X, V, II, and fibrinogen) pathway of coagulation is typically associated with a variable degree of bleeding tendency. Elevated levels of procoagulant factors such as factors VIII, IX, XI, fibrinogen, and factor VII, on the other hand, are recognized risk factors for vascular disease and thrombosis. Deficiency of natural anticoagulant proteins such as protein C, protein S, antithrombin, or heparin cofactor II is associated with venous thromboembolic disease; a natural anticoagulant protein excess state associated with bleeding has not been described to date. Reduced circulating levels of protein Z have been suggested to play a role in abnormal bleeding and venous thrombosis. Deficiency of a profibrinolytic cascade component, such as tissue-type plasminogen activator (t-PA) or plasminogen, and excess plasma levels of the fibrinolytic inhibitor, plasminogen activator inhibitor-1 (PAI-1), have been linked to hypercoagulability and thrombosis. Deficiency of fibrinolytic inhibitors such as α_2-antiplasmin and PAI-1 may precipitate a hyperfibrinolytic bleeding state. Deficiency of endothelial cell–derived von Willebrand factor is associated with altered primary and secondary hemostasis due to deficient platelet anchoring at sites of vascular injury and shortened factor VIII survival characteristic of von Willebrand disease. Deficient endothelial cell production of thrombomodulin or release of t-PA may be associated with a thrombotic tendency.

NORMAL HEMOSTASIS

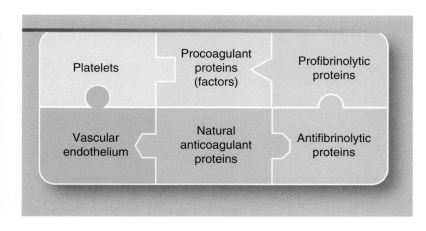

Figure 5-1. Major components of the hemostatic system. The hemostatic system is composed of six major components: platelets, vascular endothelium, procoagulant plasma protein "factors," natural anticoagulant proteins, profibrinolytic proteins, and antifibrinolytic proteins. Each of these six components must be present in a fully functional form and in an adequate quantity to prevent excessive blood loss following vascular trauma and at the same time prevent pathologic thrombosis.

Major Components of the Hemostatic System (Normal Functions)

Platelets

  Primary hemostasis (platelet plug formation)

  Provides a phospholipid surface to concentrate and facilitate thrombin and fibrin generation

Vascular endothelium

  Anticoagulant barrier between blood and subendothelial connective tissues

  Produces and stores von Willebrand factor, plasminogen activators (PAs) and PA inhibitors

  Expresses thrombomodulin, which mediates the activation of protein C

Procoagulant proteins (factors)

  Secondary hemostasis (promotes the formation of thrombin and fibrin to stabilize platelet plugs)

Natural anticoagulant proteins

  Regulates thrombin and fibrin formation to localize and limit thrombus to sites of vascular injury

Profibrinolytic proteins

  Localizes and limits thrombus deposition and degrade thrombus when no longer needed

Antifibrinolytic proteins

  Regulates endogenous plasminogen activators and plasmin activity

Figure 5-2. The major "normal" functions of the six hemostatic components outlined in Figure 5-1.

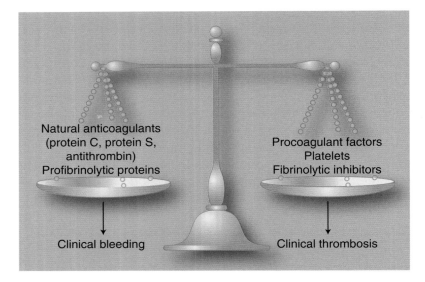

Figure 5-3. The hemostatic balance. The hemostatic system is highly regulated and maintains a delicate balance between a prohemorrhagic state and a prothrombotic state. Any significant acquired or congenital imbalance in the hemostatic "scales" may lead to a pathologic outcome. The balance between these opposing groups of proteins and not the level of any individual factor seems most critical to hemostatic regulation.

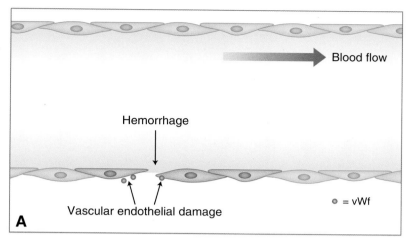

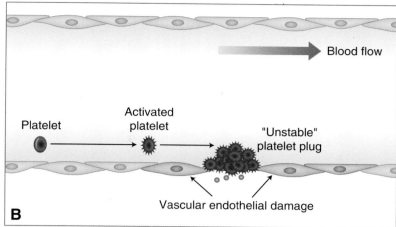

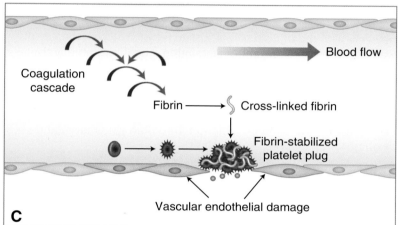

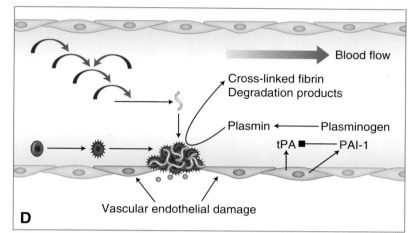

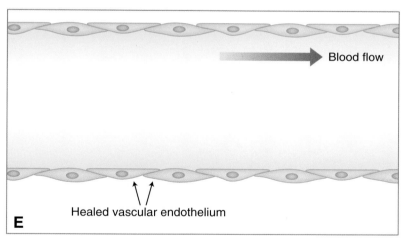

Figure 5-4. The classical process of normal hemostasis. Hemostasis is a multistep process that can be divided into primary hemostasis and secondary hemostasis. Primary hemostasis comprises the reactions needed to form a platelet plug at a site of vascular damage, and combined with vessel vasoconstriction, constitutes our initial defense against bleeding. Secondary hemostasis comprises the reactions needed to generate cross-linked fibrin required to stabilize the platelet plug and form a durable thrombus.

Primary hemostasis consists of three major and not necessarily sequential events. **A**, Platelet adhesion. Following vascular injury, platelets rapidly attach to exposed subendothelial collagen and von Willebrand factor (vWf). **B**, Platelet activation. After adhering to a site of injury, platelets are stimulated by various agonists (collagen, thrombin, epinephrine, ADP, and thromboxane A$_2$) to release their α- and dense-granule contents, which further promote platelet recruitment, activation, and aggregation. **C**, Secondary hemostasis. A series of reactions (coagulation cascade) are triggered concomitantly with platelet plug formation, resulting in the generation of cross-linked fibrin that interlaces the platelet plug. Efficient secondary hemostasis requires a phosphatidylserine-rich phospholipid surface, such as that provided by activated platelets. **D** and **E**, The endogenous fibrinolytic system (plasminogen system) produces plasmin that degrades the cross-linked fibrin, limits thrombus size, and degrades the thrombus following vessel healing. PAI-1—plasminogen activator inhibitor-1; t-PA—tissue-type plasminogen activator.

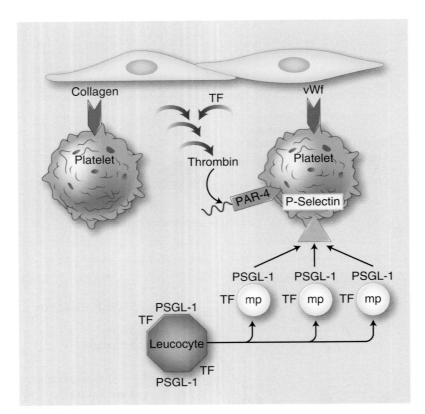

Figure 5-5. Cell-mediated initiation of coagulation. Based on cutting-edge studies using intravital high-speed widefield and confocal microscopy, we have a better understanding of the steps involved in experimental arterial thrombosis. Endothelial von Willebrand factor (vWf) and subendothelial collagen mediate the interaction of platelets with the injured vessel. Tissue factor (TF) from the vessel wall promotes local thrombin generation. Local thrombin activates platelets via protease-activated receptor-4 (PAR-4) cleavage. Platelet activation leads to recruitment of additional platelets. Platelets express P-selectin, and hematopoietic cell–derived microparticles (mp) expressing P-selectin glycoprotein ligand-1 (PSGL-1) and TF accumulate. TF initiates coagulation, thrombin generation, and thrombus propagation.

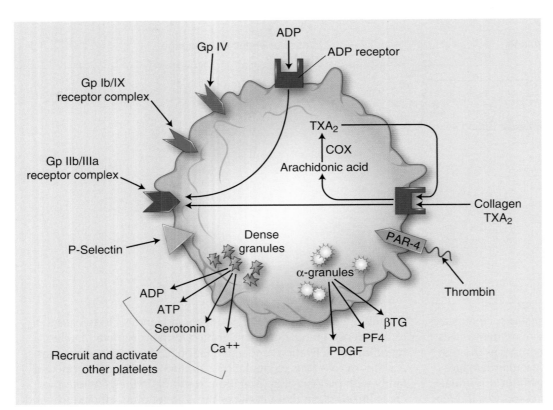

Figure 5-6. Platelet receptors and agonists. Several platelet receptors (glycoprotein [Gp] Ib/IX, Gp IV, Gp Ia/IIa, and Gp VI) are instrumental in platelet adhesion under varying conditions. Other platelet receptors (ADP receptor, protease-activated receptor-4 [PAR-4], and P-selectin) are key to platelet activation by agonists such as ADP, thrombin, and P-selectin glycoprotein ligand-1 (PSGL-1). Common events of platelet activation include Gp IIb/IIIa surface expression and cytoplasmic granule content release. α-Granules contain platelet-derived growth factor (PDGF), platelet factor 4 (PF4), β-thromboglobulin (βTG), thrombospondin, factor V, and von Willebrand factor. Dense granules contain calcium, serotonin, and adenine nucleotides (ADP and ATP). COX—cyclo-oxygenase; TXA_2—thromboxane A_2.

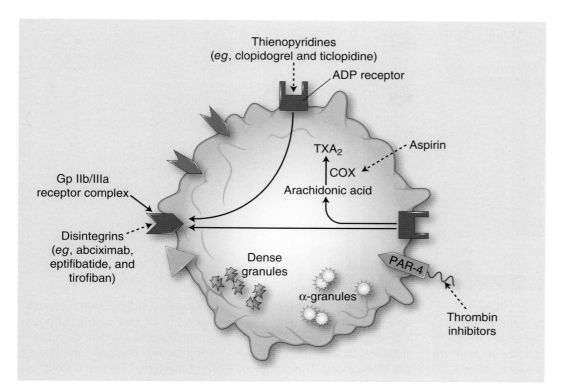

Figure 5-7. Antiplatelet therapy targets. Oral aspirin and thienopyridine antiplatelet agents target cyclo-oxygenase (COX) and the ADP receptor, respectively. Therapies that target the glycoprotein (Gp) IIb/IIIa receptor are highly effective inhibitors of platelet aggregation. PAR-4—protease-activated receptor-4; TXA_2—thromboxane A_2.

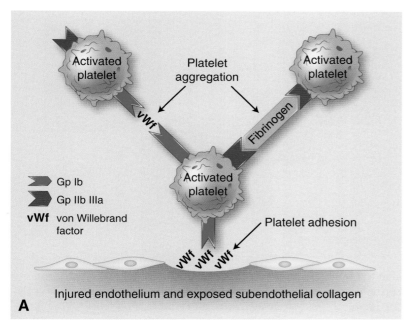

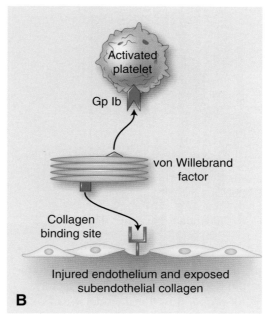

Figure 5-8. Platelet adhesion and aggregation. **A,** Under low shear stress conditions, platelet adhesion is likely mediated by platelet glycoprotein (Gp) Ia/IIa–, Gp IV-, and Gp VI-mediated binding to subendothelial collagen. Platelet aggregation (bridging) under low shear stress is mediated by fibrinogen and Gp IIb/IIIa. **A** and **B,** Under conditions of high shear stress, such as at a site of high-grade arterial stenosis, platelet adhesion is mediated by platelet Gp Ib/IX with von Willebrand factor (vWf) serving as a bridge between the platelet receptor and subendothelial collagen. Under high shear stress, platelet aggregation is mediated by vWf and Gp Ib/IX. Deficiency of endothelial cell–derived vWf is associated with altered primary and secondary hemostasis due to deficient platelet adhesion and aggregation as well as shortened factor VIII survival, characteristic of von Willebrand disease.

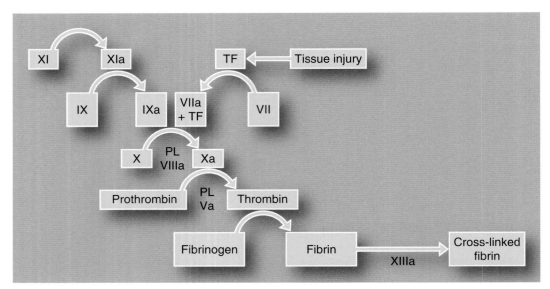

Figure 5-9. Coagulation cascade. Factors XI, IX, and VIII form the intrinsic pathway, whereas factor VII and tissue factor form the extrinsic pathway (tissue factor constituting the "extrinsic" trigger to coagulation). Factors X, V, and II (prothrombin) and fibrinogen form the common pathway of coagulation. Factor VIIIa functions as a cofactor during the activation of factor X to Xa. Factor Va functions as a cofactor during the activation of prothrombin to thrombin. Both the "tenase" (factors VIIIa, IXa, and X) and "prothrombinase" (factors Xa, Va, and II) complexes require a phospholipid-rich surface, such as a platelet, to facilitate efficient reactions. Once formed, thrombin converts fibrinogen to fibrin, activates additional factor VIII and V, activates factor XIII (fibrin cross-linking factor), and participates as a platelet agonist. The pivotal role of thrombin highlights the potency of antithrombotics such as indirect (heparin, low molecular weight heparin, and fondaparinux) and direct (argatroban, bivalirudin, and lepirudin) thrombin inhibitors.

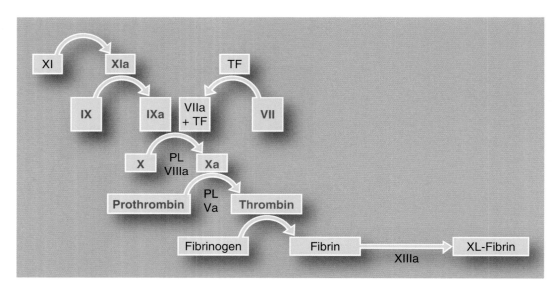

Figure 5-10. Procoagulant vitamin K–dependent (*green*) and serine protease factors (*red*). Vitamin K–dependent coagulation factors require reduced vitamin K for proper post-translational γ-carboxylation of select N-terminal glutamic acid residues and are thus affected by the vitamin K epoxide reductase antagonist warfarin. Serine proteases are targets for heparins. PL—phospholipid; TF—tissue factor.

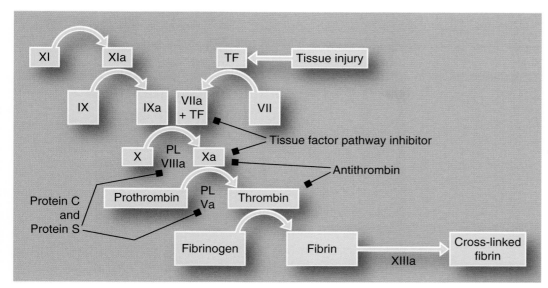

Figure 5-11. Natural anticoagulants. Natural anticoagulants function to prevent pathologic thrombus formation, confine thrombus formation to the sites of vascular injury, and limit thrombus size. The two major natural anticoagulants are antithrombin (formally antithrombin III) and the activated form of protein C (APC). The activity of antithrombin is greatly enhanced by endothelial cell surface heparan sulfate and pharmacologic heparins (unfractionated heparin, low molecular weight heparin, and fondaparinux).

The activity of APC is enhanced by its cofactor, protein S. Antithrombin directly binds and inactivates serine proteases such as factor Xa and thrombin (factor IIa). Activated protein C regulates thrombin generation by cleaving the procoagulant cofactors, factor Va and factor VIIIa, into inactive moieties (factors Vi and VIIIi, respectively). Tissue factor (TF) pathway inhibitor inhibits factor Xa and, when bound to factor Xa, can inhibit the factor VIIa–tissue factor complex. PL—phospholipid.

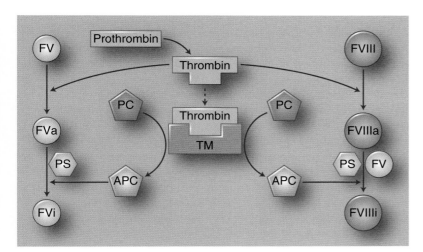

Figure 5-12. The pivotal role of thrombin. The pivotal role of thrombin is in controlling its own generation by both activating procoagulant factors and cofactors (factors [F] V and VIII) and, in conjunction with endothelial thrombomodulin (TM), activating the natural anticoagulant protein C (PC) into activated protein C (APC). Excess prothrombin, protein C deficiency, protein S (PS) deficiency, and factor V resistance to the neutralizing effect of APC all may lead to pathologic thrombosis.

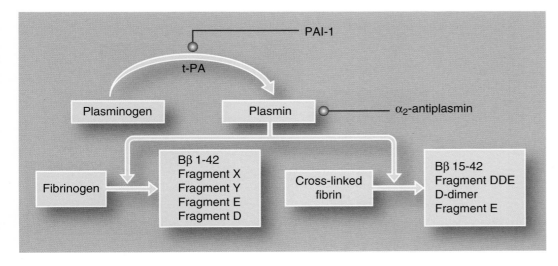

Figure 5-13. Physiologic fibrinolysis. This process is initiated primarily by endothelial cell–derived tissue-type plasminogen activator (t-PA) that converts plasminogen to plasmin (see Fig. 5-4D). Plasmin degrades fibrinogen and fibrin, limits thrombus size, and helps clear thrombus once the inciting vascular injury has been repaired. Plasmin-mediated fibrinogenolysis yields fibrinogen degradation products including fragment X, fragment E, and fragment D. Plasmin-mediated cross-linked fibrinolysis yields degradation products including fragment DDE and D-dimer. The fibrinolytic system itself is regulated by α_2-antiplasmin and endothelial cell– and platelet-derived plasminogen activator inhibitor-1 (PAI-1).

The Clinical Presentation of Bleeding Disorders

Mucocutaneous bleeding
Prolonged bleeding from cuts
Surgical bleeding
Easy and spontaneous bruising
Petechiae
Purpura
Hemarthroses
Deep muscle hematomas
Intracranial hemorrhage
Delayed post-trauma bleeding
Heavy menses
Asymptomatic

Figure 5-14. The clinical presentation of bleeding disorders. Bleeding disorders can range from asymptomatic to fatal hemorrhage. The clinical presentation varies somewhat based on the nature of the underlying hemostatic defect. Patients with thrombocytopenia, qualitative platelet dysfunction, and disorders of small blood vessels often present with petechiae, purpura, spontaneous mucocutaneous bleeding, and prolonged bleeding following minor trauma. It may be difficult to differentiate between platelet-related and vascular bleeding disorders. Abnormal uterine bleeding is often described by women with underlying thrombocytopenia or von Willebrand disease. Deep muscular hematomas, hemarthroses, and excessive post-traumatic bleeding are most commonly linked to coagulation factor or cofactor deficiencies. Delayed bleeding following trauma and surgery has been described in patients with coagulation factor deficiencies, in those with factor XIII deficiency, and in association with excessive endogenous fibrinolytic activity, such as antiplasmin deficiency. The clinical presentation of antithrombotic drug–related bleeding correlates with the primary target and mechanism of action of the particular drug. Bleeding secondary to antiplatelet agents mimics thrombocytopenia, whereas bleeding due to heparin and other anticoagulants mimics coagulation factor deficiencies.

The Clinical Presentation of Thrombotic Disorders

Superficial venous thrombosis
Deep venous thrombosis
Pulmonary embolism
Portal vein thrombosis
Retinal vein thrombosis
Sagittal sinus thrombosis
Myocardial infarction
Intracardiac chamber thrombosis
Stroke
Acute limb or gut ischemia
Vascular access thrombosis
Asymptomatic

Figure 5-15. The clinical presentation of thrombotic disorders. Thrombotic disorders can range from asymptomatic to fatal arterial or venous thrombosis. Any and all vascular beds may be affected by thrombosis. The most common arterial thrombotic events include coronary artery thrombosis (myocardial infarction), cerebral vascular thrombotic occlusion (stroke), and peripheral arterial thrombosis resulting in acute limb ischemia. Peripheral arterial thrombosis may present with limb swelling, coolness, and discoloration. The affected limb may appear pale, hyperemic, or ecchymotic (gangrenous). The most common venous thrombotic events include lower extremity and pelvic deep vein thrombosis and pulmonary embolism. Venous thromboses in unusual sites, such as the mesenteric veins, intracranial venous sinuses, and vena cava, pose unique diagnostic and therapeutic challenges. Extremity deep venous thrombosis may present as a combination of limb pain, swelling, redness, and collateral vein engorgement. Extensive and complete venous thrombotic occlusion may lead to increased limb compartment pressures, arterial compromise, limb ischemia (phlegmasia cerulea dolens), and venous limb gangrene.

Definitions of Cutaneous Lesions Seen in Hemostatic and Thrombotic Disorders

Type of Lesion	Description
Petechiae	Pinpoint red lesions < 2 mm in diameter reflecting small extravasations of blood into skin and subcutaneous tissues; often present as clusters or showers of lesions distributed in dependent parts of the body.
Purpura	Extravasations of blood into the skin and underlying subcutaneous tissues measuring between 2 mm and 1 cm in diameter. Nonpalpable purpura often results from decreased mechanical integrity of the microcirculation and supporting connective tissues and direct microvascular trauma. Palpable purpura describes purpuric lesions that are palpable at the bedside. The palpable component of the lesion may represent a small fibrin clot underlying or associated with the extravasated blood.
Ecchymoses	Extravasation of blood into the skin and subcutaneous tissues measuring > 1 cm in diameter. Fresh bruises associated with bleeding tend to be dark purple lesions that evolve into shades of green and yellow as they resolve over the course of 10 to 14 days. Ecchymoses may actually enlarge and spread as they resolve. A palpable and very tender central hemorrhage may develop within very large ecchymoses. Prominently red ecchymoses may represent steroid-induced or senile purpura, whereas dark black bruises surrounded by erythema and often presenting with bullous regions may represent venous limb gangrene or warfarin-induced skin necrosis.
Telangiectasias	Cutaneous vascular lesions that blanch when compressed, range in size from pinpoint to several cm in diameter, and range in color from intense red to deep blue. Unlike purpura, the blood remains confined within the vasculature in cases of telengectasia. Partial blanching may be observed in cases of true purpura.

Figure 5-16. Cutaneous lesions in hemostatic and thrombotic disorders. Both bleeding and thrombotic disorders may clinically manifest as cutaneous lesions. These lesions include petechiae, purpura, ecchymoses, and telangiectasias. Unfortunately, what is often called *purpura* may have nothing to do with a coagulation or vascular process and is not true purpura. What may be viewed as being ecchymosis due to a bleeding tendency may actually be a manifestation of vascular thrombosis and associated ischemia or gangrene. A definition of these terms seems appropriate before discussing individual disorders.

Quantitative Platelet Disorders

Causes of Thrombocytopenia
Insufficient platelet production
Multilineage bone marrow failure, *eg*, leukemia, lymphoma, carcinoma, myelodysplasia, aplastic anemia, myelofibrosis, megaloblastic anemia, cytomegalovirus infection
Selective megakaryocyte disruption, *eg*, amegakaryocytic ITP, viral infections, gold therapy, alcohol intoxication
Hereditary thrombocytopenia, *eg*, Bernard-Soulier syndrome, May-Heglin syndrome, Wiskott-Aldrich syndrome
Platelet sequestration
Hypersplenism due to portal hypertension or infiltrative disease
Increased peripheral platelet destruction
Autoimmune, *eg*, ITP, systemic lupus erythematosus, lymphoid malignancies, HIV-associated, postinfectious
Alloimmune, *eg*, post-transfusion purpura, neonatal
Drug-induced, *eg*, heparin-induced thrombocytopenia, antibiotics
Overt consumption, *eg*, disseminated intravascular coagulation, thrombotic thrombocytopenic purpura, hemolytic-uremic syndrome, Kasabach-Merritt syndrome, extracorporeal circulation
Other
Dilution associated with massive transfusion of packed red blood cell units or plasma
Artifactual thrombocytopenia (in vitro platelet clumping)

Figure 5-17. Causes of thrombocytopenia. Hemorrhagic platelet disorders are caused by a quantitative deficiency of circulating platelets (thrombocytopenias), a qualitative defect in platelet function, or a combination of both. The hemorrhagic presentation of myeloproliferative disorders such as essential thrombocythemia may occur despite platelet counts well in excess of 1 million per microliter because of associated platelet dysfunction. Thrombotic platelet disorders may be associated with thrombocytopenia (eg, thrombotic thrombocytopenic purpura and heparin-induced thrombocytopenia), increased platelet counts (eg, polycythemia vera), and excess in vitro platelet aggregation (ie, the "sticky platelet" syndrome).

Thrombocytopenia reflects an imbalance between the rates of platelet production and platelet consumption, clearance, or destruction. Insufficient platelet production may result from gener-

alized bone marrow failure due to bone marrow infection, hematologic malignancy, chemotherapeutic medications, or infiltration by metastatic carcinoma or myelofibrosis. Selective reduction in megakaryocytes may be caused by medications such as gold, toxins such as alcohol, and viral infections. Increased peripheral platelet destruction is typically drug induced or immune mediated. Alloimmune thrombocytopenia may develop following transfusion in PA[1A]-negative patients. A wide spectrum of medications can induce thrombocytopenia by inducing immune clearance or enhanced aggregation of platelets. Thrombocytopenia due to peripheral platelet destruction and consumption is a major element of disseminated intravascular coagulation and thrombotic thrombocytopenic purpura. ITP—immune-mediated thrombocytopenic purpura.

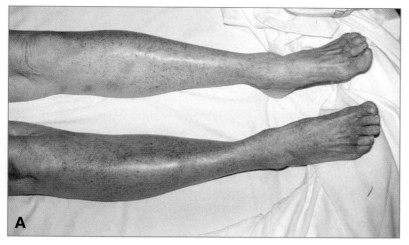

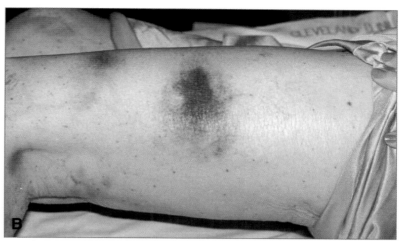

Figure 5-18. Clinical presentation of immune-mediated thrombocytopenic purpura (ITP). Acute ITP is primarily a self-limited disease of children. Acute ITP often follows a viral illness, is associated with profound thrombocytopenia, and uncommonly requires specific therapeutic intervention. Adults usually develop chronic ITP with serum platelet–associated immunoglobulin G (IgG) antibodies. These antibodies may be directed against membrane glycoproteins such as Gp IIIa, IIb, or Ib. These antibodies are therefore able to induce a qualitative platelet disorder in addition to inducing accelerated platelet clearance and thrombocytopenia. Platelet production may also be inappropriately decreased in ITP. The clinical presentations of ITP include petechiae (**A**) and ecchymoses (**B**). Platelet-associated IgG is not specific for chronic ITP but may be detected in settings such as solid tumors and lymphoproliferative disorders as well as in normal individuals. Antiplatelet antibody testing is not generally recommended. The diagnosis of ITP requires the exclusion of other disorders associated with immune thrombocytopenia, such as connective tissue diseases, lymphoproliferative disorders, and HIV infection. Consumption of drugs associated with immune thrombocytopenia should also be excluded. A peripheral blood smear review is required to rule out artifactual thrombocytopenia due to in vitro platelet clumping. A bone marrow examination allows one to confirm the presence of megakaryocytes and rule out bone marrow failure.

Drug-induced Thrombocytopenia

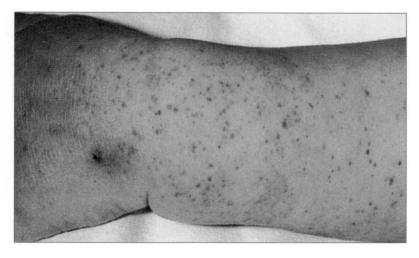

Figure 5-19. Cutaneous hemorrhage and purpura in a patient with drug-induced thrombocytopenia. Drug-induced thrombocytopenia may result from bone marrow suppression or peripheral immune destruction and clearance. Most patients with drug-induced thrombocytopenia present with mucocutaneous hemorrhage and purpura as shown here, similar to that of immune-mediated thrombocytopenic purpura. Immune thrombocytopenia induced by heparin and heparin-derived drugs rarely produces signs and symptoms suggestive of a bleeding diathesis; rather, there is a profound hypercoagulable state often associated with manifestations of venous and arterial thrombosis.

Heparin-induced Thrombocytopenia

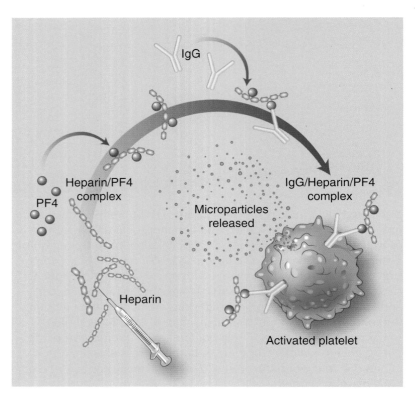

Figure 5-20. Pathogenesis of heparin-induced thrombocytopenia (HIT). Heparin-induced thrombocytopenia with thrombosis (HITT), also known as the "white clot" syndrome, constitutes the major life- and limb-threatening complication of the far more common clinical syndrome known as HIT. Prompt consideration of these paradoxic, thrombotic, adverse drug reactions in patients who develop thrombocytopenia, with or without new or propagating venous and arterial limb thromboses during heparin therapy, is the cornerstone to appropriate HIT/HITT diagnosis and limb salvage. Immediate discontinuation of all forms and routes of heparin exposure remains the essential component of HIT/HITT treatment. The pathogenesis of HIT/HITT involves the formation of complexes between heparin and platelet factor 4 (PF4). PF4 is a normal platelet α-granule moiety released by platelets when they are activated by agonists including heparin. Immune complexes composed of heparin, PF4, and anti-heparin:PF4 immunoglobulin G (IgG) antibodies interact with platelet FcγII receptors, leading to potent platelet activation, aggregation, microparticle formation, and a marked increase in thrombin generation. HIT-associated IgG may activate the endothelium by interacting with heparan/PF4 complexes and lead to increased tissue factor synthesis, which may further contribute to excess thrombin generation and thrombosis formation. HITT constitutes a more severe form of HIT, with evidence of macrovascular thrombosis or thrombus-induced end-organ dysfunction.

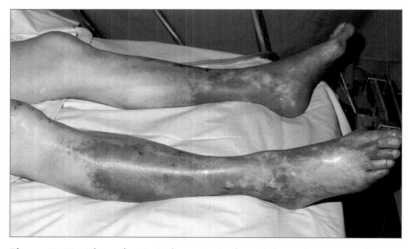

Figure 5-21. Thrombosis in heparin-induced thrombocytopenia (HIT). HIT typically develops between 5 and 14 days after the commencement of heparin therapy and produces a variable but often profound thrombocytopenia. A platelet count fall that begins before day 5 of heparin is not likely to represent HIT, except in patients with a recent (within 3 months) heparin exposure. These patients may experience an abrupt onset of thrombocytopenia upon reexposure to heparin as a result of acute platelet activation secondary to circulating HIT–immunoglobulin G. The thrombotic tendency associated with HIT may last for at least 30 days, and HIT with thrombosis (HITT) may develop well after the discontinuation of heparin and platelet count recovery.

Thrombosis is the major complication of HIT. Venous thrombosis is more common than arterial thrombosis in HIT patients, especially in patients who receive heparin for postoperative deep vein thrombosis prophylaxis. Extremity deep vein thrombosis is the most frequently encountered venous thrombotic complication in HIT patients, followed in frequency by pulmonary embolism and cerebral sinus thrombosis. Most HIT-associated arterial thromboses involve the extremities, but stroke, myocardial infarction, and renal artery thrombosis related to heparin infusion have been described. HITT following coronary artery bypass grafting may present as bypass graft occlusion, left atrial thrombus formation, valvular thrombosis, or pulmonary embolism.

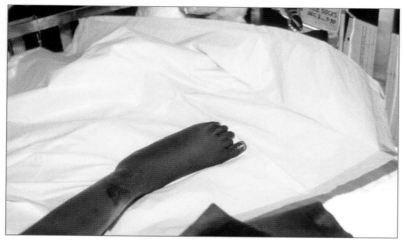

Figure 5-22. Venous limb gangrene. Warfarin anticoagulation may be desired for long-term therapy, but should never be used as the sole alternative anticoagulant in patients with heparin-induced thrombocytopenia (HIT) and heparin-induced thrombocytopenia with thrombosis (HITT). Warfarin has the disadvantage of requiring 5 or more days to achieve full therapeutic effect and has been associated with venous limb gangrene when used alone. Warfarin treatment is the major factor contributing to limb amputation caused by progression of otherwise unremarkable deep vein thromboses to phlegmasia cerulea dolens in HIT patients. The combination of HIT-associated hypercoagulability and warfarin-induced protein C deficiency most likely produces a profound procoagulant state that causes venous limb gangrene. The existence of this syndrome justifies the absolute need for systemic anticoagulation with an alternative anticoagulant such as argatroban, bivalirudin, lepirudin, or possibly fondaparinux during the initiation of warfarin anticoagulation in patients with HIT and HITT.

Thrombotic Thrombocytopenic Purpura

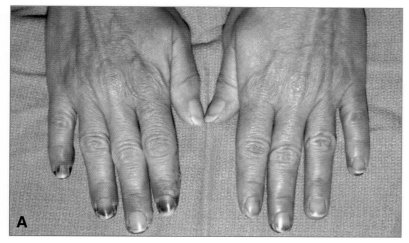

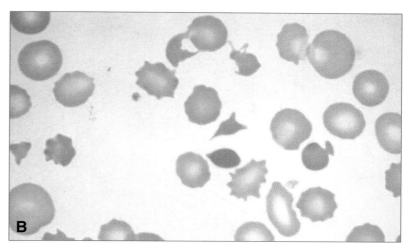

Figure 5-23. Thrombotic thrombocytopenic purpura (TTP). TTP is a multisystem disorder characterized by disseminated microvascular thrombotic phenomenon including digital ischemia (**A**). TTP is characterized by varying degrees of thrombocytopenia, microangiopathic hemolytic anemia, fever, renal dysfunction, and neurologic symptoms. TTP is most common in adults in whom neurologic symptoms predominate. The hemolytic-uremic syndrome refers to the pediatric disorder in which renal failure predominates. Because the anemia in TTP is associated with mechanical red blood cell damage caused by microthrombi, schistocytes are easily identified on the peripheral smear (**B**). An elevated lactate dehydrogenase, indirect bilirubin, aspartate aminotransferase (serum glutamic-oxaloacetic transaminase), and reticulocyte count usually accompany the hemolytic anemia. Thrombocytopenia is universally present and often severe. TTP is most commonly wrongly identified as vasculitis, catastrophic antiphospholipid antibody syndrome, HELLP syndrome (hemolysis, elevated liver enzymes, and low platelets), sepsis, immune-mediated thrombocytopenic purpura, and disseminated intravascular coagulation (DIC). TTP, unlike DIC, does not result in abnormal screening coagulation times and fibrinogen levels. TTP has been associated with HIV infection and the use of drugs such as cyclosporine, mitomycin C, and thienopyridine antiplatelet agents. Mutations in or autoantibodies against the von Willebrand factor (vWf)-cleaving protease ADAMTS13 (A Disintegrin And Metalloproteinase with a ThromboSpondin type 1 motif, member 13) may result in ADAMTS13 deficiency, accumulation of unusually large vWf multimers, and clinical TTP.

Disseminated Intravascular Coagulation

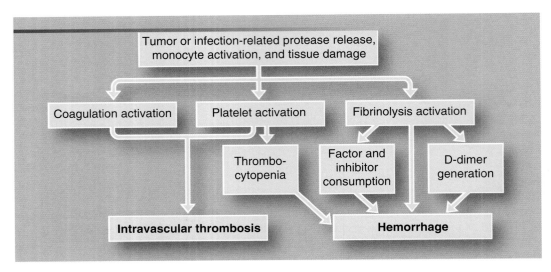

Figure 5-24. Processes involved in disseminated intravascular coagulation (DIC). DIC is a potentially lethal complex consumptive coagulopathy associated with a variety of medical and surgical disease states. DIC is not a disease in itself, but, like fever, it is a manifestation of a multitude of underlying disorders. Unlike normal localized coagulation in response to focal vascular injury, DIC represents an exaggerated, poorly controlled systemic response to illness. Whatever the inciting event, procoagulant mechanisms are activated, intravascular fibrin is produced, small vessel thrombosis occurs, and ischemic organ damage results. A compensatory fibrinolysis develops and combined with the exhaustion of coagulation factors and thrombocytopenia contributes to a concomitant hemorrhagic diathesis.

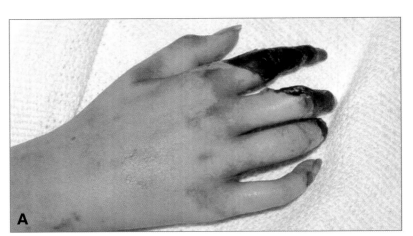

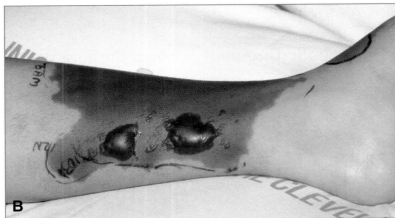

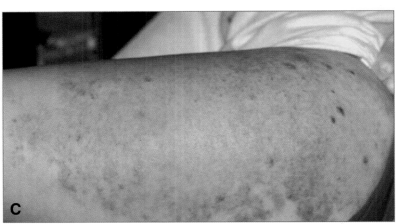

Figure 5-25. Disseminated intravascular coagulation (DIC). Acute (overt or uncompensated) DIC is associated with obstetric accidents, bacterial sepsis, tissue injury secondary to trauma or burns, and acute myelogenous leukemia. The bleeding observed in acute DIC stems from factor deficiencies and thrombocytopenia caused by diffuse organ-based and peripheral microvascular thromboses (**A**). Skin necrosis due to thrombosis of cutaneous vessels may be difficult to differentiate from large ecchymoses related to thrombocytopenia (**B**). More indolent, chronic DIC is associated with solid tumors, connective tissue disorders, aortic aneurysms, and giant hemangiomas (Kasabach-Merritt syndrome; **C**). Because increased factor consumption is balanced by a compensatory increase in production, chronic DIC is also known as "compensated" DIC. When screening tests are normal, chronic DIC is called "non-overt." In chronic DIC, thrombotic complications may predominate. The prothrombin time and the activated partial thromboplastin time are usually prolonged in patients with DIC. The fibrinogen level is either low or found to be decreasing on serial measurements. Fibrin(ogen) degradation products (FDPs) are increased. The most specific fibrin degradation product is the cross-linked FDP, D-dimer. Natural anticoagulants are consumed, leading to a prothrombotic state. Red blood cells that encounter strands of fibrin laid across the vessel lumen are sheared, and microangiopathic hemolysis results (*see* Fig. 5-23B).

Thrombocytosis and Thrombocythemia

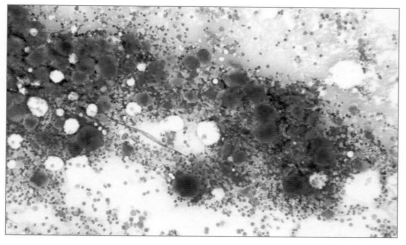

Figure 5-26. Expanded megakaryocyte population. Platelet counts may be increased as the result of a primary bone marrow disorder, such as a myeloproliferative syndrome or the 5q⁻ syndrome, or secondary to iron deficiency, inflammation, or infection. In cases of secondary thrombocytosis, the platelet count is rarely greater than 1 million per microliter and usually not directly linked to bleeding or thrombosis. In secondary thrombocytosis, the increased platelet count corrects once the underlying pathologic process is resolved. In cases of primary thrombocytosis related to essential thrombocythemia, the platelet count usually exceeds 1 million per microliter and a bone marrow aspirate contains an expanded megakaryocyte population.

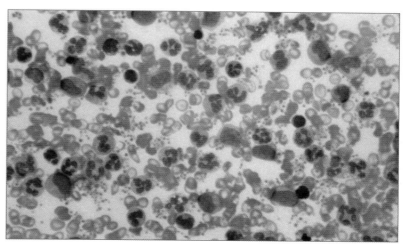

Figure 5-27. Polycythemia vera. In polycythemia vera, thrombocythemia is usually accompanied by leukocytosis, leukocyte left shift, and an expanded red blood cell mass. The degree of platelet count excess may actually correlate more with an associated bleeding tendency than a thrombotic tendency.

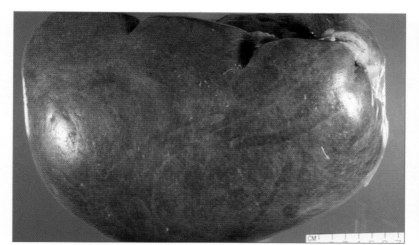

Figure 5-28. Severe splenomegaly. Myeloproliferative syndromes like polycythemia vera, myeloid metaplasia with myelofibrosis (MMM), and chronic myelogenous leukemia can be associated with massive splenomegaly, which may warrant splenectomy to control symptoms and cytopenias in MMM.

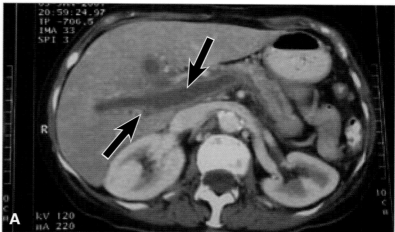

Figure 5-29. Acute venous thrombosis in unusual locations. Acute venous thrombosis that occurs in an unusual location, such as the portal vein (*arrows* in **A**)

Continued on the next page

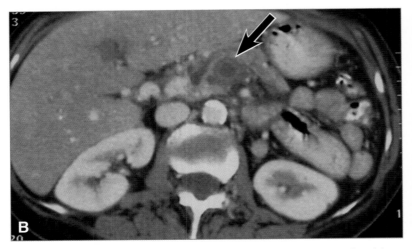

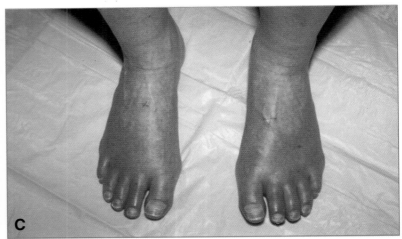

Figure 5-29. *(Continued)* or mesenteric vein (*arrow* in **B**), should prompt an evaluation for a myeloproliferative syndrome in addition to testing for a natural anticoagulant deficiency and paroxysmal nocturnal hemoglobinuria. Painful, intense redness of the hands and/or feet (erythromelalgia; **C**) should prompt an evaluation for essential thrombocythemia.

QUALITATIVE PLATELET DISORDERS

Disorders that Affect Platelet Function

Inherited	Acquired
Adhesion defects	Adhesion defects
von Willebrand disease	Acquired von Willebrand syndrome
Bernard-Soulier syndrome	Activation defects
Activation defects	Cyclooxygenase inhibitors, *eg*, ASA
Storage pool deficiency	Thienopyridines, *eg*, clopidogrel
Dense granule deficiency	Phosphodiesterase inhibitors
α-Granule deficiency	Myelodysplastic syndromes
Signal transduction disorders	Acquired storage pool deficiency, *eg*, DIC and TTP
Agonist receptor abnormalities	Aggregation defects
G-protein defects	Gp IIb/IIIa inhibitor therapy
Cyclooxygenase and thromboxane synthase deficiencies	Abciximab
Wiskott-Aldrich syndrome	Tirofiban
Aggregation defects	Eptifibatide
Hypofibrinogenemia	Myeloproliferative syndromes
Dysfibrinogenemia	Uremia
Glanzmann's thrombasthemia	

Figure 5-30. Disorders that affect platelet function. Drugs are the most common cause of acquired platelet dysfunction, with aspirin being the most common offender. Common drugs that interfere with platelet membrane function include tricyclic antidepressants, chlorpromazine, cocaine, lidocaine, propranolol, cephalosporins, penicillins, and alcohol. Common drugs that interfere with platelet prostaglandin synthesis include aspirin, the nonsteroidal anti-inflammatory drugs (NSAIDS), furosemide, verapamil, hydralazine, methylprednisolone, and cyclosporine. Aspirin irreversibly impairs platelet function for the life of the platelet, whereas NSAIDS reversibly impair platelet function. Drugs that inhibit platelet phosphodiesterase activity include caffeine, dipyridamole, aminophylline, and theophylline. Drugs that irreversibly block the platelet ADP receptor include ticlopidine and clopidogrel. Platelet glycoprotein (Gp) IIb-IIIa inhibitors, such as abciximab, tirofiban, and eptifibatide, have a dramatic effect on platelet aggregation.

Platelet Gp IIb-IIIa is absent in Glanzmann's thromboasthenia. Because Gp IIb-IIIa interacts with fibrinogen to produce platelet aggregation, its deficiency results in a bleeding disorder. In the Hermansky-Pudlak syndrome, a platelet aggregation defect is associated with oculocutaneous albinism and an increased quantity of ceroid-like pigment in bone marrow macrophages. Secondary disorders causing acquired platelet dysfunction include uremia, liver disease, myeloproliferative and myelodysplastic disorder, paraproteinemias, autoimmune disorder, and cardiopulmonary bypass. ASA—acetylsalicylic acid; DIC—disseminated intravascular coagulation; TTP—thrombotic thrombocytopenic purpura.

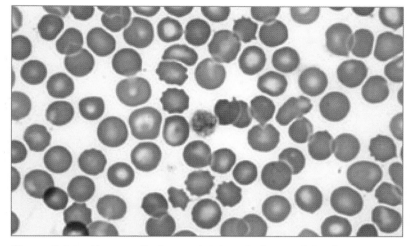

Figure 5-31. Abnormally large platelets. In Bernard-Soulier syndrome, the platelets are abnormally large, and platelet glycoprotein Ib molecules, which function as receptors for von Willebrand factor, are absent and, accordingly, a deficiency in platelet adhesion results.

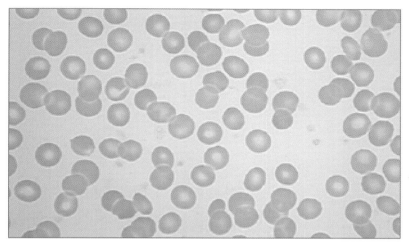

Figure 5-32. "Gray" platelets. Sufficient platelet production of ADP and its subsequent release is necessary for normal aggregation. Storage pool disease may result from a decrease in the number of platelet-dense granules, which are ADP-storage granules. This may result in circulating, granule-deficient, "gray" platelets that can be easily overlooked on a peripheral smear.

COAGULATION DISORDERS

Hemorrhagic Coagulation Disorders

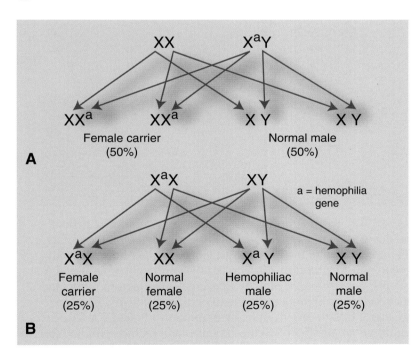

Figure 5-33. Hemophilia. Hemophilia A and B result from functional deficiencies of the intrinsic coagulation pathway proteins factor VIII and factor IX, respectively. Hemophilia A and B are X-linked recessive disorders, making it a disease of males, all of whose sons will be normal and daughters will be obligatory carriers of the trait (A). Women who are hemophilia A or B carriers are not usually symptomatic but have a 50% likelihood of having an affected son (B). In the general population, hemophilia A and B affect one in every 10,000 and one in every 30,000 live male births, respectively. There is a relatively high spontaneous mutation rate for this disease, and as many as one quarter to one third of hemophiliacs may not have a family history of the disorder. Diagnosis of the carrier state for hemophilia A may be made by analyzing familial restriction fragment length polymorphisms, factor VIII to von Willebrand factor activity ratios, or the ratio of antigenic factor VIII to factor VIII functional activity. Women can have "true" hemophilia A or B only in the setting of Turner's syndrome (XO) and extreme lyonization and if their father is a hemophiliac and their mother is a hemophilia carrier. Unlike hemophilia A patients, those with hemophilia B rarely develop inhibitors.

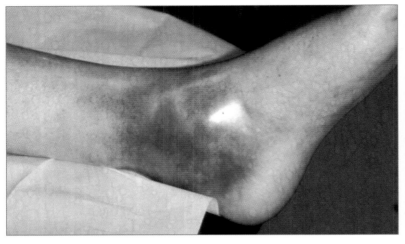

Figure 5-34. Acute hemarthroses. Hemophiliacs with a factor VIII or IX activity level of less than 1% (0.01 U/mL) are classified as having "severe" disease, those with a level between 1% and 5% have "moderate" disease, and those with levels greater than 5% have "mild" disease. The severity of disease remains uniform among a kindred. Patients with "severe" hemophilia experience spontaneous bouts of hemorrhage in the absence of any provocation. Patients with "moderate" or "mild" disease usually bleed only as a result of trauma or surgery. Acute hemarthroses and muscle hematomas are the most common bleeding manifestations of hemophilia A.

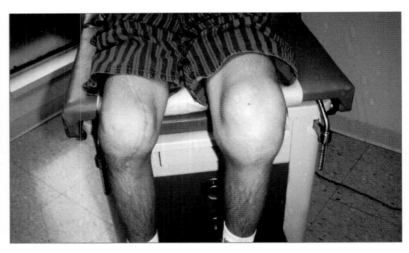

Figure 5-35. Chronic arthropathy. As a result of repeated episodes of hemarthrosis, patients develop a chronic arthropathy with notable cartilage destruction and synovial lining hyperplasia. The resultant joint destruction results in chronic pain, deformity, disability, and a joint even more susceptible to bleeding (target joint). The joints most frequently involved are the knees, elbows, ankles, and shoulders. Small intramuscular hematomas are common and may resolve spontaneously. Large intramuscular bleeds involving the psoas muscles or thigh muscles may result in pseudocyst formation and compression of vital structures, that is, compartment syndrome.

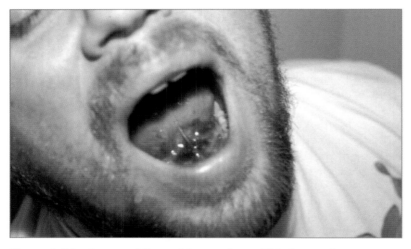

Figure 5-36. Acute sublingual hemorrhage. This hemorrhage may result in submandibular swelling.

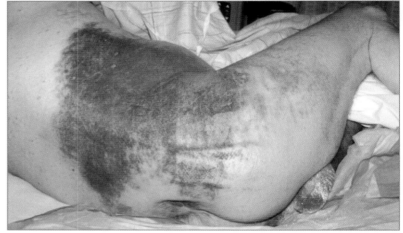

Figure 5-37. Retroperitoneal hemorrhage in an inhibitor patient. The development of a neutralizing alloantibody (inhibitor) to factor VIII remains one of the most devastating complications of severe hemophilia A. Inhibitors develop in at least 21% of hemophilia A patients, after as few as nine to 30 exposures to factor VIII replacement therapy, and predominantly in pediatric patients. Transient low-titer inhibitors are most likely of minimal clinical consequence. High-titer (greater than 5 Bethesda units) and high-responding (brisk amnestic response following factor VIII reexposure) inhibitors place patients at risk for significant morbidity and increased mortality related to bleeding. In this inhibitor patient, acute retroperitoneal bleeding resulted in visible subcutaneous bruising days following the original bleed.

ACQUIRED HEMOPHILIA

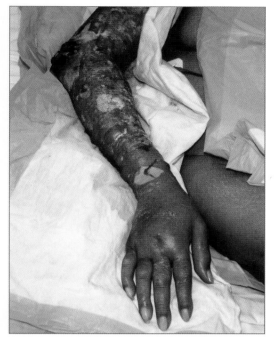

Figure 5-38. Extremity compartment syndrome. Acquired hemophilia A is a serious immune-mediated hemorrhagic diathesis caused by the development of neutralizing and clearing antifactor VIII (FVIII) antibodies in individuals without a preexistent congenital FVIII deficiency. Acquired hemophilia A is an uncommon disorder, with an incidence of 0.2 to 1.0 case per million population per year. Individuals over the age of 50 years are most often affected and typically present with an unexplained prolongation of the activated partial thromboplastin time accompanied by large ecchymotic lesions, melena, hematuria, deep hematomas, hemarthroses, extremity compartment syndrome, and retroperitoneal or intracranial hemorrhage. Approximately 50% of patients who develop autoimmune anti-FVIII antibodies have an underlying medical condition, such as an autoimmune disease (eg, rheumatoid arthritis, systemic lupus erythematosus), inflammatory bowel disease, malignancy, or pregnancy. Medications such as sulfonamides, phenytoin, and penicillins have also been implicated. The remaining 50% have idiopathic acquired hemophilia A. Mortality associated with major bleeding episodes approximates 22%. Inhibitors to other coagulation factors, including von Willebrand factor, factor V, and factor IX, have been described but are relatively rare.

VON WILLEBRAND DISEASE

Classification of von Willebrand Disease

Type 1 vWD accounts for 80% of cases and represents a partial quantitative deficiency of vWf. Levels of vWf and factor VIII are usually reduced in parallel and all multimer sizes are reduced in concentration.
Type 2 vWD represents a series of qualitative disorders in which levels of vWf and factor VIII are normal or only slightly reduced
Type 2A variants have decreased platelet-dependent function associated with absence of high molecular weight multimers
Type 2B variants have increased affinity for platelet glycoprotein Ib-IX, resulting in variable degrees of platelet agglutination and thrombocytopenia
Type 2M variants have decreased platelet-dependent function not caused by the absence of high molecular weight multimers
Type 2N variants have markedly decreased affinity for factor VIII caused by a mutation in the factor VIII binding domain (can be confused with hemophilia A in males)
Type 3 vWD represents a profound deficiency of vWf inherited as an autosomal recessive disorder associated with severe bleeding

Figure 5-39. Revised classification of von Willebrand disease (vWD). In 1924, Dr. Eric von Willebrand described features that differentiated a newly identified bleeding disorder from classic hemophilia. Bleeding was primarily mucocutaneous rather than the hemarthroses or deep muscle hematomas seen in hemophilia. Inheritance was autosomal dominant (involved both sexes) rather than X linked. Finally, patients in his described kindred had prolonged bleeding times rather than the normal bleeding times seen in hemophilia. He hypothesized that a qualitative disorder of platelet function existed. The abnormality in platelet function was not the result of a defect in the platelet itself but rather a deficiency of a plasma factor ultimately named von Willebrand factor (vWF). vWD is the most common inherited bleeding disorder, with an estimated prevalence between one in 1000 to one in 100. Mucocutaneous bleeding in the form of epistaxis, menorrhagia, gingival bleeding, or easy bruising is the most common symptom in vWD. Most patients with vWD do not have frequent bleeding episodes, except following trauma or surgery. Spontaneous hemarthroses are unusual and occur almost exclusively in patients with severe disease (type 3 vWF). Unlike hemophilia, affected members of the same family may have very variable manifestations of this bleeding disorder ranging from easy bruising to life-threatening hemorrhages.

Various Laboratory Tests Used to Differentiate Among Bleeding Disorders

Bleeding Disorder	aPTT	PT	TT	Fibrinogen	BT
Hemophilia A	↑	↔	↔	↔	↔
Hemophilia B	↑	↔	↔	↔	↔
Factor XI deficiency	↑	↔	↔	↔	↔
von Willebrand disease	↔↑	↔	↔	↔	↑
Factor XIII deficiency	↔	↔	↔	↔	↔
Bernard-Soulier syndrome	↔	↔	↔	↔	↑
Glanzmann's thrombasthenia	↔	↔	↔	↔	↑

↔ indicates within the normal range; ↑ indicates increased.

Figure 5-40. Laboratory tests used to differentiate among bleeding disorders. Readily available coagulation tests such as the activated partial thromboplastin time (aPTT) and bleeding time (BT) aid in the initial evaluation of patients with suspected bleeding disorders. Although von Willebrand disease (vWD) is common, its laboratory evaluation may be challenging. Test results may vary in a patient at different times. If an initial battery of tests is normal but clinical suspicion remains high, testing should be repeated. There is a relationship between von Willebrand factor (vWF) levels and ABO blood groups. Type O patients have the lowest levels, followed by types A, B, and AB. Stress and exercise transiently increase vWF levels, and hormonal changes in pregnancy may normalize vWF levels, even in severely deficient patients. The bleeding time is usually prolonged. The aPTT is often prolonged yet may be normal in patients with mild disease. Depending on subtype and severity of disease, accelerated factor VIII clearance results in decreased levels of factor VIII coagulant activity, which in turn result in aPTT prolongation. vWf activity, measured as ristocetin cofactor activity, and antigenic levels are sensitive and specific tests for the detection of vWD. Multimer analysis allows differentiation of the various types of vWD. PT—prothrombin time; TT—thrombin time.

ANTICOAGULATION-ASSOCIATED BLEEDING

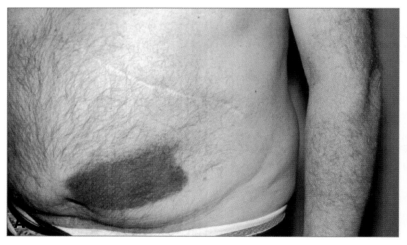 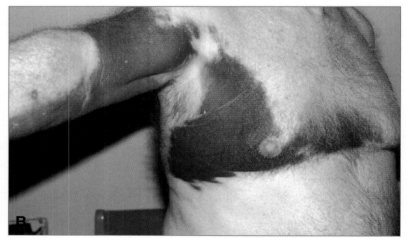

Figure 5-41. Anticoagulation-associated bleeding. Bleeding remains the major complication associated with antithrombotic therapies. Bleeding may be localized to the site of drug administration (*ie*, subcutaneous injection site cutaneous bleeding [**A**]) or may occur at a distant site (**B**). The bleeding associated with antiplatelet medications mimics the type and degree of bleeding observed in patients with quantitative and qualitative platelet disorders. The bleeding associated with anticoagulants is similar to that seen in patients with coagulation factor deficiencies. Spontaneous hemarthrosis is rare in the setting of anticoagulation. Gastrointestinal tract, genitourinary tract, and central nervous system bleeding are more commonly encountered presentations.

A Candidate Hypercoagulable States

Protein C deficiency

Protein S deficiency

Antithrombin deficiency

Heparin cofactor II deficiency

α_2-Macroglobulin deficiency

Plasminogen deficiency

Dysfibrinogenemia

Factor XI excess

Factor VIII excess

Factor V deficiency/excess

Hyperfibrinogenemia

Thrombomodulin deficiency

TFPI deficiency

t-PA deficiency

PAI-1 excess

Factor VII excess

Activated protein C resistance

Factor V Leiden

Prothrombin G20210A/C20209T

Hyperhomocysteinemia

Lupus anticoagulants

Anticardiolipin antibodies

"Sticky platelet" syndrome

B Prevalence of Major Thrombosis Risk Factors

Patient Type	Protein C Deficiency, %	Protein S Deficiency, %	AT Deficiency, %	APCR, %	PGM, %	tlMTHFR, %
Healthy	0.2–0.4	1–3	0.02	3–7	2	5–10
First VTE	3	2	1	> 20	6.2	5–10
Recurrent VTE	5–10	5–10	5–10	> 50	18	10

Figure 5-42. Hypercoagulable states. The term *hypercoagulable state* and its synonym, *thrombophilia*, refer to any inherited or acquired abnormality of the hemostatic system that places an individual at an increased risk for thrombosis. **A**, Candidate hypercoagulable states. These abnormalities include elevated levels of selected procoagulant factors, deficiencies of natural anticoagulant proteins, resistance to the anticoagulant activity of activated protein C, thrombocythemia, "sticky" platelets, fibrinolytic system derangements, and endothelial cell dysfunction. **B**, The prevalence rates of several important inherited hypercoagulable states in the general population, in patients with a first thrombotic event, and in those with recurrent thrombosis. The discovery of factor V Leiden, prothrombin G20210A, and inherited hyperhomocysteinemia has significantly increased the number of thrombosis patients in whom a biochemical explanation for hypercoagulability can be identified. Any approach to the hypercoagulable patient should include a comprehensive clinical evaluation and a carefully conceived laboratory evaluation. The "best" approach must be individualized to meet the specific needs of an individual patient and should have an impact on patient management or family screening. Testing rarely affects acute thrombosis management. AT—antithrombin; APCR—activated protein C resistance; PAI-1—plasminogen activator inhibitor-1; PGM—prothrombin gene mutation; tlMTHFR—thermolabile methylene tetrahydrofolate reductase; t-PA—tissue-type plasminogen activator; VTE—venous thromboembolism.

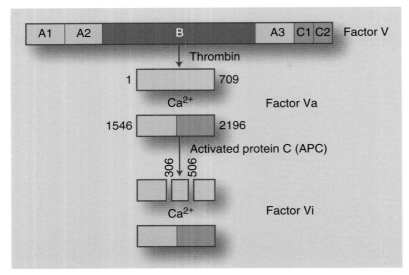

Figure 5-43. Activation and inactivation of factor V. Factor V Leiden, or factor V G1691A, is a single-point mutation in the gene that codes for coagulation factor V, which predicts the replacement of arginine at amino acid residue 506 by glutamine (Arg506Gln). This autosomal dominant mutation renders factors V and Va partially resistant to inactivation by the activated form of protein C (APC; a natural anticoagulant). APC inactivates factor Va in an orderly and sequential series of cleavages, first at Arg506 and then at Arg306 and Arg679. Partial resistance is explained by the fact that cleavage of factor Va by APC at Arg306 continues to occur, although at a slower rate. This provides a pathophysiologic explanation for why factor V Leiden, although common, is a relatively weak risk factor for venous thromboembolisms (VTEs). The mutation results in greater amounts of factor Va available for coagulation reactions, shifting the hemostatic balance toward greater thrombin generation. Factor V Leiden accounts for 92% of cases of APC resistance (APC-R), with the remaining 8% of cases resulting from pregnancy, oral contraceptive use, cancer, selected antiphospholipid antibodies, and other factor V point mutations. APC-R is an independent risk factor for VTEs, even in the absence of factor V Leiden.

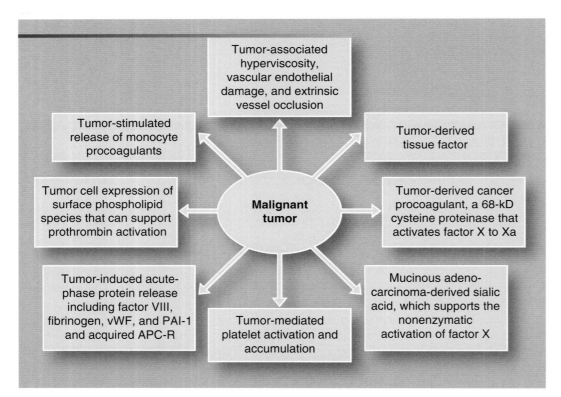

Figure 5-44. Mechanisms of cancer-associated hypercoagulability. The most important testing in patients with idiopathic thrombosis may actually be an age- and gender-appropriate cancer screening. It is well-known that cancer and cancer therapies can produce a hypercoagulable state and precipitate clinical thrombosis. It is also important to note that approximately 10% of individuals with idiopathic venous thrombosis will be diagnosed with a malignancy within 1 year of thrombosis diagnosis. Because different patients with different tumor histologies of different stages being treated with different chemotherapeutic agents can manifest very different spectrums of hypercoagulable tendencies, it is difficult to use standard laboratory testing to predict which patients will experience a clinical thrombosis. APC-R—activated protein C resistance; PAI-1—platelet activator inhibitor-1; vWF—von Willebrand factor.

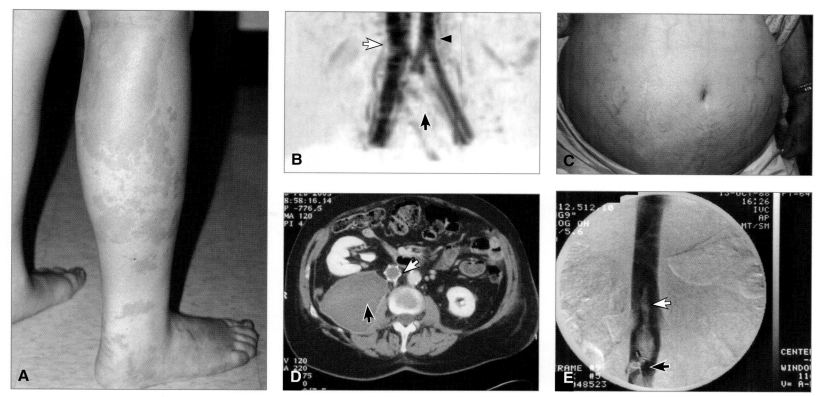

Figure 5-45. Clinical images of lower extremity and vena caval deep venous thrombosis (DVT). There are no specific signs or symptoms associated with hypercoagulable states. The most common clinical manifestation of an underlying hypercoagulable state is lower extremity DVT with or without pulmonary embolism. Because the clinical signs and symptoms associated with DVT and pulmonary embolism are insensitive and nonspecific, objective diagnostic confirmation by the use of an imaging method, such as contrast venography and duplex ultrasound, is mandatory.

Patients with acute lower extremity DVT may be asymptomatic or present with limb warmth, redness, swelling, palpable venous "cord," and pain. **A**, A patient with acute right leg DVT with associated swelling and patchy erythema. **B**, Pelvic magnetic resonance venogram of left leg DVT. Left leg DVT that develops in the setting of left iliac vein extrinsic compression by the right iliac artery is called May-Thurner syndrome. It reveals absent filling of the left iliac vein beginning at the point where the artery crosses the vein (*black arrow*). The *white arrow* indicates the inferior vena cava (IVC); the *arrowhead* indicates the aorta. **C**, IVC thrombosis. IVC thrombosis may initially present as bilateral leg swelling or the appearance of abdominal wall surface collateral vessels. For patients with acute lower extremity DVT who either cannot receive anticoagulation or develop new pulmonary emboli despite anticoagulation, treatment often involves placement of an IVC filter. These filters appear to provide short-term protection against subsequent pulmonary emboli. The decision to place a filter should not be reflexive because of cost and associated complications. **D**, The CT scan demonstrates a right-sided retroperitoneal bleed (*black arrow*) associated with IVC filter placement (*white arrow*). **E**, Thrombosis of an IVC filter (*black arrow*) in a hypercoagulable cancer patient with thrombus extension "above" the filter (*white arrow*), placing the patient at risk for massive pulmonary embolism.

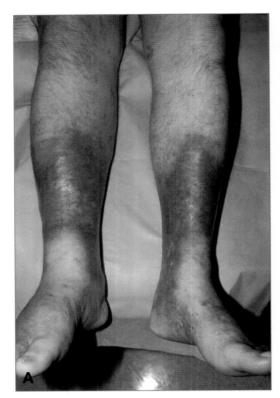

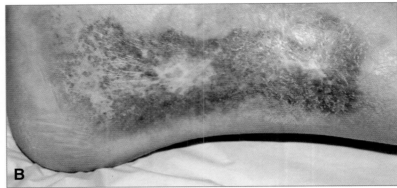

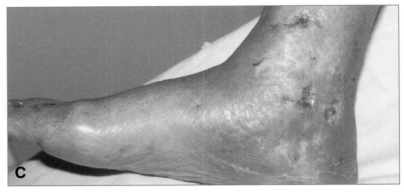

Figure 5-46. The post-thrombotic syndrome (PTS). PTS may include chronic swelling, supramalleolar skin pigmentation, subcutaneous sclerosis, venous claudication, and venous stasis ulceration (**A–C**). The skin pigmentation develops from brownish hemosiderin deposits as a result of erythrocyte extravasation from the venous circulation and subsequent degradation in the subcutaneous tissues. Up to 80% of patients with deep venous thrombosis will develop some degree of PTS, with most patients developing PTS within 2 years after the thrombosis. In select cases of chronic venous insufficiency, livedo reticularis with ulceration called livedoid vasculitis or atrophie blanche forms. Atrophie blanche, as seen in **B**, represents arteriolar infarction of middle dermal vessels, resulting in a very painful, hypoperfused area of often ulcerated skin.

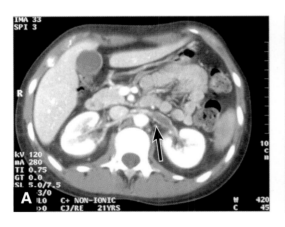

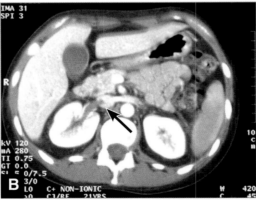

Figure 5-47. Efficacy of contrast-enhanced CT imaging to diagnose intra-abdominal venous thrombosis. **A,** Left renal vein thrombosis (*arrow*). **B,** Right renal vein thrombosis (*arrow*). Contrast-enhanced CT is very useful to diagnose intra-abdominal venous thromboses involving the portal vein (*see* Fig. 5-29*A*) and mesenteric vein as well (*see* Fig. 5-29*B*).

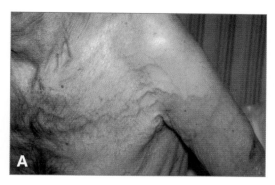
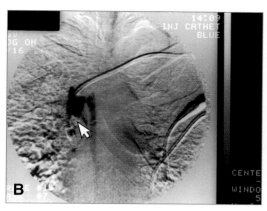
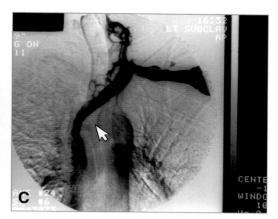

Figure 5-48. Upper extremity deep vein thrombosis (DVT). Upper extremity DVT may present as arm or neck swelling, pain, or redness as well as prominent visible venous collaterals involving the anterior chest, upper arm, and axilla (**A**). A major risk factor for axillosubclavian vein, internal jugular vein, and superior vena cava (SVC) thrombosis is the presence of an indwelling central venous access device. **B,** Central venous access device inserted through the left subclavian vein with its tip within the SVC. Injection of contrast media through the catheter reveals complete SVC thrombotic occlusion (*arrow*). **C,** Restoration of SVC patency (*arrow*) following a catheter-directed infusion of a thrombolytic agent.

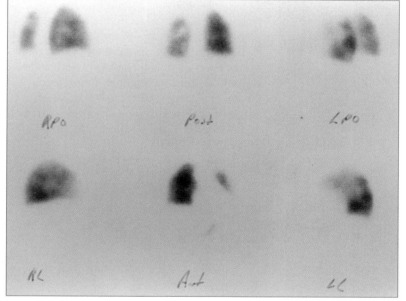

Figure 5-49. Perfusion study. An initial objective evaluation for pulmonary embolism (PE) usually involves ventilation/perfusion lung scintigraphy (V/Q lung scan) or contrast-enhanced helical CT. V/Q lung scanning combines ventilation and perfusion nuclear medicine imaging techniques. The ventilation (V) study involves the inhalation of a radioactive gas (typically ^{133}Xe or ^{127}Xe, ^{81}Kr, or aerosolized ^{99m}Tc), which provides an image of all ventilated portions of the lung. The perfusion (Q) study consists of an intravenous injection of ^{99m}Tc-labeled macroaggregated human serum albumin particles with the patient in supine position. Any obstruction to arterial flow is viewed as an area of "perfusion defect" on gamma camera images. This perfusion study shows several views of the lungs demonstrating subsegmental absence of tracer, suggestive of PE. The presence of multiple segmental perfusion defects increases the test specificity for PE. Based on the presence and extent of matched (absence of both perfusion and ventilation) and unmatched (absence of perfusion but preserved ventilation) defects, the V/Q scan can be interpreted as either normal or low, intermediate, or high probability for PE. Contrast-enhanced helical CT is performed by scanning a distance of 10 to 12 cm from the aortic arch to 2 cm below the inferior pulmonary veins during a single 30-second breath hold while the pulmonary vasculature is opacified by the automated injection of iodinated contrast medium. The major strengths of helical (spiral) CT include the rapid nature of data acquisition and the lower percentage of nondiagnostic studies owing to its ability to simultaneously evaluate vascular as well as nonvascular intrathoracic structures (*see* Fig. 5-50).

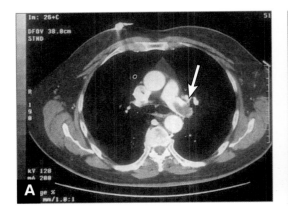 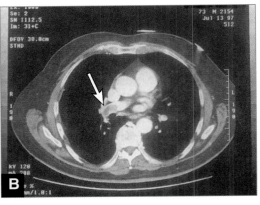

Figure 5-50. Helical CT images of left (**A**) and right (**B**) pulmonary artery thromboses (*arrows*). Helical CT is very effective for detection of segmental or more proximal pulmonary embolism, including these arteries.

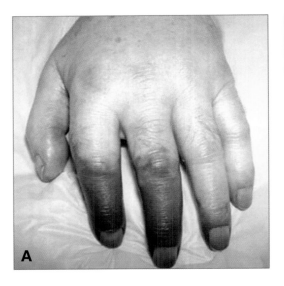 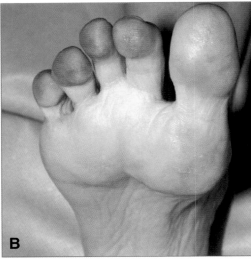

Figure 5-51. Digital ischemia associated with adenocarcinoma of the lung. The hypercoagulability of malignancy can manifest as deep venous thrombosis, superficial venous thrombosis, catheter-associated thrombosis, arterial thrombosis, disseminated intravascular coagulation, or marantic endocarditis. **A**, Ischemia affecting the fingers. **B**, Ischemia affecting the toes.

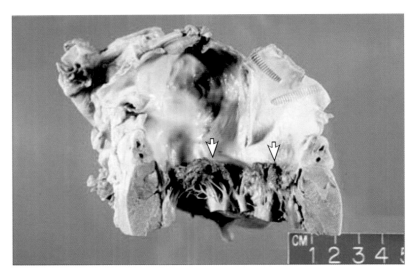

Figure 5-52. Gross image of marantic endocarditis. This patient with metastatic melanoma presented with widespread arterial emboli. *Arrows* indicate the valve thromboses.

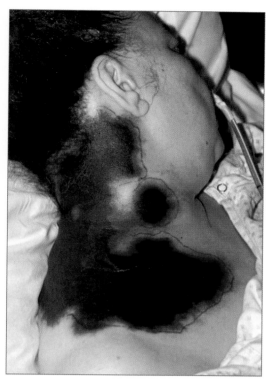

Figure 5-53. Warfarin-induced skin necrosis involving the right shoulder and neck. Warfarin-induced skin necrosis is an unusual but devastating complication of warfarin therapy, occurring within the first week of initiating therapy. Affected patents have usually received large loading doses of warfarin, perhaps in the absence of therapeutic heparin, low molecular weight heparin, or fondaparinux anticoagulation. Many patients with this syndrome have been found to have heterozygous protein C deficiency. The basis for this complication is thought to be a warfarin-induced rapid reduction in protein C levels in patients with a preexisting inherited protein C deficiency that results in a hypercoagulable state and thrombosis. Clinically, the skin lesions usually begin on certain subcutaneous areas of the body (breasts, abdomen, and thighs) as erythematous patches. Lesions progress to blebs followed by demarcated skin necrosis. Skin biopsy reveals generalized thrombosis of skin vessels.

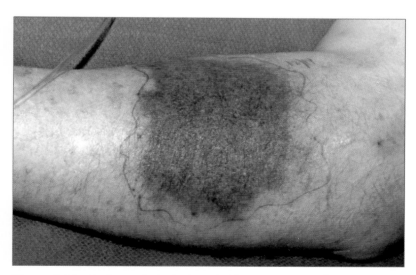

Figure 5-54. Early warfarin-induced skin necrosis involving a patient's extremity.

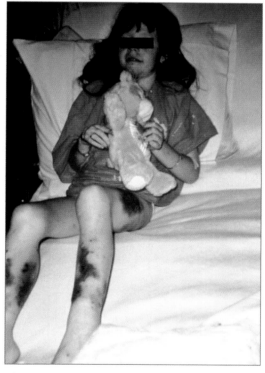

Figure 5-55. Skin necrosis in a pediatric patient. This child with antiphospholipid antibody syndrome and acute pulmonary embolism developed skin necrosis during the initiation of oral warfarin anticoagulation.

Vascular Disorders Associated with Purpura and Bleeding

Hereditary
Hereditary hemorrhagic telangiectasia (Osler-Weber-Rendu)
Ehlers-Danlos syndrome
Marfan syndrome
Fabry syndrome
Osteogenesis imperfecta
Allergic
Henoch–Schönlein purpura
Leukocytoclastic vasculitis (drug-related)
Atrophic
Senile purpura
Cushing syndrome
Steroid-induced bruising
Amyloidosis
Paraproteinemia, *eg*, myeloma and Waldenström's macroglobulinemia
Scurvy
Infectious
Viral infections
Bacterial infections
Rickettsial infections

Figure 5-56. Vascular disorders associated with purpura and bleeding. Several vascular disorders are associated with purpura and bleeding in the absence of a true platelet or hemostatic disorder. Some vascular disorders, such as senile purpura, drug-related allergic purpura, and calciphylaxis, produce nonpalpable purpura. Disorders such as cryoglobulinemia and Henoch–Schönlein purpura produce palpable purpura. Other vascular disorders are not associated with purpura and bleeding but have an appearance that may be mistaken for a bleeding disorder or limb thrombosis and prompt a useless laboratory and vascular evaluation.

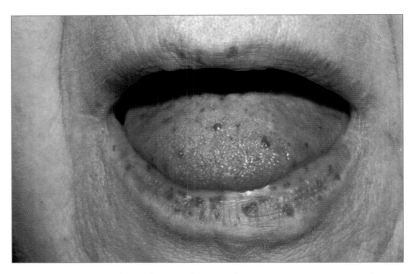

Figure 5-57. Hereditary hemorrhagic telangiectasia (HHT or Osler-Weber-Rendu syndrome). HHT is an autosomal dominant disorder with an estimated frequency of one in 50,000 that presents with widespread cutaneous, mucosal, and visceral telangiectasias. Patients may present with gastrointestinal bleeding due to mainly gastric and duodenal arteriovenous malformations (AVMs) or symptomatic pulmonary AVMs. Pulmonary AVMs may lead to hypoxemia due to shunting and embolic stroke or brain abscess related to paradoxic embolism. HHT has been identified as being caused by mutations affecting the endothelial protein endoglin, which mediates endothelial cell response to transforming growth factor-β (TGF-β). A second form of HHT has been linked to mutations affecting the TGF-β II receptor. A third form has been linked to a cell-surface receptor for the TGF-β superfamily called activin receptor–like kinase 1.

Papular, punctate, and linear telangiectasias are predominantly found involving the tongue, lips, digit tips, perioral region, and trunk. Epistaxis is the most common bleeding manifestation and may result in significant anemia. The signs and symptoms of HHT progressively worsen with aging. The bleeding tendency is related to vascular mechanical fragility that is related to a discontinuous endothelium and smooth muscle layer plus elastin deficiency.

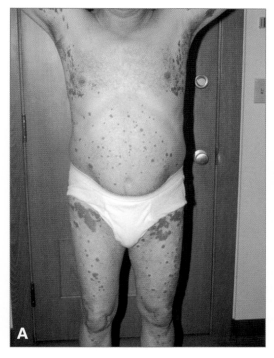

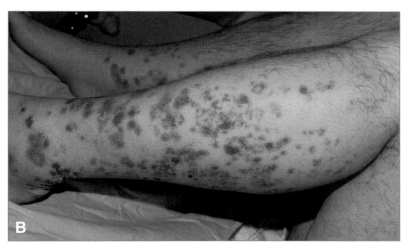

Figure 5-58. **A** and **B**, Henoch-Schönlein purpura (HSP). HSP is an allergic vasculitis that most commonly affects children. HSP causes palpable purpuric lesions, pruritic papules, and plaques involving the legs and buttocks. The lesions are frequently symmetric and may be accompanied by erythema, urticarial swelling, and tingling sensations. Intestinal submucosal hemorrhage, hematuria, and arthritis may accompany the cutaneous manifestations.

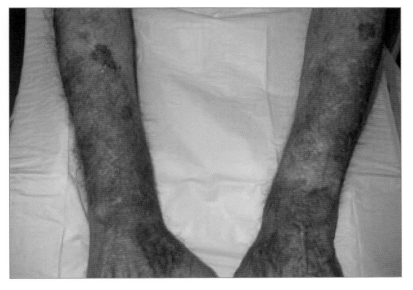

Figure 5-59. Senile purpura. Senile purpura is characterized by red and purple purpuric and ecchymotic patches mainly on the extensor surface of the arms and hands. Aging-related decreases in collagen, elastin, and subcutaneous fat combined with years of sunlight-induced damage likely result in senile purpura. The affected skin is thin, lacks elasticity, tears easily, and heals poorly following trauma. Senile purpura has a similar appearance to that of steroid-induced and Cushing syndrome–related purpura.

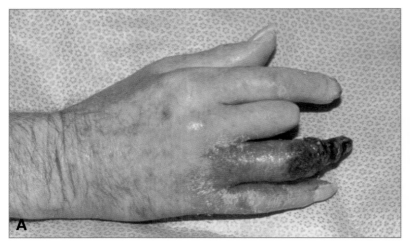

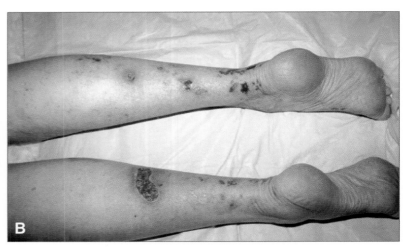

Figure 5-60. Cryoglobulinemia. Cryoglobulins are cold-precipitable proteins in serum. Cryoglobulins may be idiopathic in nature or related to an underlying lymphoproliferative syndrome or plasma cell dyscrasia. Cryoglobulins may be IgG, IgM, or IgA. Mixed cryoglobulins are usually composed of rheumatoid factor IgM complexed with a monoclonal or polyclonal IgG and may be idiopathic or secondary to a disorder such as hepatitis C infection. The immune complexes may interfere with normal platelet function and fibrin polymerization. Hyperviscosity and direct vascular trauma from the circulating cryoglobulin cause small vessel hemorrhage. Cryoglobulinemia may present with acral hemorrhagic necrosis (**A**), palpable purpura (**B**), livedo reticularis, and frank leg ulcerations.

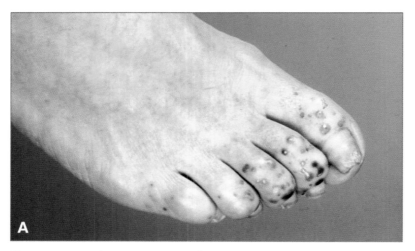

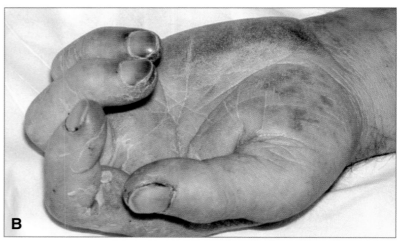

Figure 5-61. Infection-associated purpura. Infectious purpura may involve direct vascular invasion by the organism, immune-complex vasculitis, disseminated intravascular coagulation, and septic emboli. These images show digital (**A**) and palmar (**B**) septic emboli in patients with bacterial endocarditis. These lesions may be confused with atheroemboli and aseptic thromboembolic disease.

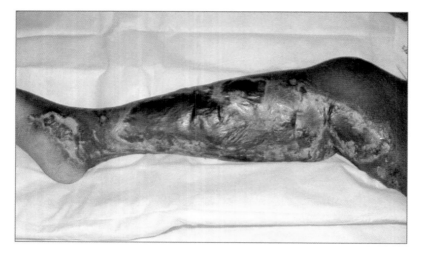

Figure 5-62. Calciphylaxis. Calciphylaxis describes patients with systemic calcinosis often in the setting of renal failure and deficiencies of natural anticoagulants such as protein C. Patients develop soft tissue and arterial calcium deposition due to a high calcium–phosphorus product greater than 70. Severe pain and ischemic tissue necrosis are major challenges of calciphylaxis management.

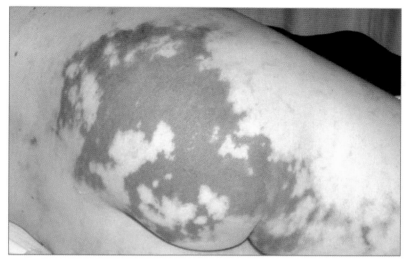

Figure 5-63. Atheroemboli. Atheroemboli containing cholesterol crystals usually originate from atherosclerotic plaques located in the aorta. The emboli often develop following vascular manipulation, such as that which occurs during cardiac catheterization. Atheroemboli may also develop following surgical vascular manipulation and following the initiation of warfarin therapy in older individuals. Showers of atheroemboli may result in digital petechiae, purpura, cyanosis, and gangrene. The lesions may be very painful. This patient had atheroemboli involving the right buttocks with an appearance that could be confused with that of anticoagulation-related bleeding and ecchymosis.

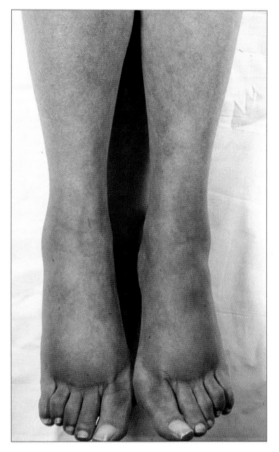

Figure 5-64. Acrocyanosis. Acrocyanosis signifies persistent cyanosis and coldness of the digits, hands, and feet. The face and ears may also be involved. The blueness of acrocyanosis intensifies in cold environments and lessens on warming. This blueness must be differentiated from extensive ecchymosis.

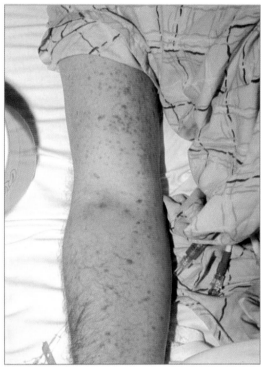

Figure 5-65. Leukemia cutis. Myeloid precursors in patients with acute myelogenous leukemia can infiltrate the skin, gingiva, and central nervous system as well as form head and neck myeloblastomas. These lesions may be widespread and vary in size from several millimeters to several centimeters in diameter. They are often palpated as freely mobile subcutaneous nodules with overlying discoloration ranging from red-brown to blue-gray in appearance. Confusion with petechiae and purpura, especially in a thrombocytopenic patient, is understandable.

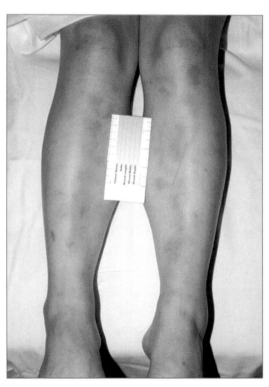

Figure 5-66. Cutaneous vascular malformations. This young woman was referred to several hematologists for evaluation of a bleeding disorder manifesting as bilateral below-knee "extensive bruising" that never healed. Further evaluation including magnetic resonance imaging revealed what appeared to be a very superficial network of venovenous malformations. Screening laboratory testing failed to reveal any evidence of a hemorrhagic disorder.

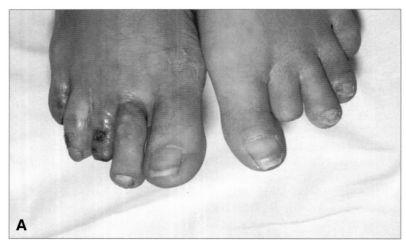

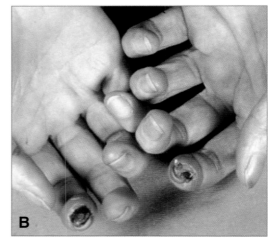

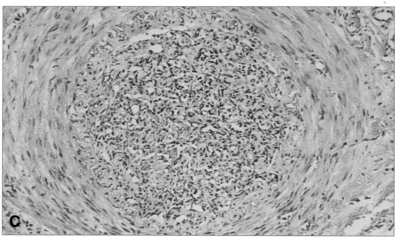

Figure 5-67. Thromboangiitis obliterans (Buerger disease). Intermittent claudication in a young male smoker should alert physicians to possible Buerger disease. This vasculopathy mainly affects distal arteries, resulting in digital ulceration, gangrene, and autoamputation (**A** and **B**).

Upper extremities are involved in approximately 40% of cases. Thrombophlebitis develops at some point in roughly 40% of patients. Histologic examination of amputated limbs may reveal vascular lumens occluded by a highly cellular thrombus with characteristic microabscesses (**C**).

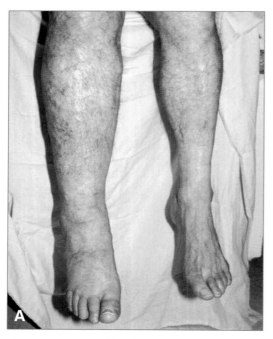

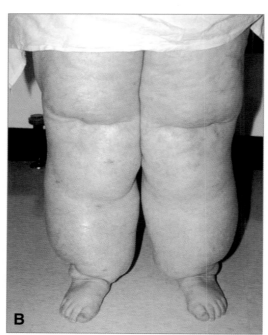

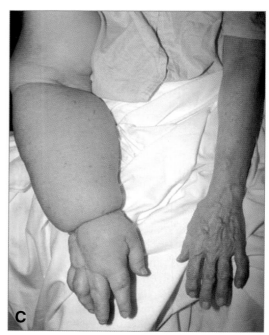

Figure 5-68. Swollen limbs. An acutely swollen limb warrants an evaluation for venous thrombosis. Chronically swollen limbs may reflect remote venous thrombosis with resultant chronic venous insufficiency. Other causes of enlarged limbs that have been clinically mistaken for acute venous thrombosis include Klippel-Trenaunay-Weber syndrome (**A**), lipedema (**B**), and lymphedema (**C**). Klippel-Trenaunay-Weber syndrome consists of a triad of cutaneous capillary hemangioma (port-wine stain), bone and soft tissue (muscular) hypertrophy, and varicose veins. Most patients have lower extremity involvement with an oversized limb and a prominent varicose vein network. Lipedema is bilateral and symmetric deposition of fat in the legs that spares the feet and is nonpitting. Extremity lymphedema is caused by the inability of the lymphatic system to normally carry lymph, leading to lymph fluid stasis. Lymphedema may be primary or secondary to obstruction, interruption, or replacement of lymphatic channels. Secondary lymphedema may develop following surgery in relation to lymph node invasion by tumor or recurrent skin or soft tissue infections. The patient shown in **C** has severe postmastectomy lymphedema.

RECOMMENDED READING

Collins PW: Treatment of acquired hemophilia A. *J Thromb Haemost* 2007, 5:893–900.

Deitcher SR: Antiplatelet, anticoagulant, and fibrinolytic therapy. In *Harrison's Principles of Internal Medicine*, edn 16. New York: McGraw-Hill; 2004:687–693.

Deitcher SR: Disorders of platelets and coagulation. In *The Cleveland Clinic Foundation Intensive Review of Internal Medicine*, edn 4. Philadelphia: Lippincott Williams & Wilkins; 2005: 282–297.

Deitcher SR, Gomes MPV, Haire WD: Diagnosis, treatment, and prevention of cancer-related venous thrombosis. In *Clinical Oncology*, edn 3. Philadelphia: Elsevier; 2004:891–924.

Deitcher SR, Rogers G: Thrombosis and antithrombotic therapy. In *Wintrobe's Clinical Hematology*, edn 11. Philadelphia: Lippincott Williams & Wilkins; 2004:1713–1758.

Franchini M: Advances in the diagnosis and management of von Willebrand disease. *Hematology* 2006, 11:219–225.

Furie B, Furie BC: Thrombus formation in vivo. *J Clin Invest* 2005, 115:3355–3362.

George JN: Clinical practice: thrombotic thrombocytopenic purpura. *N Engl J Med* 2006, 354:1927–1935.

George JN: Managment of patients with refractory immune thrombocytopenic purpura. *J Thromb Haemost* 2006, 4:1664–1672.

Levi M: Pathogenesis and treatment of DIC. *Thromb Res* 2005, 115(Suppl 1):54–55.

CHAPTER 6

Anemias

Ayalew Tefferi and Chin-Yang Li

Anemia is defined as a decrease in hemoglobin (or hematocrit) level from an individual's baseline value. Because individual baseline hemoglobin levels are often not available during routine clinical practice, physicians use gender- and race-specific reference ranges to make a working diagnosis of anemia. In general, "normal" hemoglobin levels are approximately 1 to 2 g/dL lower in women and African-American men compared with white men. It is important to keep in mind that anemia itself is often not a disease but a marker of one. However, independent of the underlying disease, severe anemia per se can either be life-threatening or significantly compromise quality of life.

There are numerous ways of classifying the causes of anemia, and no particular way is necessarily superior to another. It is equally important to appreciate the difference in the approach to diagnosis between children and adults, men and women, and two persons of different ethnic backgrounds. Regardless of the specific algorithm one chooses to follow in the evaluation of anemia, it is essential that easily remediable causes such as nutritional deficiencies, hemolysis, and anemia of renal insufficiency be identified early and treated appropriately. In this chapter, we have taken the approach that is most helpful in routine clinical practice.

In general, one can substantially narrow the differential diagnosis of anemia by subcategorization into "microcytic," "macrocytic," and "normocytic" subtypes based on the mean corpuscular volume (MCV). Such classification is, however, a starting point and not exact. Once a particular anemic process has been classified into microcytic, macrocytic, or normocytic subtype, the next step would be to examine the red blood cell (RBC) indices (MCV, RBC count, and RBC distribution width) in order to obtain additional clues to a specific diagnosis. The peripheral smear examination serves a similar purpose and final diagnosis is made based on specific laboratory tests.

Practical Classification of Anemia

Microcytic Anemias (MCV < 80 fL)	Macrocytic Anemias (MCV > 100 fL)	Normocytic Anemias (MCV 80–100 fL)
Iron deficiency anemia	Megaloblastic macrocytic anemia (MCV can be > 110 fL)	Stem cell defect/decreased erythropoiesis
Thalassemia	B$_{12}$/folate deficiency	Intrinsic causes
α-Thalassemia	Hydroxyurea treatment	Idiopathic aplastic anemia
β-Thalassemia	Myelodysplastic syndrome	PNH-associated aplastic anemia
Thalassemic hemoglobinopathy (*eg*, hemoglobin E)	Large granular lymphocyte disorder	Diamond-Blackfan syndrome
Microcytic anemias not related to iron deficiency or thalassemia	Round macrocytic anemia (MCV is often < 110 fL)	Fanconi's anemia
X-linked sideroblastic anemia	Excess alcohol usage	Congenital dyserythropoietic anemia (CDA types I, II, III)
Lead poisoning	Liver disease	Ineffective erythropoiesis associated with MDS and other CMD
Few instances of anemia of chronic disease (*eg*, rheumatoid arthritis)	Reticulocytosis	Extrinsic causes
Hodgkin lymphoma		Drug associated
Castleman disease		Toxin associated
Myelofibrosis with myeloid metaplasia		Radiation associated
		Renal insufficiency associated
		Endocrinopathy associated
		Immune mediated (*eg*, pure red cell aplasia)
		Cytokine mediated (*eg*, anemia of chronic disease)
		Marrow infiltrative process such as metastatic cancer and lymphoma
		Hemolytic anemias
		Red cell intrinsic causes
		Membranopathies (*eg*, hereditary spherocytosis)
		Enzymopathies (*eg*, G6PD deficiency)
		Hemoglobinopathies (*eg*, sickle cell disease)
		Red cell extrinsic causes
		Immune mediated (autoimmune): drug associated, virus associated, lymphoid disorder associated, idiopathic
		Immune mediated (alloimmune): immediate transfusion reaction, delayed transfusion reaction, neonatal hemolytic anemia
		Microangiopathic (*eg*, TTP/HUS)
		Infection associated (*eg*, falciparum malaria)
		Chemical agent associated (*eg*, spider venoms)
		Red cell intrinsic causes
		Membranopathies (*eg*, hereditary spherocytosis)
		Enzymopathies (*eg*, G6PD deficiency)
		Hemoglobinopathies (*eg*, sickle cell disease)

Figure 6-1. Practical classification of anemia. The mean red blood cell corpuscular volume (MCV) is used to classify anemia into microcytic, macrocytic, and normocytic subtypes. In the context of macrocytic anemia, subclassification into marked (MCV > 110 fL) and mild to moderate (MCV 100–110 fL) macrocytosis allows further refinement of the differential diagnosis, because marked macrocytosis is almost always associated with megaloblastic (oval macrocytosis) anemia, whereas the MCV in round macrocytic anemia is often below 110 fL. CDA—congenital dyserythropoietic anemia; CMD—chronic myeloproliferative disorders; G6PD—glucose-6-phosphate dehydrogenase; HUS—hemolytic-uremic syndrome; MDS—myelodysplastic syndrome; PNH—paroxysmal nocturnal hemoglobinuria; TTP—thrombotic thrombocytopenic purpura.

Normal Complete Blood Cell Count and Red Cell Indices		
	Normal Ranges in Whites According to Sex	
	Male	Female
Hemoglobin, g/dL	13.5–17.5	12.0–15.5
Hematocrit, %	38.8–50	34.9–44.5
Red blood cell count, $\times 10^{12}/L$	4.32–5.72	3.9–5.03
Mean corpuscular volume, fL	81.2–95.1	81.6–98.3
Red cell distribution width	11.8–15.6	11.9–15.5
Leukocyte count, $\times 10^9/L$	3.5–10.5	3.5–10.5
Platelet count, $\times 10^9/L$	150–450	150–450

Figure 6-2. Normal complete blood cell count and red cell indices. Once a particular anemic process has been classified into microcytic, macrocytic, or normocytic subtype, the next step would be to examine the red blood cell indices (mean corpuscular volume, red blood cell count [RBCC], and red blood cell distribution width [RDW]) to obtain additional clues to specific diagnosis. For example, RDW is typically increased in iron deficiency anemia and megaloblastic macrocytic anemia, whereas it is normal in anemia of chronic disease and round macrocytic anemia. Similarly, an increased RBCC suggests thalassemia.

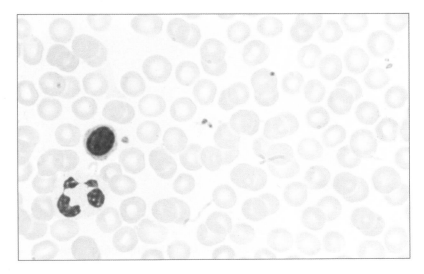

Figure 6-3. A normal peripheral blood smear. The peripheral blood smear examination is readily available in routine clinical practice and provides substantial morphologic information that aids in the specific diagnosis of anemia. A drop of blood is applied against a glass slide that is subsequently stained with polychrome stains (Wright-Giemsa) to permit identification of the various cell types. These stains are mixtures of basic dyes (methylene blue) that are blue and acidic dyes (eosin) that are red. As such, acid components of the cell (nucleus, cytoplasmic RNA, basophilic granules) stain blue or purple, and basic components of the cell (hemoglobin, eosinophilic granules) stain red or orange. In addition to the polychrome stains, monochrome stains are sometimes used to visualize young red cells (reticulocyte stain), denatured hemoglobin (Heinz body stain), or cellular iron (Prussian blue stain).

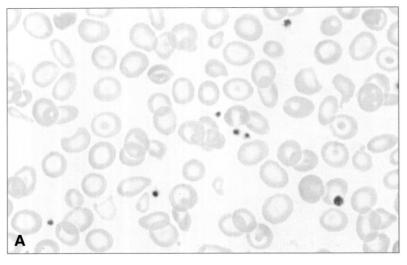

A

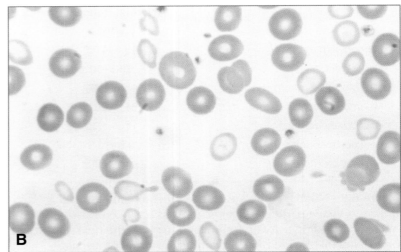

B

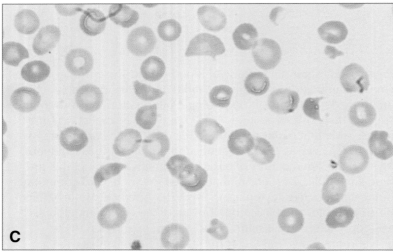

C

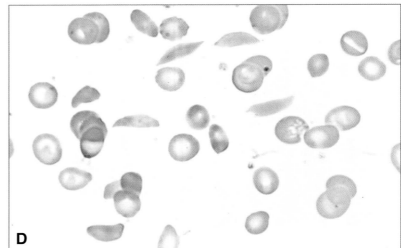

D

Figure 6-4. Red cell shape changes. Changes seen in the peripheral smear. **A**, Target cells characterize thalassemia but also may be seen after splenectomy and in liver disease. **B**, Dimorphic red blood cells (two distinctly sized red cell populations) may be seen in myelodysplastic syndrome and in patients who have had trans- fusions (**C**). The smear is also critical for revealing schistocytes (microangiopathic hemolytic anemia, including thrombotic throm- bocytopenic purpura/hemolytic uremic syndrome and valvular hemolysis). **D**, Sickle cells.

Continued on the next page

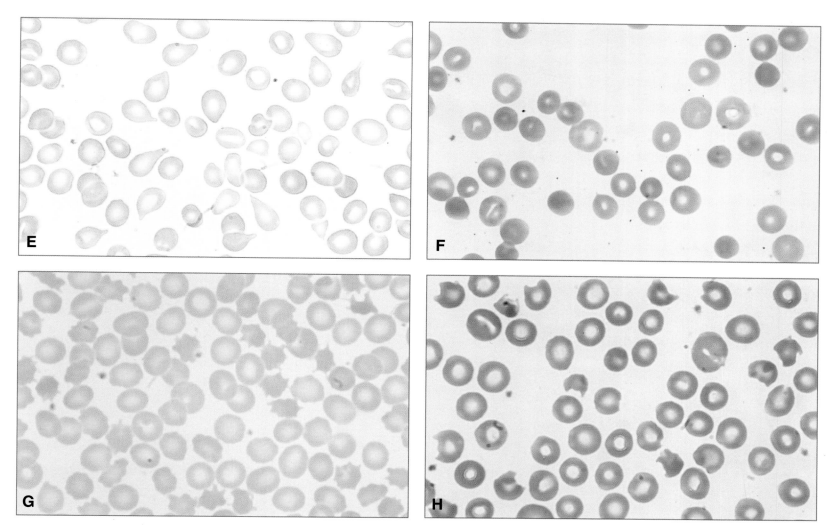

Figure 6-4. *(Continued)* **E**, Tear drop–shaped cells (dacryocytes; associated with a bone marrow infiltrative process including metastatic cancer and bone marrow fibrosis). **F**, Spherocytes (hereditary spherocytosis, autoimmune hemolytic anemia). **G**, Acanthocytes (liver disease, abetalipoproteinemia, asplenia). **H**, Bite cells (drug-induced hemolysis, glucose-6-phosphate dehydrogenase deficiency, unstable hemoglobinopathies).

A

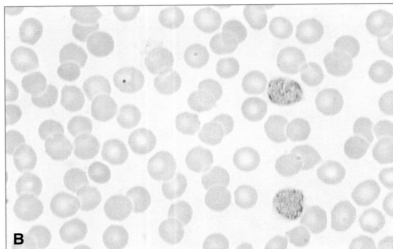

B

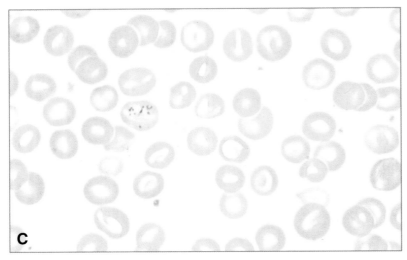

C

Figure 6-5. Red blood cell inclusion bodies seen in the peripheral smear. **A,** Howell-Jolly bodies (nuclear remnants) are present in both anatomic (surgical splenectomy) and functional (sickle cell disease, amyloidosis, celiac sprue) asplenia. Heinz bodies (not shown) represent denatured hemoglobin and are present in drug-induced hemolytic anemias, thalassemias, unstable hemoglobinopathy, and glucose-6-phosphate dehydrogenase deficiency. **B,** A well-prepared smear may reveal intra-erythrocyte parasites, including malaria and *Babesia*. **C,** Aggregates of ribosomes are sometimes visible and stain with the Wright-Giemsa stain as punctate basophilia and are seen as basophilic stippling. Basophilic stippling that is coarse rather than punctate implies lead poisoning or thalassemia.

MICROCYTIC ANEMIA: IRON DEFICIENCY ANEMIA

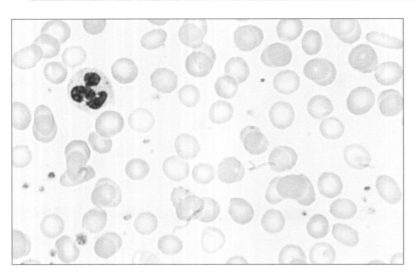

Figure 6-6. Peripheral blood smear showing iron deficiency anemia (IDA). The first step in the evaluation of microcytic anemia is to rule out IDA. Microcytic anemia from IDA is often associated with increased red blood cell distribution width and sometimes with reactive thrombocytosis. The peripheral smear in IDA (*see* Fig. 6-5) usually shows anisocytosis and poikilocytosis. In severe cases, cigar-shaped red blood cells and elliptocytes are characteristically present. Conversely, polychromasia (the Wright-Giemsa stain equivalent of reticulocytosis) and basophilic stippling are conspicuously absent.

Iron Studies in the Evaluation of Anemia

Iron Studies	Iron Deficiency Anemia	Anemia of Chronic Disease	Thalassemia
Serum ferritin	Low	Normal or increased	Normal or increased
Serum iron	Low	Low or normal	Normal or increased
Transferrin (TIBC)	Normal or increased	Normal	Normal
Transferrin saturation	Low	Low or normal	Normal or increased

Figure 6-7. Iron studies in the evaluation of anemia. The diagnosis of iron deficiency anemia (IDA) is confirmed by demonstrating a low serum ferritin level (normal range, 20–300 µg/L). The other serum iron studies (serum iron, total iron binding capacity [TIBC], transferrin saturation) lack either specificity or sensitivity and therefore have limited value in the evaluation of IDA. If the serum ferritin value is low, it is diagnostic of an iron-depleted state. IDA is unlikely in the presence of a normal serum ferritin level.

Causes of Iron Deficiency Anemia

Cause	Comments
Menstrual bleeding	Most frequent cause in young women
Pregnancy	Diversion of iron to the fetus and placenta
Children	Increased demand during growth
Upper GI bleeding	Many causes including ulcer, varices, hiatal hernia, gastritis, HHT
Lower GI bleeding	Colon cancer, angiodysplasia
Intestinal malabsorption	Crohn's disease, celiac sprue, intestinal surgery, hookworm infestation
Urogenital	Urolithiasis, bladder cancer, prostate pathology, schistosomiasis
Factitious bleeding	

Figure 6-8. Causes of iron deficiency anemia (IDA). In developing countries, the major causes of IDA include inadequate nutrition and intestinal parasitosis (hookworm infestation). In the more developed countries, the most common causes include gastrointestinal (GI) and menstrual blood loss. In a young woman, IDA can be attributed to menstruation, under the proper clinical context. Otherwise, quantification of stool blood and full GI work-up may be required to identify the source of bleeding in most patients. A small number of patients may have no historical clue for malabsorption and may have negative results after extensive GI work-up. In this situation, it should be remembered that the clinical presentation of sprue may be subtle and the measurement of serum carotene, stool fat, and serum antigliadin, antiendomysial, and tissue transglutaminase antibodies is a reasonable next step. The antibody tests have high prediction accuracy. HHT—hereditary hemorrhagic telangiectasia.

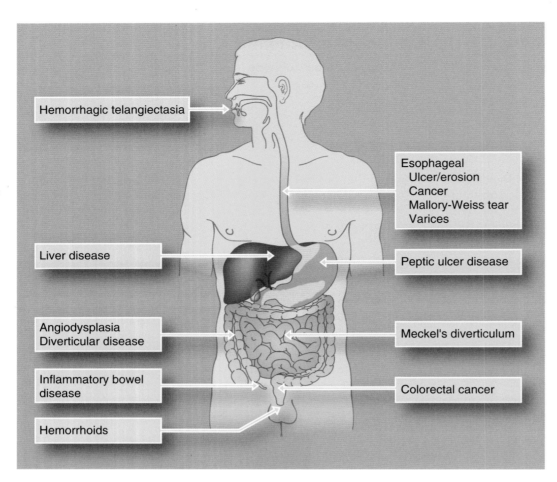

Figure 6-9. Gastrointestinal (GI) work-up for iron deficiency anemia. The GI investigation starts with colonoscopy in most patients. A negative colonoscopy is usually followed by an upper endoscopy. If both are negative, then a small intestinal barium study is performed to look for tumors or intestinal wall abnormalities. Additional evaluation techniques for a bleeding source include extended upper endoscopy (push or capsule enteroscopy), a Tc-labeled Meckel scan (to look for Meckel's diverticulum), a bleeding scan (Tc-tagged autologous red cells), angiography, and perioperative enteroscopy.

Management of Iron Deficiency Anemia

Preparation	Strength	Elemental Iron	Ascorbic Acid
Ferrous sulfate tablet	324 mg	65 mg	0
Ferrous sulfate elixir (Feosol*)	220 mg/5 mL	44 mg/5 mL	0
Ferrous sulfate solution (Fer-in-sol†)	125 mg/mL	25 mg/mL	0
Ferrous fumarate tablet (Vitron-C‡)	200 mg	66 mg	125 mg
Ferrous gluconate tablet	300 mg	35 mg	0
Ferrous gluconate elixir (Fergon§)	300 mg/5 mL	35 mg/5 mL	0
Polysaccharide iron (Niferex¶)	150 mg	150 mg	0

*GlaxoSmith Kline, Research Triangle Park, NC.
†Mead Johnson, Evansville, IN.
‡Gemini Pharmaceuticals, Commack, NY.
§Bayer, Morristown, NJ.
¶Ethex Corp., St. Louis, MO.

Figure 6-10. Management of iron deficiency anemia. The three iron salts (sulfate, fumarate, gluconate) are roughly equivalent in both efficacy and side effects. The addition of ascorbic acid is of dubious value. Iron supplements are preferably taken before meals, two to four times a day. Taking the iron pills with meals alleviates gastrointestinal side effects but absorption is compromised. Enteric-coated or sustained-release preparations are more expensive and their possible benefit in reducing side effects is countered by reduced absorption due to retarded dissolution. For patients who cannot tolerate oral iron or for those who have intestinal malabsorption, parenteral iron dextran preparation is available (InFeD, Watson Pharmaceuticals, Corona, CA) and may be administered carefully.

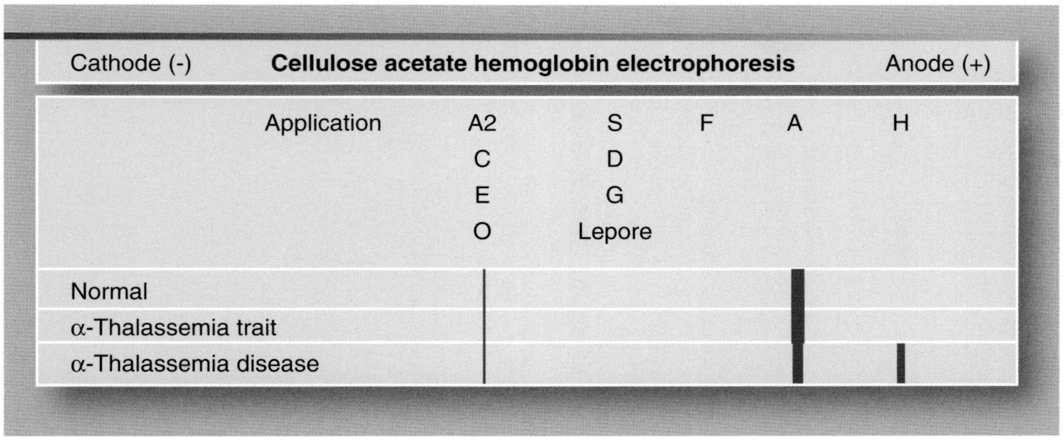

Figure 6-11. Hemoglobin electrophoresis in α-thalassemia. If the serum ferritin level in microcytic anemia is normal, the next step is to determine the onset of microcytosis. If the microcytosis is newly acquired, investigation for thalassemia is unwarranted. Otherwise, hemoglobin electrophoresis is in order. This test is helpful for revealing the presence of some, but not all, thalassemic syndromes (hemoglobin disorders characterized by decreased globin-chain synthesis). Most thalassemia syndromes (α and β) do not involve structural variants of the hemoglobin molecule. As such, hemoglobin electrophoresis may not detect an abnormality. This is especially true for α-thalassemia. Like any other thalassemia syndrome, α-thalassemia may exist as either the trait (two of four allele deletion) or the disease (three of four allele deletion). In the former instance, the result of hemoglobin electrophoresis is normal. In the latter instance (hemoglobin H disease), the presence of β-chain tetramers (hemoglobin H) is revealed by hemoglobin electrophoresis (5%–30%).

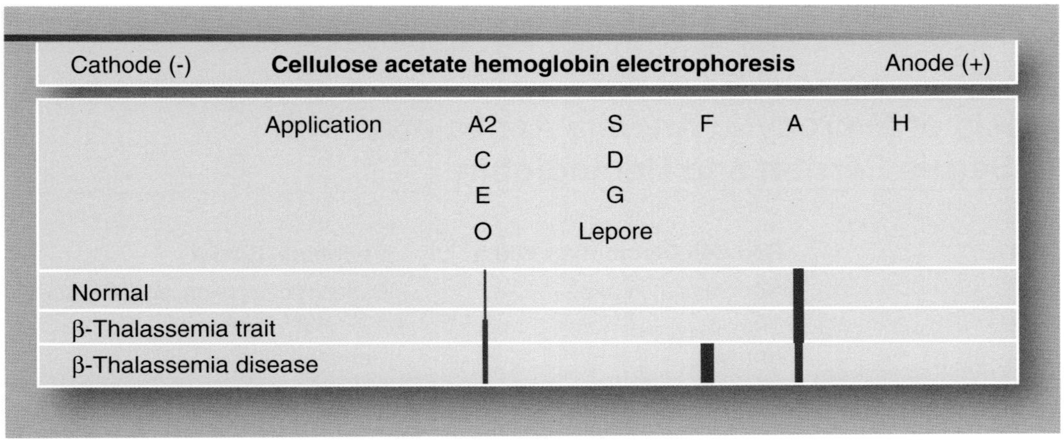

Figure 6-12. Hemoglobin electrophoresis in β-thalassemia. *See* Figure 6-11 legend.

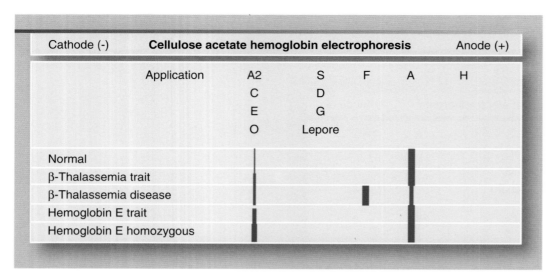

Cathode (−)	Cellulose acetate hemoglobin electrophoresis					Anode (+)
	Application	A2 C E O	S D G Lepore	F	A	H
Normal						
β-Thalassemia trait						
β-Thalassemia disease						
Hemoglobin E trait						
Hemoglobin E homozygous						

Figure 6-13. Hemoglobin electrophoresis in thalassemic hemoglobinopathies. Rare microcytic thalassemia disorders that result from structural hemoglobin variants are directly identified by hemoglobin electrophoresis. These include β (hemoglobin Lepore) and α (hemoglobin Constant Spring) structural variants. Hemoglobin Lepore results from a nonhomologous crossover of β and δ gene sequences that creates a fusion β-chain variant (δβ), resulting in a disorder that is clinically similar to β-thalassemia. Similarly, hemoglobin Constant Spring is clinically similar to α-thalassemia and is a result of termination codon mutation that creates an elongated α chain. Finally, hemoglobin E (a structural hemoglobinopathy that is prevalent in Southeast Asia) is also characterized by microcytosis because of a decreased synthesis of the abnormal β chain. This results from an RNA splice site mutation associated with the production of an alternative messenger RNA that is not effectively translated.

MICROCYTIC ANEMIA: NOT ASSOCIATED WITH EITHER IRON DEFICIENCY OR THALASSEMIA

Differential Diagnosis of Microcytic Anemia Associated with Normal Serum Ferritin and Hemoglobin

Electrophoresis			
	Molecular Test	Red Cell Distribution Width	Peripheral Smear
α-Thalassemia trait	Positive	Normal or increased	Basophilic stippling, polychromasia, target cells
Anemia of chronic disease	Negative	Normal	Unremarkable
Sideroblastic anemia	Negative	Increased	Dimorphic red blood cells

Figure 6-14. The differential diagnosis of microcytic anemia associated with normal serum ferritin and normal hemoglobin electrophoresis. Currently, there exists a molecular genetic test (polymerase chain reaction–based assay) that may detect the deletion defect in most patients with α-thalassemia. However, the test is expensive and suspected cases may be managed without laboratory confirmation. The information on ethnic origin and family history is often adequate to establish a working diagnosis and provide genetic counseling for affected patients. Similarly, there is no positive blood test that confirms anemia of chronic disease or sideroblastic anemia. These are often considered based on the basis of the clinical presentation, peripheral smear examination, and, if indicated, bone marrow examination. The microcytosis in sideroblastic anemia is accompanied by red cell dimorphism and coarse basophilic stippling, whereas the bone marrow reveals ringed sideroblasts. The peripheral smear in anemia of chronic disease is unremarkable. Moderate to severe microcytic anemia might accompany chronic infections (endocarditis), Hodgkin disease, Castleman disease (angiofollicular lymph node hyperplasia), temporal arteritis, rheumatoid arthritis, and other connective tissue diseases.

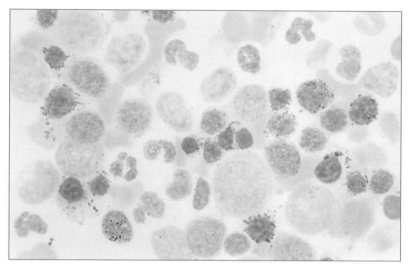

Figure 6-15. Bone marrow showing ring sideroblasts (RS) in sideroblastic anemia (SA). RS are erythroid precursors whose mitochondria, which are located around the nucleus, are loaded with nonheme iron. RS is secondary to defective iron utilization that results from a hereditary impairment of heme synthesis (aminolevulinic acid synthase deficiency in hereditary SA) or an acquired pathology that results from either chemical toxicity (lead, isoniazid, alcohol) or a clonal stem cell disease (refractory anemia with RS). Hereditary SA is usually X-linked recessive. Patients with hereditary SA present early in childhood with severe microcytic anemia and over many years develop hemochromatosis. Fifty percent of the cases may respond to high doses of oral pyridoxine (200 mg/d).

NORMOCYTIC ANEMIA

Differential Diagnosis of "Normocytic" Anemia	
Non-nutritional Causes of Normocytic Anemia	**Examples**
Anemia of chronic disease	Connective tissue disorders, chronic inflammation, diabetes
Renal anemia	
Ineffective erythropoiesis	Myelodysplastic syndrome
Marrow infiltrative process	Lymphoma, multiple myeloma, metastatic cancer, myelofibrosis
Marrow failure	Aplastic anemia, pure red cell aplasia, drug-induced aplasia
Hemolytic anemia	Immune-mediated, membranopathies, enzymopathies, hemoglobinopathies, microangiopathic

Figure 6-16. The differential diagnosis of "normocytic" anemia, including causes that are listed with both microcytic and macrocytic anemia. The critical issue in the evaluation of any form of anemia is to recognize treatable causes early. In a patient with normocytic anemia, iron and vitamin B_{12} deficiencies are possible causes despite their usual association with microcytic and macrocytic anemia, respectively. Other treatable causes of normocytic anemia include anemia of renal insufficiency, bleeding, and hemolysis.

As such, the initial investigation of normocytic anemia should include determination of serum ferritin and B_{12}/folate levels (to address nutritional causes) and the serum creatinine level (to address anemia of renal insufficiency). If the serum creatinine level is increased, determination of serum erythropoietin may be helpful for confirming relative hypoerythropoietinemia. If these initial tests are unrevealing and bleeding is not clinically suspected, then the possibility of hemolysis is considered.

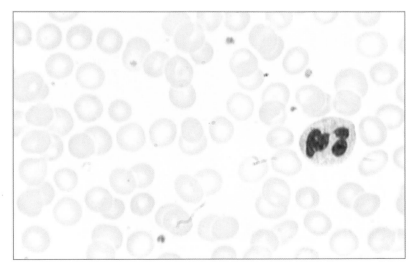

Figure 6-17. Anemia of chronic disease (ACD). Any infectious or inflammatory process is capable of inducing ACD. The measurement of serum ferritin level is the single best noninvasive test to differentiate iron deficiency anemia (IDA) from ACD. A low serum ferritin is diagnostic of IDA. Another concern during the evaluation of ACD is the possible presence of a primary bone marrow disease. In this regard, the decision to obtain a bone marrow biopsy should take into account the likelihood of discovering a primary bone marrow disease and the therapeutic and prognostic value of the information from the procedure. Some patients with ACD may respond to exogenous administration of erythropoietin.

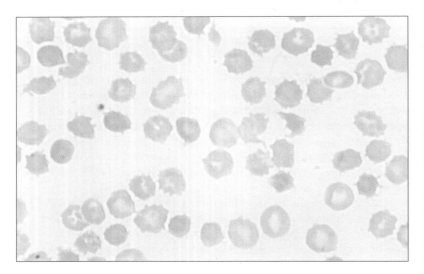

Figure 6-18. Anemia associated with renal insufficiency. Erythropoietin (EPO) production is compromised in the presence of kidney disease. Although baseline production may not be substantially affected, the physiologically appropriate anemia-induced increase in EPO production is suboptimal. Although anemia is severe and symptomatic only with advanced kidney disease (serum creatinine > 3 mg/dL), mild to moderate anemia may be seen in moderate renal insufficiency (serum creatinine 1.5–3 mg/dL), especially in diabetic patients with nephrotic syndrome. Exogenous administration of EPO is the treatment of choice.

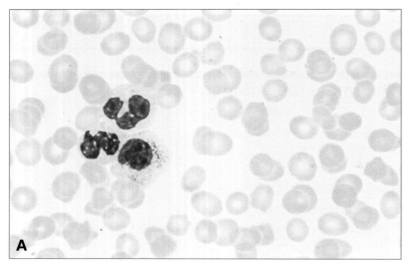

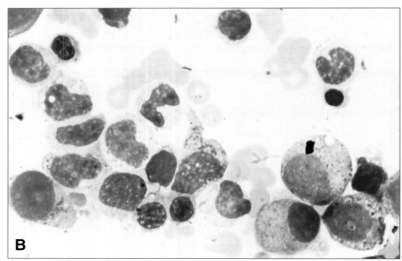

Figure 6-19. The myelodysplastic syndrome (MDS). MDS represents an example of anemia associated with ineffective hematopoiesis. Although mostly normocytic, the anemia in MDS is macrocytic in a substantial minority of the patients. **A**, The peripheral blood smear is characterized by oval macrocytes, red blood cell dimorphism, monocytosis, and pseudo–Pelger-Huet anomaly (granulocyte nuclear hypolobulation). **B**, The bone marrow aspirate shows asynchrony in nuclear-cytoplasmic maturation, erythroid nuclear dysplasia (multinucleation, nuclear budding), hypogranular myeloid cells, left-shifted myelopoiesis, and dysplastic megakaryopoiesis.

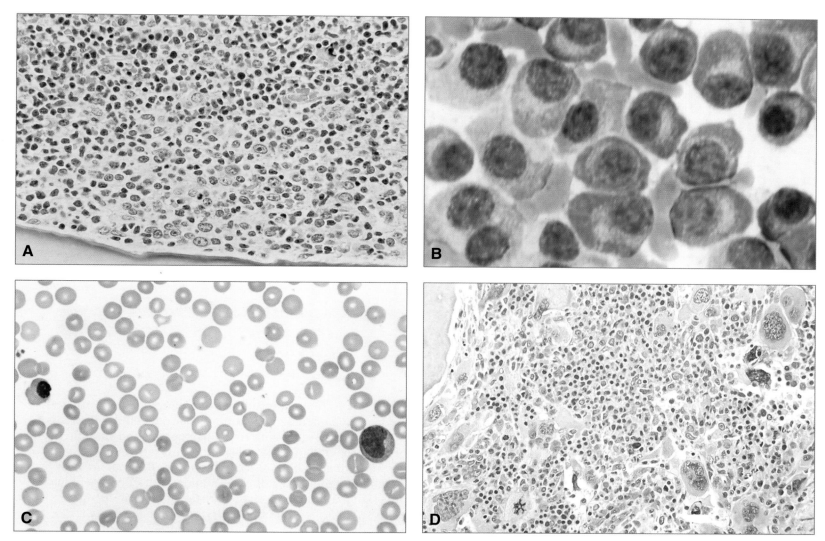

Figure 6-20. Processes that lead to decreased bone marrow. A decreased bone marrow reserve can result from a variety of infiltrative processes, including lymphoma (**A**), multiple myeloma (**B**), metastatic cancer (**C**), and bone marrow collagen deposition seen in myelofibrosis with myeloid metaplasia (**D**). Most of these conditions are associated with normocytic anemia and the presence of nucleated red blood cells, immature myeloid cells, and dacryocytosis in the peripheral smear (leukoerythroblastosis) (**C**).

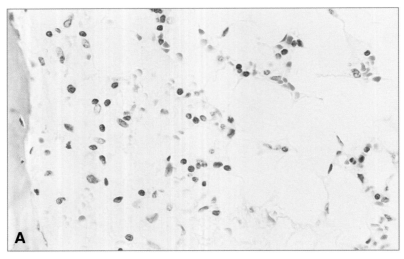

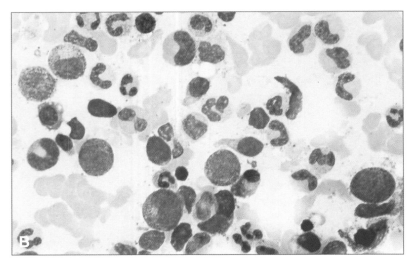

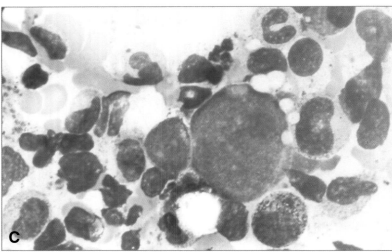

Figure 6-21. Anemia resulting from marrow failure. Aplastic anemia is characterized by a bone marrow cellularity of less than 20% associated with reticulocytopenia and variable degrees of pancytopenia (**A**). The aplastic process is selective to the erythroid lineage in pure red cell aplasia (**B**). Both aplastic anemia and pure red cell aplasia may result from a parvovirus infection that produces characteristic changes in the bone marrow, including vacuolated erythroid precursors (**C**).

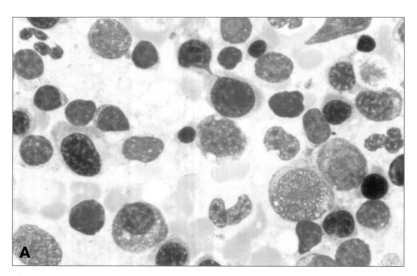

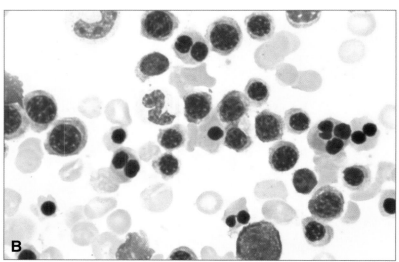

Figure 6-22. Anemia resulting from congenital dyserythropoietic anemia (CDA). CDA is a congenital anemia disorder that is characterized by marked erythroid dysplasia, ineffective erythropoiesis, and secondary hemochromatosis. In CDA type I, multinucleated erythroid precursors and internuclear chromatin bridges are seen (**A**). A similar histology is noted in CDA type II (**B**), also known as hereditary erythroblastic multinuclearity with positive acidified serum. Erythroid multinuclearity is marked in CDA type III.

The Hemolysis Work-up			
	All Types of Hemolytic Anemias	**Intravascular Hemolytic Anemia**	**Extravascular Hemolytic Anemia**
Reticulocyte count	Increased	Increased	Increased
LDH	Increased	Increased	Increased
Indirect bilirubin	Increased or normal	Increased	Increased or normal
Haptoglobin	Decreased	Decreased	Decreased
Urine hemosiderin	Present or absent	Present	Absent

Figure 6-23. The hemolysis work-up. The hemolytic anemias can be broadly divided into extravascular hemolytic anemia occurring in the monocyte-macrophage system of the spleen and intravascular hemolytic anemia occurring by lysis inside the blood vessels. During both processes, laboratory evidence of increased cell destruction (increased lactic dehydrogenase [LDH]), increased hemoglobin catabolism (increased levels of indirect bilirubin), and bone marrow regenerative effort (reticulocytosis) may be appreciated. Similarly, serum haptoglobin is expected to be low in both processes because of hemoglobin spillage from macrophages during extravascular hemolysis. On the other hand, the demonstration of hemosiderinuria or free plasma and urine hemoglobin is relatively specific for intravascular hemolytic anemia.

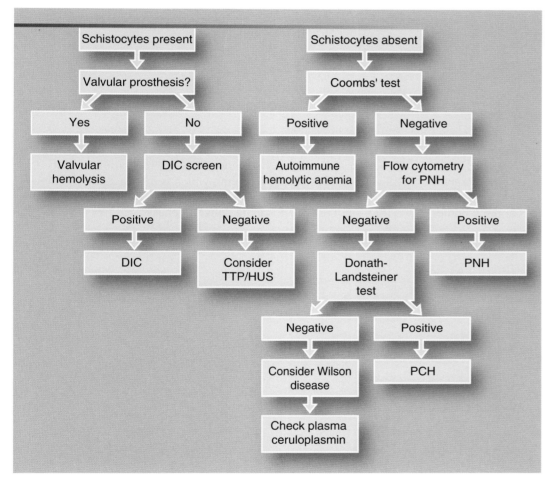

Figure 6-24. An algorithm for the evaluation of intravascular hemolysis. In intravascular hemolytic anemia, free hemoglobin in the plasma readily dissociates into β hemoglobin dimers. These are promptly picked up by haptoglobin and are carried to the liver, where they undergo intrahepatocyte degradation. The leftover hemoglobin dimers (unbound to haptoglobin) in the plasma are either filtered by the kidneys (32 kD) or the iron in the dimers is oxidized into the ferric state (methemoglobin). The methemoglobin in the plasma splits into globin and ferriheme. Ferriheme is picked up by either albumin (methemalbumin) or hemopexin (another plasma protein that binds ferriheme) and carried to the liver (hepatocytes) for the usual heme degradation process. The hemoglobin dimers excreted by the kidneys are resorbed by the proximal tubular cells, where they are degraded into hemosiderin, bilirubin, and globin. The tubular cells are shed every 2 to 7 days and the cellular iron deposits can be demonstrated with a Prussian blue stain of spun urine sediment (hemosiderinuria). In severe intravascular hemolytic anemia, excess filtered hemoglobin appears in the urine (hemoglobinuria). DIC—disseminated intravascular coagulation; HUS—hemolytic-uremic syndrome; PCH—paroxysmal cold hemoglobinuria; PNH—paroxysmal nocturnal hemoglobinuria; TTP—thrombotic thrombocytopenic purpura.

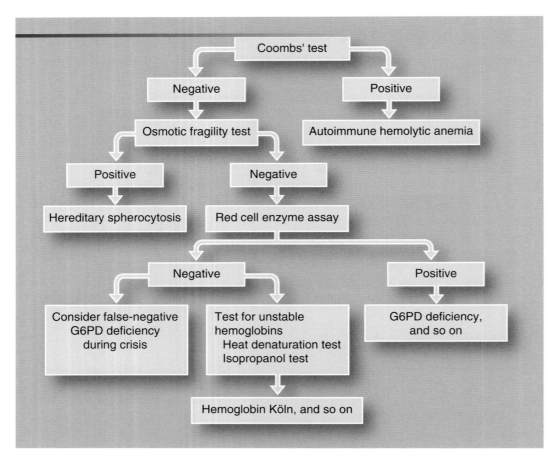

Figure 6-25. Evaluation of extravascular hemolytic anemia. In extravascular hemolytic anemia, the red cell is first phagocytosed into the macrophage (mostly in the spleen), where the cell membrane is disrupted and the hemoglobin separates into heme and globin. The globin disintegrates into its constituent amino acids and the heme is oxidized (heme oxygenase) by cleavage of the porphyrin ring into biliverdin, iron, and carbon monoxide. The biliverdin is reduced (biliverdin reductase) to bilirubin, which is released into the bloodstream, picked up by albumin, and carried to the liver (hepatocytes). G6PD—glucose-6-phosphate dehydrogenase.

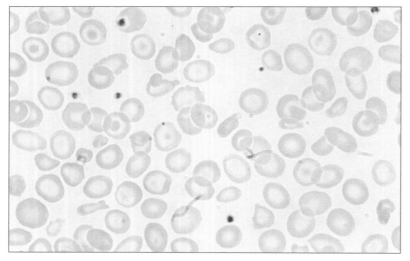

Figure 6-26. Peripheral smear from a patient with thalassemia major. In the evaluation of extravascular hematopoiesis, the ethnic origin from Southeast Asia, Africa, or the Mediterranean basin suggests the presence of a hemoglobinopathy such as thalassemia major or enzymopathy such as glucose-6-phosphate dehydrogenase (G6PD) deficiency (not shown). G6PD synthesis is under an X chromosome gene control and is therefore an X-linked trait affecting primarily males. The normal G6PD in whites is denoted as G6PD B+ (the wild type) and is found in 70% of blacks. Fifteen percent of the latter have the variant G6PD A+. Both these variants are functionally normal variants. Ten percent of blacks carry the defective allele and experience intermittent episodes of hemolysis. The G6PD variant in people of Mediterranean origin is G6PD B-, which has even lower enzyme activity and causes more severe and sometimes chronic hemolysis. In the latter group, the ingestion of uncooked fava beans (broad beans) may cause acute hemolysis (favism). The precipitation of the denatured product on the red cell membrane (Heinz body inclusions) is sometimes noted on the peripheral smear under special basic stain.

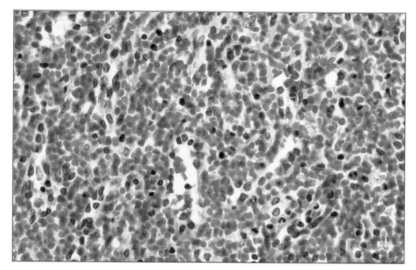

Figure 6-27. Spleen histology in a patient with hereditary sphero-cytosis (HS). The cause of hemolysis in HS is a defect in the skeletal proteins (spectrin, ankyrin, band 3 protein, protein 4.2) of the red cell membrane, which results in a spherocytic shape. As a result, they are trapped in the microcirculation of the spleen and are destroyed by the macrophages of the spleen. This leads to functional splenomegaly in the majority of the patients. Similarly, the chroni-cally increased production of bilirubin results in clinical jaundice and pigmented gall stone formation. Additional clinical features include periods of severe hypoproliferative anemia from either folate deficiency (megaloblastic crisis) or parvovirus B19 infection (aplastic crisis).

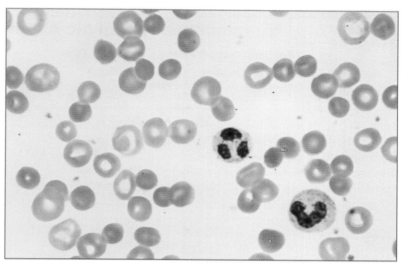

Figure 6-28. Spherocytic hemolytic anemia. The presence of spherocytes in the peripheral blood smear suggests either heredi-tary spherocytosis (HS) or autoimmune hemolytic anemia (AIHA). Spherocytes have increased osmotic fragility (because of decreased distensibility associated with reduced surface membrane) in hypo-tonic saline and this test (the osmotic fragility test) is positive in both HS and AIHA. The two are distinguished by the Coombs' test, which is positive in AIHA and negative in HS.

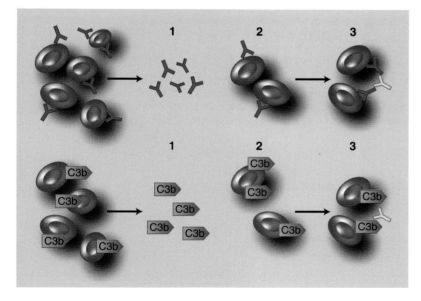

Figure 6-29. The Coombs' test. The purpose of the Coombs' test is to determine whether red cell–binding antibody (IgG) or comple-ment (C3) is present on the red cell membrane (the direct Coombs' test) or sera (the indirect Coombs' test). In the direct test, the patient's red cells are incubated with polyspecific rabbit antihuman IgG and anticomplement. In the presence of red cell–bound antibodies or complement, red cell agglutination occurs (positive Coombs' test). In the indirect test, another person's red cells (heterologous red cells) are first incubated with the patient's serum (to allow circulat-ing antibodies to bind to the red cells), and then a direct Coombs' test is performed. Monospecific sera can be used to detect only IgG or complement on the red cell. However, the Coombs' test does not detect IgM antibody and its presence is surmised by the detection of complement only on the red cells. A positive direct Coombs' test suggests the presence of autoantibodies to red cells. A positive indirect Coombs' with a negative direct test suggests the presence of alloantibodies to red cells. The indirect Coombs' test is also helpful for determining red cell antigen specificity to antibody.

Autoimmune Hemolytic Anemia

	Reaction Temperature	Antibody Type	Site of Hemolysis
Warm AIHA	Body temperature	IgG usually	Extravascular
Cold AIHA	4°–30°C	IgM usually, IgG in PCH	Intravascular

Figure 6-30. Autoimmune hemolytic anemia (AIHA). The red cell antibodies in AIHA may react best at body temperature (warm AIHA) or at temperatures between 4° and 30° C (cold AIHA). The antibody in warm AIHA is usually IgG and does not bind complement. As such, red cell destruction in warm AIHA is primarily extravascular and involves antibody-mediated phagocytosis by the reticuloendothelial system. Cold AIHA, in contrast, is usually IgM mediated and involves complement fixation and complement-mediated intravascular red cell lysis. IgG-mediated cold AIHA is represented by paroxysmal cold hemoglobinuria (PCH).

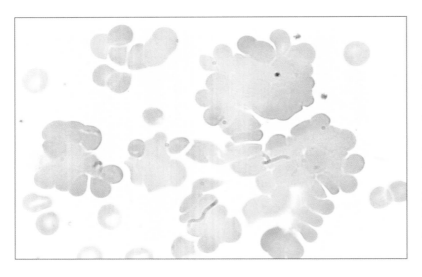

Figure 6-31. Red cell agglutination in a patient with cold agglutinin disease. Cold autoimmune hemolytic anemia (AIHA) may be either IgM or IgG mediated. IgM-mediated cold AIHA may be idiopathic or associated with infections (Epstein-Barr virus, mycoplasma), lymphoma, or autoimmune diseases. The Coombs' test is positive (anticomplement only) and the blood smear may show red cell agglutination. The cold agglutinin titer is often greater than 1:1000. IgG-mediated cold AIHA is represented by paroxysmal cold hemoglobinuria (PCH). The direct Coombs' test is positive (due to the presence of complement only) during or following an acute hemolytic episode. However, the test can be negative during remission. The cold agglutinin titer is usually low (< 1:64). The diagnosis of PCH is confirmed by the Donath-Landsteiner test.

Terms with Relevance to the Cold Agglutinin Test

Term	Definition
Cold agglutinin	An immunoglobulin (antibody) that causes red cell agglutination in lower than body temperature conditions. The clinical phenotype includes cold-induced hemolytic anemia and acral symptoms. The red cell epitope is "I" in idiopathic CAD and either "I" (mycoplasma pneumonia) or "i" (infectious mononucleosis) in secondary CAD. The anti "P" antibody that causes hemolysis in paroxysmal cold hemoglobinuria is IgG instead of IgM and causes hemolysis (cold hemolysin) rather than agglutination in the cold.
Cryoglobulin	An immunoglobulin or immunoglobulin–immunoglobulin complex that undergoes reversible precipitation in lower than body temperature conditions.
Cryoglobulinemia	A condition characterized by the presence of cryoglobulin (cold-induced acral symptoms and immune complex–mediated vasculitis).
	Type I: monoclonal, usually vasculitis
	Type II: monoclonal (usually IgM) associated with polyclonal (usually IgG)
	Type III: polyclonal, associated with polyclonal (usually IgM against IgG)

Figure 6-32. Cold agglutinin titer and the Donath-Landsteiner test. The cold agglutinin titer test is used to detect and quantify cold-reacting immunoglobulins (mostly IgM). Red cells from affected patients are incubated at 4° C overnight in serially diluted autologous serum. The dilution factor that results in red cell agglutination is reported as the cold agglutinin titer. Clinically relevant hemolysis occurs at titers of more than 1:256. Most cold autoimmune hemolytic anemia is IgM-mediated, whereas paroxysmal cold hemoglobinuria is IgG-mediated. The laboratory diagnosis of paroxysmal cold hemoglobinuria involves the Donath-Landsteiner test. This test involves preincubation of a patient's red cells with autologous serum at 4° C followed by the addition of complement at 37° C. A positive test is characterized by visible hemolysis. Antigen specificity in cold autoimmune hemolytic anemia is labeled "i" for infectious mononucleosis and "P" for paroxysmal cold hemoglobinuria. CAD—cold agglutinin disease.

Alloimmune Hemolytic Anemia

Subtypes	Antibody Type	Type of Hemolysis	Frequent Cause
HDN	IgG	Extravascular	Previous pregnancy or transfusion
IHTR	IgM	Intravascular	Clerical error
DHTR	IgG	Extravascular	Recent RBC transfusion

Figure 6-33. Alloimmune hemolytic anemia. Three clinical conditions illustrate alloimmune hemolytic anemia: hemolytic disease of the newborn (HDN), immediate hemolytic transfusion reaction (IHTR), and delayed HTR (DHTR). IHTR occurs when patients are mistakenly (most frequently from clerical error) transfused with red cell antigen (ABO, Kell, Jkᵃ, Fyᵃ) mismatched blood. The recipient's preexisting, usually IgM, antibodies bind to the donor's red cells and cause a complement-mediated intravascular hemolysis. DHTR is characterized by the onset of anemia after 5 to 10 days following red blood cell (RBC) transfusion. DHTR is an extravascular hemolysis that results from an anamnestic response in a presensitized patient in whom pretransfusion antibody testing missed identification because of low antibody titers. HDN represents hemolysis in the fetus or newborn by antibodies produced by the mother.

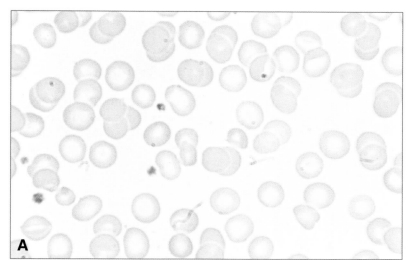

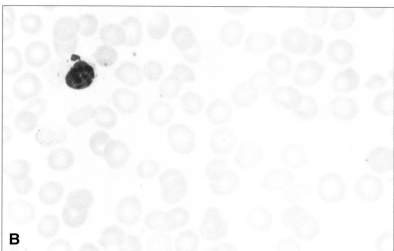

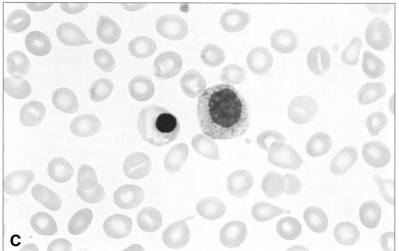

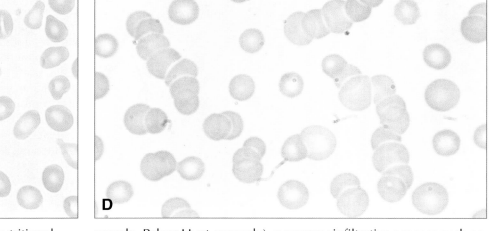

Figure 6-34. Normocytic anemia not associated with nutritional deficiency, renal insufficiency, bleeding, or hemolysis. The primary consideration in this setting is either anemia of chronic disease (ACD) or a primary bone marrow disorder. It is not always easy to differentiate the two. The peripheral smear examination is unremarkable in ACD (**A**). In contrast, characteristic changes are seen in the myelodysplastic syndrome (**B**; dimorphic red cell populations, pseudo–Pelger-Huet anomaly), a marrow infiltrative process such as metastatic cancer or bone marrow fibrosis (**C**; teardrop-shaped and nucleated red cells, immature myeloid precursors), and multiple myeloma (**D**; red cell rouleaux formation). In addition to anemia, a primary bone marrow disease also results in quantitative and qualitative abnormalities of white blood cells and platelets.

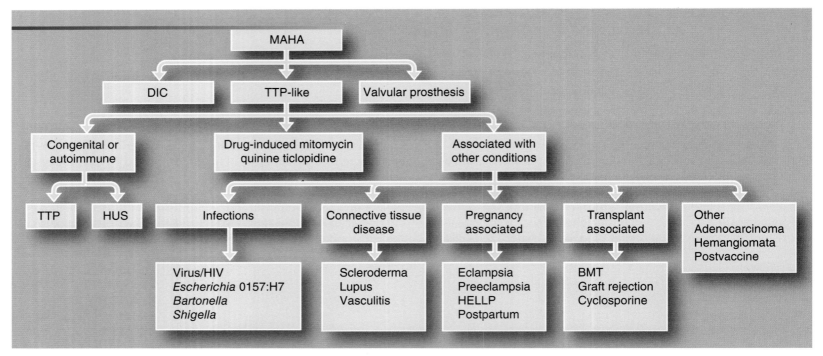

Figure 6-35. The microangiopathic hemolytic anemia (MAHA) process. MAHA is defined as an intravascular hemolytic process that is a result of red cell injury by an abnormal endothelial surface. In thrombotic thrombocytopenic purpura (TTP), the pathogenesis has been linked to severe deficiency of the enzyme (protease) that cleaves the von Willebrand factor (vWF). The protease defi-ciency is secondary to genetic mutation in familial TTP and an antibody-mediated inhibition of the enzyme in the sporadic form. BMT—bone marrow transplant; DIC—disseminated intravascular coagulation; HELLP—hemolysis, elevated liver enzymes, and low platelet syndrome; HUS—hemolytic-uremic syndrome.

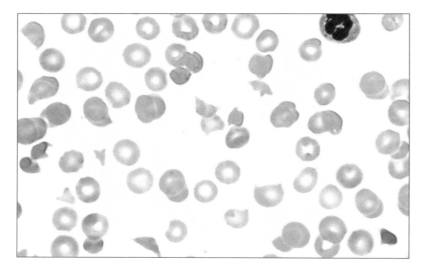

Figure 6-36. Peripheral smear showing schistocytosis and thrombocytopenia. All patients with thrombotic thrombocytopenic purpura (TTP) and hemolytic-uremic syndrome (HUS) have schistocytosis, intravascular hemolysis (high lactic dehydrogenase, low haptoglobin), and thrombocytopenia. In addition, approximately 70% of the patients with TTP may have fluctuating neurologic changes, renal insufficiency, and/or fever. Patients with HUS have renal insufficiency without neurologic disease. Plasma exchange (the combination of plasmapheresis and normal fresh frozen plasma infusion) is the cornerstone of therapy for both TTP and HUS. Platelet transfusion is best avoided unless the patient is bleeding.

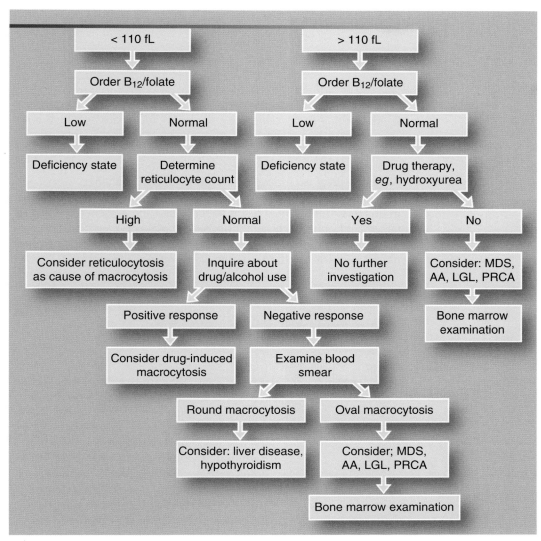

Figure 6-37. Subclassification of macrocytic anemia based on mean corpuscular volume (MCV). In general, an MCV value of above 110 fL is often associated with oval (megaloblastic) macrocytosis and the differential diagnosis with such marked macrocytosis is narrow, as indicated here. All causes of marked macrocytosis can also cause macrocytic anemia with an MCV of 100 to 110 fL. This is also the range of MCV value that is often associated with causes of round (nonmegalobalstic) macrocytosis including excess alcohol consumption, liver disease, and reticulocytosis. AA—aplastic anemia; LGL—large granular lymphocytosis; MDS—myelodysplastic syndrome; PRCA—pure red cell aplasia.

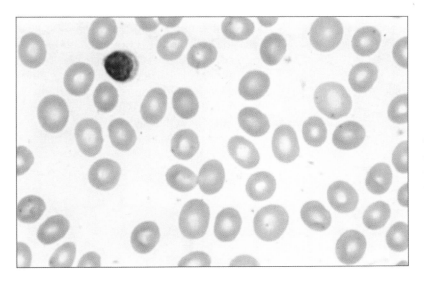

Figure 6-38. Evaluation of macrocytic anemia. The first step is to exclude substance (alcohol) or drug (eg, hydroxyurea) use that is associated with macrocytosis. Similarly, in any patient with macrocytosis, B_{12} or folate deficiency must be ruled out. In folate deficiency, serum folate levels are usually low. However, because recent dietary changes may affect the serum folate level, the serum homocysteine level may be used, instead, to evaluate folate deficiency (the serum homocysteine level is increased during folate deficiency as a result of impaired folate-dependent conversion of homocysteine to methionine).

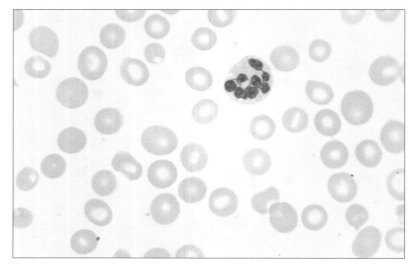

Figure 6-39. Oval macrocytes and hypersegmented neutrophils in B₁₂ deficiency. In B₁₂ deficiency, serum B₁₂ levels are usually but not always low. A more sensitive and highly specific test is measurement of serum methylmalonic acid level (B₁₂ cofactor activity is required to convert methylmalonyl coenzyme A to succinyl coenzyme A). A normal level excludes the possibility of B₁₂ deficiency. Once B₁₂ deficiency is confirmed, the next step is to determine the cause. In this regard, the initial test is to screen for the presence of intrinsic factor antibodies. If these antibodies are present, then a working diagnosis of pernicious anemia is made and additional testing may not be necessary. Otherwise, the Schilling test is performed.

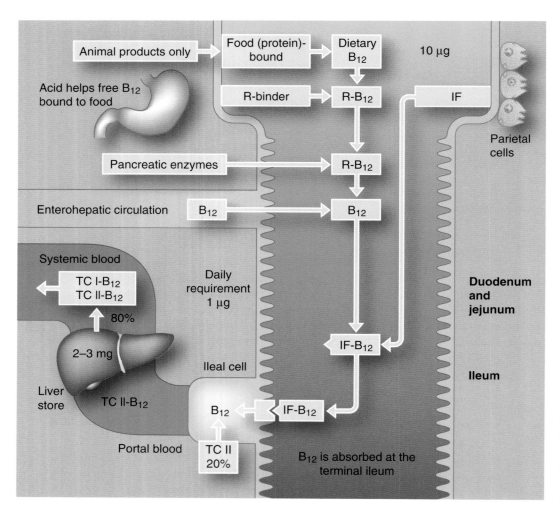

Figure 6-40. Vitamin B₁₂ absorption and transport. Vitamin B₁₂ in food is bound to protein and must undergo peptic digestion in the acidic environment of the stomach to be released. In the stomach, the food-free form initially binds to salivary haptocorrin (a vitamin B₁₂–binding protein formerly known as R-binder) only to be rereleased again in the duodenum after pancreatic enzymes degrade the haptocorrin. In the duodenum, the free vitamin B₁₂ combines with another B₁₂-binder (intrinsic factor [IF]) secreted by the parietal cells of the stomach. Vitamin B₁₂ is absorbed at the terminal ileum, and then only when it is bound to intrinsic factor. Once absorbed, vitamin B₁₂ is freed from the B₁₂-IF complex and released into the blood where it is transported by a specific carrier protein, transcobalamin II (TC II). However, 80% of plasma vitamin B₁₂ is bound to other serum haptocorrins (TC III and I). The TC II-B₁₂ complex is carried to cells and is pinocytosed via TC II receptors. Intracellularly, vitamin B₁₂ joins forces with folate and assists in DNA synthesis.

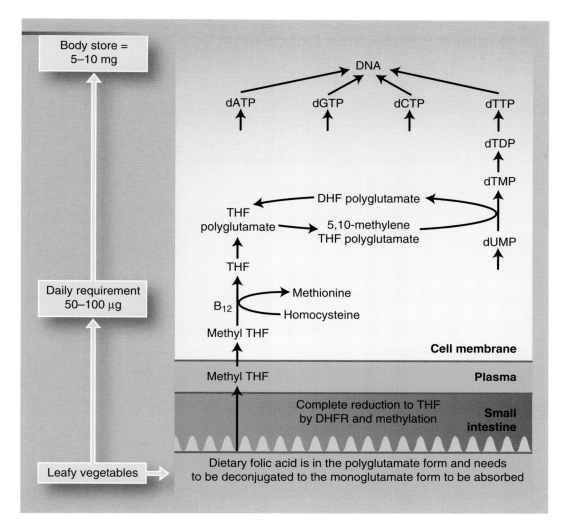

Figure 6-41. Folate digestion and absorption. Dietary folic acid is in the polyglutamate form that is deconjugated to the monoglutamate form during absorption. In the mucosa, folic acid undergoes complete reduction by dihydrofolate reductase (DHFR) into tetrahydrofolate (THF). It is then methylated and released into the blood and transported (no specific carrier protein) into the target cells where it transfers its methyl group to homocysteine to form methionine and THF. This reaction is made possible by the enzyme methionine synthetase that requires vitamin B_{12} as a cofactor. THF is used in the transfer of one-carbon fragments from donors such as serine to DNA bases.

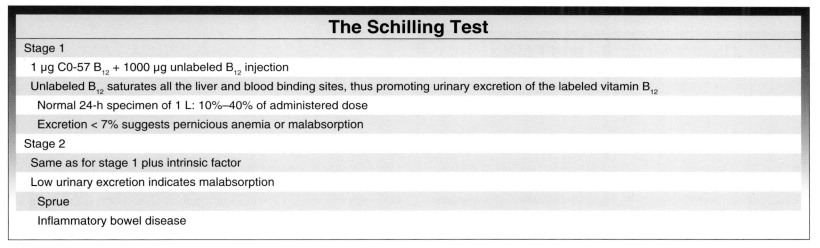

The Schilling Test

Stage 1
1 μg C0-57 B_{12} + 1000 μg unlabeled B_{12} injection
Unlabeled B_{12} saturates all the liver and blood binding sites, thus promoting urinary excretion of the labeled vitamin B_{12}
Normal 24-h specimen of 1 L: 10%–40% of administered dose
Excretion < 7% suggests pernicious anemia or malabsorption
Stage 2
Same as for stage 1 plus intrinsic factor
Low urinary excretion indicates malabsorption
Sprue
Inflammatory bowel disease

Figure 6-42. Stages of the Schilling test. The Schilling test helps differentiate pernicious anemia (PA) from primary intestinal malabsorptive disorders (celiac sprue, inflammatory bowel disease). The test is performed in two stages. In the first stage, the patient receives, simultaneously, 1 mg of unlabeled B_{12} (intramuscular injection) to saturate B_{12}-binding proteins and 1 μg of radiolabeled crystalline B_{12} (oral). A 24-hour urine collection follows immediately, and if detected radioactivity in the urine is more than 7% of the ingested load, the result is considered normal and the patient does not have problems absorbing crystalline B_{12}. Therefore, a normal stage 1 Schilling test rules out PA but not malabsorption from gastric atrophy (elderly patients may have difficulty absorbing food-bound B_{12}, which requires gastric acid and pepsin to release B_{12}). However, an abnormal stage 1 test suggests either PA or a primary intestinal malabsorption disorder. Correction of an abnormal stage 1 result by the addition of intrinsic factor to the oral B_{12} dose (stage 2 Schilling test) establishes the diagnosis of PA. However, an abnormal stage 2 test does not rule out the possibility of PA because the disease may secondarily affect the intestinal epithelium and mimic a primary malabsorptive syndrome. Therefore, the best time to do the Schilling test is after 2 weeks of treatment with B_{12}, which allows healing of the absorptive surface.

Causes of Vitamin B$_{12}$ and Folate Deficiency

Folate Deficiency	B$_{12}$ Deficiency
Inadequate diet	Inadequate diet
Alcoholism and drug addiction	Strict vegetarians
Malnourished elderly	
Parenteral nutrition	
Increased requirement	Malabsorption due to IF deficiency or achlorhydria
Hemolytic anemia	Pernicious anemia
Exfoliative dermatitis	Gastric surgery
Pregnancy	Proton pump inhibitor therapy
Hemodialysis	Food-bound B$_{12}$ deficiency
Malabsorption due to intestinal disease	Malabsorption due to competing intestinal flora
Sprue	*Diphyllobothrium latum* (fish tapeworm)
Inflammatory bowel disease	Bacterial overgrowth (blind loop syndrome)
Small bowel resection (short bowel syndrome)	
Drug-induced low serum folate levels	Malabsorption due to intestinal disease
Phenytoin (mechanism unknown)	Celiac sprue
Sulfasalazine (impairs intestinal deconjugation)	Inflammatory bowel disease
Oral contraceptives	Small bowel resection
Alcohol (inhibits folate release from liver to bile)	
Folate antagonists	Intracellular unavailability (very rare)
Methotrexate (DHF reductase inhibitor)	TC II deficiency
Pentamidine	Nitrous oxide (oxidizes B$_{12}$)
Trimethoprim	Imerslund-Graesbeck syndrome (*ie*, absence of B$_{12}$ binders)
Pyrimethamine	

Figure 6-43. Causes of vitamin B$_{12}$ and folate deficiency. IF—intrinsic factor; DHF—dihydrofolate; TC—transcobalamin.

Daily Vitamin B$_{12}$ and Folate Requirements and Body Stores

	Vitamin B$_{12}$	Folic Acid
Daily requirements	0.5–1 µg	50–100 µg
Body stores	2000–5000 µg	5000–10,000 µg

Figure 6-44. Daily vitamin B$_{12}$ and folate requirements and body stores. Leafy vegetables are rich in folate, whereas animal products are the only sources of dietary B$_{12}$ (cyanocobalamin). The average daily Western diet contains approximately 5 to 10 times the daily requirements of each vitamin. The principal storage site for both vitamins is the liver. One can thus appreciate that it only takes 1 to 3 months to deplete the folate store while it may take several years to deplete the vitamin B$_{12}$ store. In general, diet is important in folate deficiency, whereas intestinal malabsorption is the usual cause of vitamin B$_{12}$ deficiency. Excessive cooking reduces available folate in the diet.

Clinical and Laboratory Effects of Vitamin B$_{12}$ and Folate Deficiency

	Vitamin B$_{12}$ Deficiency	Folate Deficiency
Megaloblastic anemia	Yes	Yes
Glossitis	Yes	Yes
Cheilitis	Yes	Yes
Intestinal malabsorption	Yes	Yes
Neurologic complications	Yes	No
Elevated serum homocysteine	Yes	Yes
Elevated serum methylmalonic acid	Yes	No

Figure 6-45. Clinical and laboratory effects of B$_{12}$ and folate deficiency. A deficiency in either folate or vitamin B$_{12}$ results in impaired DNA synthesis affecting all actively replicating cells. This is clinically manifested, usually, as megaloblastic anemia. In addition, the gastrointestinal system is often involved and the pathologic lesions include atrophic tongue, glossitis, cheilosis, and secondary intestinal malabsorption. The nervous system may be affected with vitamin B$_{12}$ but not folate deficiency. The pathogenesis of B$_{12}$ neuropathy is not known. Clinically, the process may affect the peripheral nerves (symmetrical mixed motor and sensory neuropathy), the spinal cord with demyelination of the posterior and the lateral columns (subacute combined system disease), and the brain.

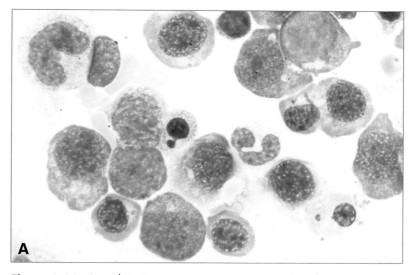

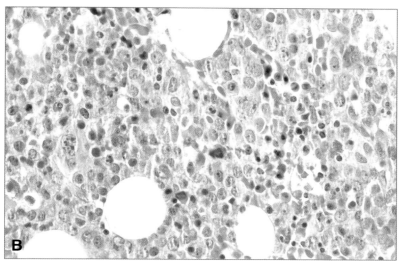

Figure 6-46. A and **B**, Pernicious anemia (PA). PA is the most frequent cause of vitamin B$_{12}$ deficiency. It is caused by idiopathic intrinsic factor (IF) deficiency. Possible autoimmune origin is suggested by the presence in most, but not all, of serum antibodies against both the parietal cells and IF, and the increased incidence of other autoimmune diseases (Hashimoto thyroiditis, vitiligo). The disease is associated with gastric mucosal atrophy and achlorhydria (since the parietal cells also produce gastric acid). Bone marrow shows nuclear-cytoplasmic asynchrony in maturation (megaloblastic changes) and giant myelocytes and metamyelocytes.

Treatment of Vitamin B$_{12}$ and Folate Deficiency

	Vitamin B$_{12}$	Folic Acid
Parenteral given either intramuscularly or subcutaneously	1000 µg/mo	Not applicable
Oral tablets	500–1000 µg/d	1 mg/d

Figure 6-47. Treatment of vitamin B$_{12}$ and folate deficiency. It is critical that accurate diagnosis be made before starting therapy. This is because folate supplementation may mask underlying B$_{12}$ deficiency by improving the anemia, but not the neurologic disease, associated with vitamin B$_{12}$ deficiency and thus allowing the neuropathy to progress. B$_{12}$ deficiency may be treated either parenterally or orally. Neurologic complications from B$_{12}$ deficiency are not always reversible with treatment.

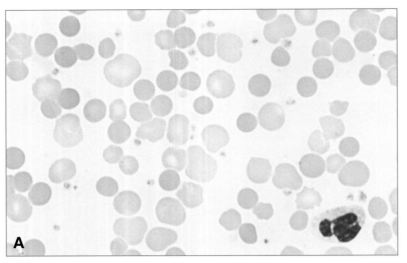

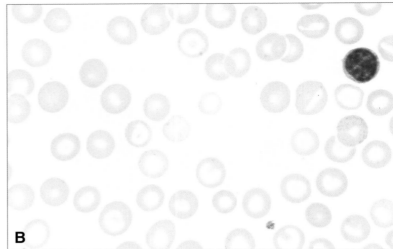

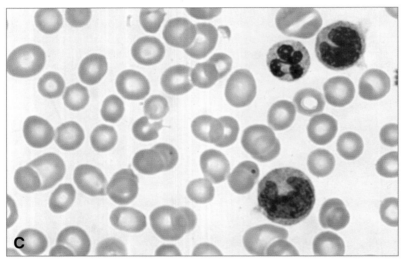

Figure 6-48. Non-nutritional macrocytic anemia that is not drug induced. Substantial polychromasia (indicative of reticulocytosis) suggests hemolysis as the cause of macrocytosis (**A**). Round morphology of the red cells, as opposed to oval macrocytosis, suggests liver disease (target cells are also evident) (**B**). Oval macrocytosis is characteristic of myelodysplastic syndrome, aplastic anemia, large granular lymphocytic leukemia, or pure red cell aplasia (**C**). Diagnosis of these disorders requires bone marrow examination with cytogenetic studies.

RECOMMENDED READING

Carmel R: Anemia and aging: an overview of clinical, diagnostic and biological issues. *Blood Rev* 2001, 15:9–18.

Fishbane S: Anemia treatment in chronic renal insufficiency. *Semin Nephrol* 2002, 22:474–478.

Gabrilove J: Overview: erythropoiesis, anemia, and the impact of erythropoietin. *Semin Hematol* 2000, 37(4 Suppl 6):1–3.

Gehrs BC, Friedberg RC: Autoimmune hemolytic anemia. *Am J Hematol* 2002, 69:258–271.

Greenberg PL, Gordeuk V, Issaragrisil S, *et al.*: Major hematologic diseases in the developing world: new aspects of diagnosis and management of thalassemia, malarial anemia, and acute leukemia. *Am Soc Hematol Educ Program* 2001, 479–498.

Means RT Jr: Advances in the anemia of chronic disease. *Int J Hematol* 1999, 70:7–12.

Paquette RL: Diagnosis and management of aplastic anemia and myelodysplastic syndrome. *Oncology (Huntingt)* 2002, 16(9 Suppl 10):153–161.

Sullivan P: Associations of anemia, treatments for anemia, and survival in patients with human immunodeficiency virus infection. *J Infect Dis* 2002, 185(Suppl 2):S138–S142.

CHAPTER 7

Hematopoietic Stem Cells and Cytokines

John G. Sharp and John D. Jackson, Jr.

Hematopoietic stem cells (HSCs) represent a hierarchy of cells resident primarily in adult bone marrow that give rise to blood cells and immune cells throughout life [1]. Several steps in these processes, including survival and the regulation of symmetric (self-renewal) divisions of undifferentiated, uncommitted HSCs and the amplification and positive and negative selection of thymus-processed lymphocytes (T cells), appear to require direct cell contact, likely integrin mediated, of the target (undifferentiated) cell with microenvironmental stromal cells of the hematopoietic microenvironment (HM) or are influenced by factors produced locally by the HM. Most proliferation (transit amplification divisions) and differentiation steps required to generate functional hematopoietic and immune cells are regulated by soluble proteins that are generically termed *cytokines*. This generic description comprises a number of structurally distinct families of glycoproteins, including colony-stimulating factors, interleukins, and chemokines, that via different families of receptors influence multiple cellular behaviors. Structurally related families of cytokines usually have multiple members. This complexity results in a dizzying array of potential regulatory interactions. The interaction of a given cytokine with its receptor initiates a pathway of signaling interactions within target cells. Cellular signaling mechanisms are "networked." Consequently, the delivery of multiple signals to a target cell with receptors for more than one cytokine not only results in a response to more than one signal, but the outcome(s) is modulated by intracellular interactions between the various signal transduction pathways activated by the original cytokine signals. Inhibitory mechanisms also exist that suppress cytokine signaling.

The differentiation of HSCs and their interactions with cells comprising the HM were diagrammed by Maximow around 1900. HMs maintain and support hematopoietic cells, and within HMs there are specialized locations that maintain HSCs; these areas are known as *stem cell niches*, a term introduced by Schofield in 1978. Currently, at this point agreement ends. Taichman and Emerson [2] proposed that osteoblasts were the primary HSC niche cells. This is supported by studies by Li's group employing bone morphogenic protein receptor (BMPR) knockout mice that have increased osteoblasts and correspondingly increased HSCs [3]. This hypothesis is also supported by the work of Scadden's group, who administered parathyroid hormone to increase osteoblast numbers (an effect described morphologically in 1950 using parathyroid extract), which concomitantly increased HSCs [4]. Other groups also favor a role for osteoblasts [5,6]. Additionally, Visnjic *et al.* [7] constructed an osteoblast-depleted mouse that was associated with a decline of HSCs. Osteopontin is implicated in these effects [8].

In contrast, Morrison's group, primarily employing immunocytochemistry for *SLAM* markers of stem cells (CD150+, CD48−), noted HSCs in bone marrow localized in proximity to endothelial cells [9]. Other data support such an association. Moreover, some endothelial cells are associated with HSCs [10]. These observations contrast with the original studies of the maintenance of HSCs in long-term bone marrow cultures [11]. In such cultures, endothelial cells are present but rare [12] and osteoblasts are absent after a week or two of culture. Rather, an undifferentiated large mesenchymal or "blanket" cell, which is associated with HSC "cobblestone areas," was proposed to be key for HSC maintenance [11]. The section on microenvironments attempts to synthesize these variant views into a rational proposition.

The molecular mechanisms that regulate HSC self-renewal and proliferation and promote or inhibit differentiation are progressively being revealed. The signaling pathways involved function during development to establish patterning and cellular systems and, in adults, to maintain stem cells. These pathways include Wnt and Wnt ligands and Frizzled and Dickkopf, which are involved in HSC self-renewal, acting via β-catenin and Tcf/Lef transcription. Bone morphogenic proteins (BMPs) and BMP antagonists function to promote stem cell differentiation and inhibit differentiation, respectively. Hedgehog proteins are expressed by some stem/progenitor cell populations, such as in multiple myeloma, and may be mitogenic. Polycomb proteins, which are involved in chromatin remodeling, eg, Bmi-1, are involved in stem cell self-renewal [13]. Potentially, part of the mechanism involves Bmi-1 down-regulation of *p16ink4a* and *p19Arf* activity. Expression of these genes is elevated in the absence of Bmi-1, and p16 is associated with cellular senescence. Knockout of *p16* may increase stem cell proliferation. In the hematopoietic system, levels of *p53* are also altered. However, in mice, removing *p16* activity can promote the onset and incidence of tumors [14], which suggests that caution will be needed in the manipulation of these genes. The notch pathway and notch ligands Delta-like and Jagged-1, together with notch inhibitor Numb, have a role in stem cell maintenance in several tissue systems and may be involved in initial differentiation of stem cells to progenitor cells. A number of other molecules, such as prostaglandin E_2 and various cytokines, influence stem cell numbers, but these likely act via secondary pathways, such as Jak/Stat.

Historically, Maximow postulated a linear branching hierarchy of connective tissue cells, also including hematopoietic cells, arising from a common precursor (monophyletic theory). Downey in the 1930s promoted a competing polyphyletic theory, which postulated that there were multiple lineage-specific stem cell populations. This issue is still not satisfactorily settled. Transplantation experiments in mouse, with implications for humans, established that a single HSC could repopulate the entire lymphohematopoietic system, compatible with the monophyletic theory. However, transplanted bone marrow cells give rise to cells in liver, lung, retina, and muscle as well as cardiomyocytes, gut cells, endothelia, and other cell types. Some but probably not all of these "transdifferentiation" or "plasticity" events arise via cell fusion [15], but the totality of mechanisms remains to be defined [16]. This continues to be a very controversial topic. However, a potential fallacy underlying the interpretation of experiments purportedly demonstrating "plasticity" is the assumption that bone marrow contains only a single stem cell population (HSCs). If marrow were to contain multiple stem cell populations, including HSCs, endothelial cells, mesenchymal stromal cells, and possibly epithelial and muscle stem cells, then the issue of plasticity might be moot and fusion a rare, probably physiologic, mechanism of rescue of damaged cells from death [17]. Instead, a "network" of multiple stem cell populations with interacting progeny could generate a functioning tissue in a manner similar to the mechanism by which interacting cytokines and signaling pathways integrate and regulate stem cell differentiation to functional progeny.

Multiple cellular interactions are required for normal functioning of the hematopoietic system. Consequently, many genes must be transcribed, or their transcription repressed, in a time-dependent manner for the system to work properly. This process involves not only cell–cell interactions and cytokine stimulation or inhibition but also small regulatory RNA species (micro RNAs). These events have to be integrated and networked to produce an appropriate type and number of blood or immune cells and to respond to demands caused by stress such as bleeding or infection. Because of its structure, the hematopoietic system is susceptible to genetic abnormalities, both inherited and acquired. If key genes are absent, or mutated, they are untranscribed or improperly transcribed and deficiencies of mature cells may result, giving rise to disorders such as aplasias or immunodeficiency diseases. Such abnormalities may arise because of a cellular defect or a cytokine abnormality. If genes are translocated, their regulation may be disrupted, leading to underproduction or, more noticeably, overproduction of stem or progenitor cell progeny. A prime example is the *bcr-abl* translocation, evident in many cases—such as the Philadelphia chromosome—that underlies chronic myelogenous leukemia. Lists of such stem cell–related diseases and cytokine abnormalities are provided.

With regard to clinical applications of HSC therapy, originally bone marrow (1968 to early 1990s) and subsequently blood stem cells have been the primary stem cell source employed clinically. Other stem cell populations including cord blood/placental cells, hepatocytes, and adipocytes have been proposed and employed. Of these, the use of cord blood/placental cells has become standard in pediatric patients and increasingly offers potential for treatment of adults. The clinical use of proposed alternative stem cell sources, such as purportedly infinitely renewable embryonic stem cells, is well in the future—provided fundamental problems such as tumorigenesis and tissue matching can be overcome. Also, issues of donor safety of some proposed sources of stem cells, such as amniotic fluid stem cells, must be addressed. In this chapter, potential sources of stem cells for transplantation are described together with diseases that might be ameliorated using cell transplants. The role of cytokines in the outcomes of cell therapies is also described.

The emphasis of this chapter is on human hematopoietic stem cells, with reference to animal data when analyses in humans would be inappropriate. Although a wide range of cytokine families are described briefly, the emphasis is on agents that have been or are currently employed clinically. Some agents with currently limited applications, such as FLT3L as a cytokine, are not discussed in detail. Additionally, reference is made briefly to topics such as hematopoiesis, cytokines and aging, anemias, and myelodysplasia, which are likely to increase in clinical prominence as baby boomers age. Nonhematopoietic uses of bone marrow cells in cardiac repair are briefly described as an example of the expanding applications of HSCs. Potential new clinical uses of nonhematopoietic—namely, mesenchymal—cells from bone marrow are mentioned. Several examples of the clinical applications of cytokines are described. The pace of innovation in this field appears to have slowed, with the emphasis shifting to generating longer-acting formulations of these agents that are easier to use in clinical practice. However, several formulations of the widely used erythropoiesis-stimulating agent erythropoietin have recently given rise to concerns over safety and efficacy [18]. This emphasizes both ongoing innovation of technologies in the application of HSCs and cytokines and the fluidity of this field of endeavor. Continuing education is an imperative. We acknowledge the availability of the first edition of this chapter by Peter Quesenberry, MD, and Mehrdad Abedi, MD. Rapid progress in the understanding of HSCs and cytokines and advances in clinical applications have necessitated significant revisions. However, the general topics and structure of the original chapter have been retained and limited, more recent references added. The emphasis is to provide a guide to the reader on a variety of topics rather than to present an exhaustive analysis. Additional reading on specific topics is therefore recommended.

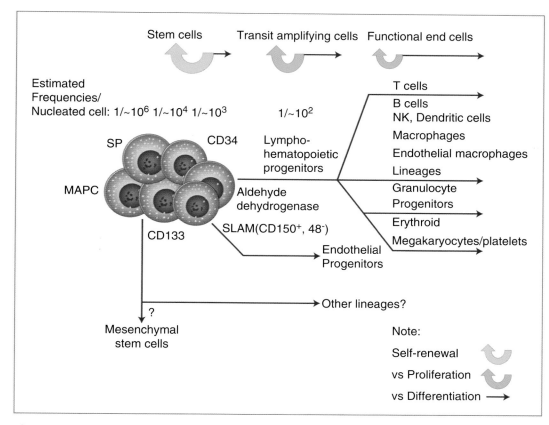

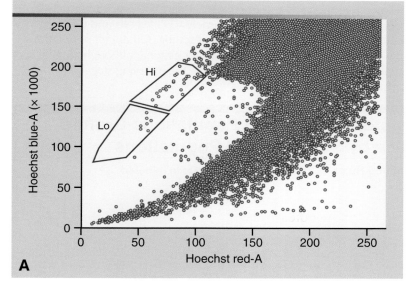

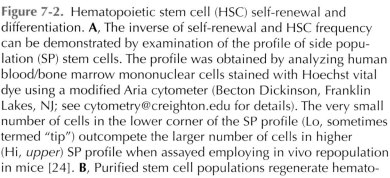

Figure 7-1. Overview of the hematopoietic stem cell (HSC) compartment. The HSC compartment, in terms of self-renewal versus differentiation, appears to consist of a hierarchy of cells whose phenotypic and functional characteristics partially overlap. Self-renewal ability declines as differentiation increases, but the frequency of cells increases. A cell with considerable potential is the multi-potential adult progenitor cell (MAPC) [19]. The ability of this cell to produce all types of hematopoietic cells has recently been verified [20], but questions remain about the ability of MAPC to generate other lineages. Other cell types in the HSC compartment are identified based primarily on alternative methods of isolation and include side population (SP) stem cells [21]. A cell identified by the Miltenyi AC133 antibody, now termed the *CD133 marker*, can give rise to both HSCs and endothelial cells [22]. Other markers of stem cells are aldehyde dehydrogenase [23] and the *SLAM* markers [9]. These self-renewing stem cells give rise to transit-amplifying lymphohematopoietic progenitor cells that show increasing lineage commitment and express lineage markers and decreasing proliferative abilities. Eventually, these progenitors differentiate terminally into specific lineages of cells, of which some, such as erythroid cells, lose proliferative ability. Other lineages, such as T cells, retain the ability to proliferate and expand as a component of their functions, even though functionally they are differentiated cells. NK—natural killer.

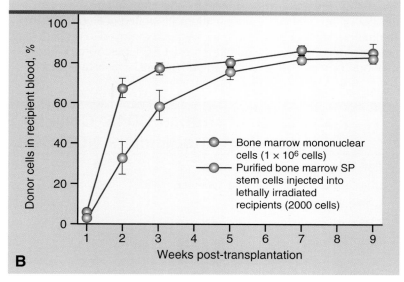

Figure 7-2. Hematopoietic stem cell (HSC) self-renewal and differentiation. **A**, The inverse of self-renewal and HSC frequency can be demonstrated by examination of the profile of side population (SP) stem cells. The profile was obtained by analyzing human blood/bone marrow mononuclear cells stained with Hoechst vital dye using a modified Aria cytometer (Becton Dickinson, Franklin Lakes, NJ; see cytometry@creighton.edu for details). The very small number of cells in the lower corner of the SP profile (Lo, sometimes termed "tip") outcompete the larger number of cells in higher (Hi, *upper*) SP profile when assayed employing in vivo repopulation in mice [24]. **B**, Purified stem cell populations regenerate hemato- poiesis in recipients undergoing myeloablative therapies almost as rapidly as whole bone marrow. For example, SP cells with a frequency of about one in 10,000 nucleated cells have the long-term repopulating abilities of the nucleated cells of whole bone marrow. There can be a slight delay in early repopulation in mice receiving SP cells, presumably because committed progenitor cells that quickly give rise to progeny are excluded. There is a great variability in the extent of self-renewal and production of clonal progeny between individual stem cells, and there is evidence of both micro-environmental and stochastic influences. (**A**, *courtesy of* G. Perry, PhD, Creighton University, Omaha, NE.)

Characteristics of Hematopoietic Stem Cells

Subpopulation	Isolation Method	Primary Characteristics	Clinical Applications	Key Studies
Multipotential adult progenitor cells	Multiple passages in culture	Multipotent, hematopoietic, and maybe other lineages	Trials proposed at University of Minnesota; licensed to Athersys (Cleveland, OH)	Verfaillie [19], Serafini et al. [20]
Side population (SP) cells	Flow cytometry by exclusion of Hoechst 33342 dye by ABCG2 transporter pump	Multipotent, hematopoietic, and other lineages; technique works for multiple species/tissues; hierarchy in that lower or "tip" SP cells outcompete upper SP cells	Primarily research applications; difficult to meet cell processing standards with flow cytometry	Goodell et al. [21], Uchida et al. [25], Abe et al. [26], Robinson et al. [24]
CD34+ cells	Magnetic beads/flow cytometry employing one of several commercial antibodies	Identifies HSCs (primarily) and precursors of some endothelial cells; potentially identifies stem cells of other tissues, eg, skin	Historically, first successful approach to clinical stem cell isolation; depletes stem cell harvest of T cells and some tumor cells	Hogan et al. [27], Ueda et al. [28]
CD133+ cells	Magnetic beads/flow cytometry employing CD133/AC133 antibody (Miltenyi)	HSCs and endothelial cells; also isolates glioma tumor stem cells	Reconstitutes recipients of high-dose therapy (eg, depletes stem cell harvests of T cells and some tumor cells)	Lang et al. [29], Bitan et al. [22]
Aldehyde dehydrogenase	Flow cytometry	Primarily employed experimentally for HSC detection and characterization	Primarily research applications, but trials in cord blood (Duke) and heart disease (Texas Heart Institute)	Storms et al. [23], Hess et al. [30]
SLAM markers (CD150+, CD48−)	Flow cytometry/immuno-histochemistry	Can simplify HSC detection/isolation compared with multiple lineage depletion; can detect HSCs in tissues	Primarily research applications	Kiel et al. [9]

Figure 7-3. Hematopoietic stem cell (HSC) populations. Characteristics of the stem cell subpopulations illustrated in Figure 7-1 are summarized here. The isolation techniques employed to prepare large numbers of cells for study differ for these HSC types. Some of these methods, primarily magnetic bead enrichment, which can be performed in closed systems are more "clinic" and regulatory friendly. Consequently, these cell types, namely CD34+ cells and CD133+ cells, are studied most in the clinical setting. Other cell populations have mostly been studied in the research arena, although clinical trials for some are under way or are in the planning stages.

Generation of Human CD45+ Cells by Selected Human Cell Populations Grafted Into Immunodeficient NOD/SCID Mice by Selected Cell Populations

Cell Type Injected Intravenously	Circulating Human CD45+ Cells per 1000 Cells Injected
Unselected G-CSF mobilized apheresis cells*	0.11 ± 0.01
CD34+ cells	20 ± 6
CD34− cells	0.09 ± 0.01
SP "stem" cells	4987 ± 2313

*A volunteer normal human donor received G-CSF 10 µg/kg daily for 5 days before apheresis. The CD34+ cells were selected using Miltenyi beads. The SP cells were isolated by flow cytometry (see Petriz [32]). The NODSCID mice were examined every 2 weeks for circulating human cells, and 77% of mice receiving 80 SP "stem" cells were chimeric with circulating human CD45+ cells > 1%. Clearly, based on the generation of progeny, CD34+ cells are more potent than CD34− cells or unseparated cells. SP cells are more potent than CD34+ cells. However, because the isolation of SP cells employs a potentially clastogenic dye and flow cytometry, this approach currently is not suitable for clinical applications. (Data collected in collaboration with M. Bishop, MD, and A. Kessinger, MD, who supervised the aphereses, and S. Pirruccello, MD, who performed the flow cytometric analyses.)

Figure 7-4. Assays of hematopoietic stem cell function. In preparation for a clinical trial, one of the standard approaches to show that a selected stem cell subpopulation will likely repopulate a damaged human hematopoietic system is to demonstrate the generation of human cells in immunodeficient mice [27]. This can also show that the cell selection process does not significantly damage the functional abilities of the selected cells. An example of such an assay is shown here, in which CD34+ versus CD34− versus side population (SP) stem cells are compared. In studying human cell production in various immunodeficient mouse models, the predominant cell type generated is significantly influenced by the genetic deficiencies of the mouse. Cytokines may be employed to amplify and expand the human cell types generated, but the genetics of the mouse model is the primary influence [31]. It is necessary to be mindful of these influences when interpreting the results of such studies. G-CSF—granulocyte colony-stimulating factor; NOD/SCID—non-obese diabetic severe combined immunodeficient.

A — Lymphohematopoietic Progenitor Cells

Name	Primary Assay	Primary Characteristics	Key Studies
T-cell precursors	Enumerated by flow cytometry	Generated primarily in thymus by HSC interaction with cortical epithelium involving notch signals; give rise to differentiated T cells	Witt and Robey [33]
B-cell precursors	Enumerated by flow cytometry	Generated primarily in bone marrow; give rise to B cells	Pelayo et al. [34]
Myeloid cells (macrophages, granulocytes, dendritic cells, NK cells)	Enumerated by flow cytometry or macrophage and granulocyte colonies in vitro when stimulated by colony-stimulating factors (see Fig. 7-5B)	NK/DC cells function in immune responses; DCs are primarily antigen-presenting cells; macrophages are primarily phagocytic cells; some macrophages can assume an endothelial phenotype	Moretta et al. [35]; Bailey et al. [36]
Erythroid progenitors	Enumerated by in vitro colony formation; small colonies in response to erythropoietin; large colonies (blast colonies) in response to erythropoietin and IL-3	Lineage-committed precursors of erythroid cells; may be depleted or increased in anemias, depending on cause	Munugalavadla and Kapur [37]
Megakaryocytes/platelets	Enumerated by counting colonies or megakaryocytes in tissue sections	Megakaryocytes are large multilobulated cells with multilobulated nuclei with variable ploidies that give rise to platelets that have pharmacologic and clotting factors	Deutsch and Tomer [38]

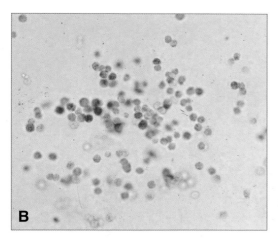

Figure 7-5. Progenitor cells. **A,** The progeny of the hematopoietic stem cell (HSC) compartment are the progenitor cell compartments, which are produced by transit amplification divisions and are characterized by increasing lineage restriction of the progeny. This is likely a continuous transition. **B,** Historically, progenitor cells were enumerated by their ability to form colonies of cells in semisolid media (plasma clot, agar, or methylcellulose) when stimulated by lineage-specific cytokines. These assays are still valid and provide quasifunctional information, that is, the progenitor cell has been demonstrated to produce progeny. Unfortunately, these assays take 7 to 14 days to complete, which limits their clinical usefulness. For immune progenitors, more rapid flow cytometric assays were developed and have become standard. Increasingly, as the flow cytometric assays of stem cell populations have been developed and their reliability demonstrated, such assays have become standard practice. Most centers characterize their transplant product based on stem cell flow cytometric evaluation, usually of CD34+ cells. Only a few centers continue to routinely perform colony-forming cell assays for clinical purposes. DC—dendritic cell; IL-3—interleukin-3; NK—natural killer.

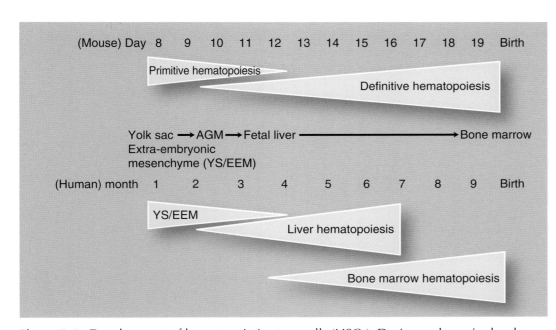

Figure 7-6. Development of hematopoietic stem cells (HSCs). During embryonic development, the first appearance of hematopoiesis consists of blood islands located in the yolk sac [39]. Early hematopoiesis has been termed *primitive* because of the presence of large nucleated erythroblasts in the circulatory system. Definitive HSCs are also believed to arise intra-embryonically in the aorta/gonad/mesonephros (AGM) region. Stem cells migrate to the liver, where they undergo expansion and differentiation into the mature lineages of the hematopoietic system, but most of the cell production at this stage is of erythrocytes. The liver is the primary site of hematopoiesis during prenatal development. HSCs also begin migrating to the bone marrow. At the time of birth, hematopoiesis has switched from the liver to bone marrow. Bone marrow is the primary site of adult hematopoiesis. The embryonic components of the newborn, the cord blood and part of the placenta, are populated by cells of hematopoietic, immune, and, likely, mesenchymal origins. Consequently, they are a tissue match to the newborn and may be collected and stored for future use. They have several attractive transplantation properties, including a lower incidence of, and less severe, graft-versus-host disease. Consequently, there is increasing interest in their collection and banking for future use.

A Functional Characteristics of Hematopoietic Stem Cells

Long-term survival
Self-renewal capacity
Considerable proliferative potential with production of a multiplicity of differentiated progeny
Generally quiescent, with an ongoing proliferative compartment, but most cells readily activatable into cell cycle, *eg*, regeneration following transplantation to lethally irradiated recipients
Possibly, and controversially, may be able to give rise to nonhematopoietic cells*

An alternative explanation is that there exist closely associated nonhematopoietic cells, eg, mesenchymal stem cells in tissues such as bone marrow, that give rise to the nonhematopoietic cells.

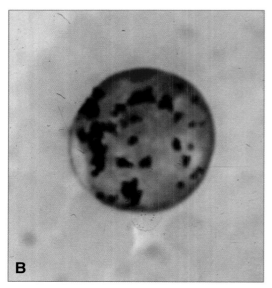

B

C Diseases Associated with Abnormal Stem/Progenitor Cell Function

Chronic myelogenous leukemia
Acute myelogenous leukemia
Myelofibrosis
Polycythemia
Aplastic anemia
Thalassemia
Sickle cell anemia
Paroxysmal nocturnal hemoglobinuria
Kostmann's neutropenia
Cyclical neutropenia
Dyskeratosis congenital/idiopathic pulmonary fibrosis

Figure 7-7. Functional properties of hematopoietic stem cells (HSCs). **A**, The functional properties of HSCs that lead to clinical interest in their application are listed here. Examples of the attraction of HSCs for therapy are their long-term survival, self-renewal, and continued production of progeny. Some patients with low granulocyte counts may benefit from granulocyte transfusions. Unfortunately, the half-life of these terminally differentiated cells is measured in hours. Although administration of amplifying cytokines helps maturing granulocyte counts in some circumstances, chronic neutropenia often presents a major therapeutic challenge. Transplantation of HSCs restores the granulocyte compartment and maintains the production of these cells long term. **B**, The quiescence of many HSCs is a major factor in their ability to regenerate following cycle specific chemotherapy; however, HSCs do divide. Their turnover in mice has been estimated at a few percent per day [40]. A stem cell isolated from a mouse administered radiolabelled (tritiated) thymidine, which was incorporated into DNA during the synthetic phase of the cell cycle, is shown. The electron emitted by the decay of tritium was detected by photographic emulsion placed over the cell on a slide and developed into silver grains (radioautography). This evidence of stem cell division indicates a need for caution when employing chemotherapeutic agents, such as busulfan, that target slowly cycling cells and may cause long-term damage to the HSC compartment [41]. **C**, Abnormalities of HSC/progenitor cell self-renewal regulation, proliferation, or differentiation are evident in a variety of diseases.

Sources of (Stem) Cells for Clinical Use

A

Currently used

Bone marrow harvest

Steady-state (nonmobilized) blood (historically; now rarely used)

Cytokine (usually G-CSF) mobilized blood (currently most used)

Umbilical cord blood and placenta (by manipulation; use two cords/adult)

Placenta (by manipulation)

Fetal liver (rarely, because of ethical issues)

Proposed

Amniotic fluid cells (there are concerns over risks to pregnant women and fetus of amniocentesis, and related cells may be present in placenta)

Embryonic stem cells: may be differentiated to blood cells (but have risks of tumorigenesis and tissue matching, as well as ethical concerns)

Diseases Potentially Amenable to Stem Cell Treatment

B

Currently used

Hematologic disorders and some connective tissue disorders are routinely treated using stem cells

Immunodeficiency disorders

Metabolic diseases

Cancer (high-dose therapy or immunotherapy)

Selected autoimmune diseases (resetting the immune system)

Cartilage damage

Nonhealing bone fractures

Osteogenesis imperfecta

Graft-versus-host disease

Cellular vehicle for gene therapy

Used in trials only

Cardiac ischemia

Peripheral vascular ischemia

Chronic obstructive pulmonary disease

Chronic skin ulcers

Central nervous system and retinal damage

Figure 7-8. Hematopoietic stem cell (HSC) transplantation. **A**, The first successful HSC transplantations were performed using bone marrow cells in mice in 1956 and in humans in 1968. For about 20 years, bone marrow was the primary clinical source of HSCs, although cord blood and fetal liver cells (rarely) were also employed. The initial attempts to employ blood mononuclear cells for transplantation were unsuccessful, although the presence of HSCs in blood had been noted. The general suspicion was that the frequency of blood HSCs was too low and they were of lower "quality." In the mid-1980s, the use of autologous blood HSCs for transplantation to patients with tumor cells in their marrow, or non-harvestable pelvic marrow due to irradiation exposure, was report-ed. Cells were collected by apheresis in steady state (no cytokines were administered). This process required, on average, about nine aphereses [42]. Other investigators used chemotherapy to mobilize more stem cells into the blood. The number of required aphereses was reduced, but there was associated uncertainty as to the optimal time of collection and some associated morbidity. HSCs harvested from blood were shown to successfully restore hematopoiesis in patients receiving marrow-ablative therapies [43]. The situation changed dramatically about 1990, when recombinant cytokines,

primarily granulocyte and granulocyte-macrophage colony-stimu-lating factors (G-CSFs and GM-CSFs), were introduced to mobilize HSCs into the circulation for collection in one to three aphereses with relative safety.

B, Diseases amenable to stem cell treatment. A wide range of diseases are potentially amenable to stem cell treatment. Stem cell therapy is standard of care for hematologic, immunodeficiency, and metabolic diseases. Clinical trials are in progress for many other diseases. The ultimate scope of successful clinical applications of stem cell therapies remains to be defined. Cytokine-mobilized blood stem cells have become the clinical standard of stem cell har-vest for autologous transplantation. Cytokine-mobilized blood stem cells from normal donors are increasingly employed for allogeneic transplantation. However, there are concerns that such transplants lead to an increased incidence of chronic graft-versus-host disease. Also, donor safety is an issue. There have been anecdotal reports of "exploding" spleens. Umbilical cord blood has growing applica-tions. The generation of HSCs from embryonic stem cells (ESCs) for clinical use, although possible experimentally [44], is likely far in the future. However, ESCs are useful for drug discovery and develop-ment and manufacture of biologicals [45].

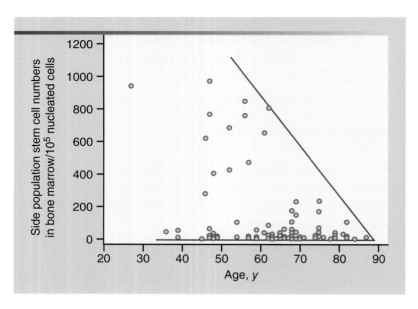

Figure 7-9. Decline of hematopoietic stem cells (HSCs) with aging. In the elderly, chemotherapy doses are frequently decreased by 25% to 33% because of concerns over comorbidities and the suspicion that HSCs may be compromised. The evidence for this is sparse, other than the decline in telomere length with age, which might compromise some HSCs. Most elderly individuals can maintain adequate steady-state hematopoiesis, but their responses to stresses may be compromised. This might relate to a decline in the number of HSCs with age (*solid lines*, indicating the wide range of individual variations). In addition to concerns over toxicity of chemotherapy, there is a growing awareness of the consequences of anemia in the elderly [46]. Anemia in the elderly not only causes physical symptoms such as fatigue, but may also amplify the symptoms of depression and dementia. The American Society of Hematology held a symposium in 2005 to raise awareness of these issues and begin planning to ameliorate this problem [47]. Stem cell homing and engraftment are also altered by aging [48]. A further consequence of the decrease in HSC numbers and function with aging is the increase in likelihood that a stem cell with genetic abnormalities, potentially as a result of accumulated mutations, will be activated to produce progeny [49]. Such progeny may have abnormal patterns of differentiation, including myelodysplasias, and may progress to leukemias [50].

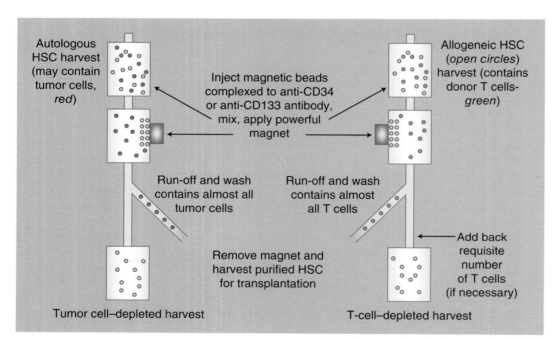

Figure 7-10. Selection of hematopoietic stem cells (HSCs) for transplantation. A concern with autologous HSCs for transplantation is that the infused harvest might contain tumor cells that can cause relapse. This is avoided in allogeneic transplantation because the harvest is obtained from a normal donor. A problem with allogeneic transplantation arises from the introduction of immunologically competent cells into immunocompromised hosts, which may result in early (acute) or delayed (chronic) graft-versus-host disease (GVHD). Relapse is lower in allogeneic transplant recipients, especially those who experience some GVHD. Unfortunately, GVHD may result in approximately the same proportion of deaths as relapse. A potential solution is to select CD34+ HSCs [51] or, more recently, CD133+ HSCs from either autologous stem cell harvests (thereby depleting, ie, "purging" tumor cells) or allogeneic harvests (thereby depleting GVHD-causing immune cells). Considerable effort was expended from 1980 to 1995 to purge tumor cells from autologous graft products [52]. However, it was difficult to demonstrate significant improvements in clinical outcomes [53,54]. It was realized that more commonly, tumor cells in the recipient that survived high-dose therapy were the likely source of relapse. This renewed interest in the concept of "cancer stem cells" with the property of therapy resistance [55]. It also promoted the notion that immunologic mechanisms of tumor destruction provided by allogeneic transplantation might provide better outcomes than attempting to purge autologous harvests. Depletion of T cells to decrease GVHD has been more successful, although a small number of T cells may need to be added back to a highly purified HSC population to prevent graft rejection. In the new strategy of allografting, so called mini-allografts, the chemo-(radio)therapy is designed primarily to be immunosuppressive so as to permit the transplanted HSC product to engraft, albeit more slowly than a full allograft, and create a chimeric recipient. This, in turn, creates a platform for additional antitumor immunotherapeutic procedures [56].

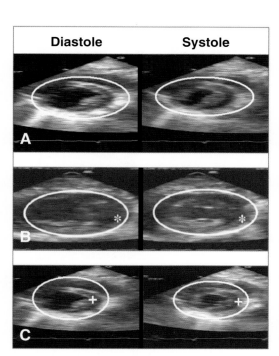

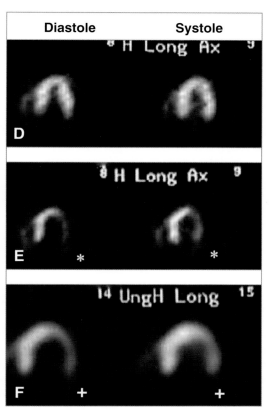

Figure 7-11. An example of nonhematopoietic applications of bone marrow mononuclear cells (BMs) and hematopoietic stem cells (HSCs): repair of ischemic heart disease. This is a relatively new and expanding application of BM or various HSC (CD34+ or CD133+) populations for therapy. The heart has a small population of CD34+ stem/progenitor cells that participate in the repair of damage. These cells, or skeletal muscle precursors (myoblasts), are difficult to harvest for therapy. Alternatively, autologous BMs/HSCs can be readily obtained in significant quantities and present no rejection problems. In a collaboration with K. Franco, MD, BMs were injected into areas of ischemic heart wall in pigs and improved wall motion. **A**, Echocardiographic image of control pig heart in diastole and systole. **B**, Thirty days after restriction of blood flow in the circumflex artery, a defect in wall contraction was detected (*asterisks*). **C**, Thirty days following BM cell injection into the defective heart wall, improved contraction was evident (*plus signs*). This correlated with improved blood perfusion of the heart wall as shown using the vascular tracing agent Cardiolite (Bristol-Myers Squibb Medical Imaging, North Billerica, MA). **D**, Perfusion scan in a control pig. **E**, Decreased perfusion was seen in the ischemic area of the heart wall (*asterisks*). **F**, Thirty days after BM cell infusion, a small improvement in perfusion was evident (*plus signs*). Several clinical trials have reported small but significant improvements, whereas others have shown no change [57–59]. (**A**, *courtesy of* T. Porter, MD; **D**, *courtesy of* J. Hankins, MD.)

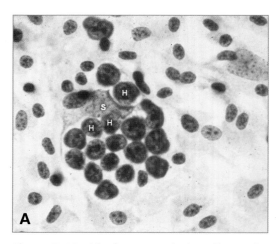

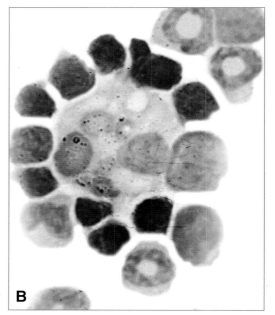

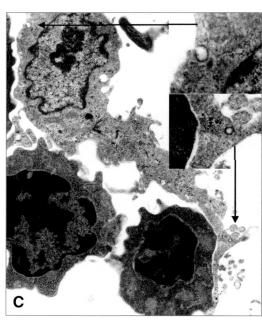

Figure 7-12. Nonhematopoietic cell populations and cellular interactions in bone marrow. **A,** In addition to hematopoietic stem cells (HSCs; *H* in the figure), bone marrow contains other cell populations, including some with characteristics of stem cell populations that give rise to nonhematopoietic cell populations [60]. These cells, historically, have been referred to as stromal cells (*S*). Stromal cells interact closely, likely via integrin and other ligand receptor interactions with hematopoietic cells [61], and in culture maintain HSC function for more than a year for mouse and 6 months for human HSC. Stromal cells are heterogeneous (blanket cells, endothelial cells, osteoblasts) with multiple functions, including participation in the HSC niche. Also, cell–cell interactions are important for normal hematopoietic cell differentiation. Erythroblasts develop in erythroblastic islets that contain a central macrophage. **B,** An erythroblastic islet at the light microscopic level. The erythroblasts have been stained for hemoglobin and appear brown. **C,** Part of a similar structure at the electron microscopic level. The intimate associations of the erythroblasts with the central macrophage are visible. Additionally, the macrophage is involved in receptor-mediated uptake of material from its surroundings, evident by the coated pit and coated vesicle. In bone marrow, megakaryocytes are located in association with sinusoidal endothelium (not shown). The megakaryocyte cytoplasm protrudes through the sinusoidal endothelium and breaks up into platelets in the vessel [38].

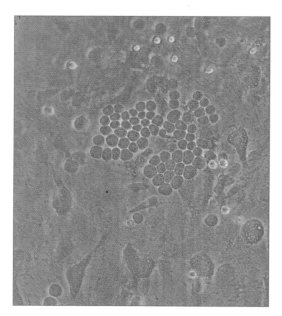

Figure 7-13. Hematopoietic cobblestones and mesenchymal cells. Hematopoietic stem cells (HSCs) associate with mesenchymal cells to generate "cobblestone areas." Cultured bone marrow aspirates generate cobblestone areas spontaneously after 1 to 3 weeks. When purified HSCs are added to stromal cells, they form cobblestones. In cobblestone areas, the HSCs migrate under the stromal cells and form a tight aggregate of flattened adjacent cells that resemble the cobblestone streets of historic old towns, hence the name. More differentiated cells remain attached, often by a thin strand of extracellular matrix material, to the upper surface of the stromal cells and therefore are refractile in phase-contrast microscopy. Such cells can be decanted from the cultures without significant effects on the HSCs, which then generate additional progeny. Often, the end of HSC maintenance is associated with a burst of production of mature cells. This hints that a function of the stroma is to maintain HSCs in a quiescent or undifferentiated state. Some mesenchymal stromal cell lines, but not all, support HSC maintenance and cobblestone formation. Formation of cobblestones serves as a quantitative assay of HSCs, and the duration of maintenance of cobblestones is an inverse measure of the primitiveness, that is, an indicator of the ability of HSCs to generate progeny [24]. The cobblestone area–forming assay is best performed as a limiting dilution assay of HSC frequency. This is the most relevant in vitro assay of HSC. Unfortunately, this evaluation takes 5 weeks or longer and is not clinically useful, except in a research setting.

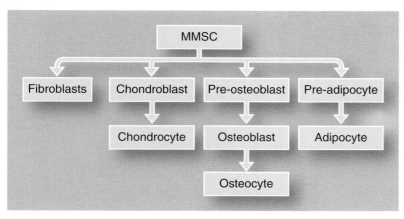

Figure 7-14. Multipotential mesenchymal stromal cells (MMSCs). MMSCs are a stromal cell population that meets the criteria of a stem cell population. Previously termed *mesenchymal stem cells*, or MSCs, this new classification [62] addresses a number of concerns, including limited evidence for self-renewal potential of the majority of cells in this compartment. Many of the cells obtained by culture and classified as MSCs appear to be transit-amplifying cells. There may be subpopulations of MMSCs. These cells express many of the markers of bone lineage cells and can repair bone defects. Some express CD51 and CD143 and may be part of a local renin-angiotensinogen system. These cells appear to have a role in effecting, or promoting, tissue repair and are beginning to be employed clinically. The proposed differentiation potential of MMSCs is outlined in the figure. In addition to producing cells of connective tissues, targets for repair appear to include skin wound healing, which is accelerated when bone marrow cells are added, and potentially lung and other tissues. MMSCs can be employed in cardiac repair as shown in Figure 7-11. The mechanism(s) of this effect is currently ill-defined. However, there is evidence that the donor cells activate, or promote repair by, endogenous cells. In such a schema, a relatively small number of cells, designated "tissue repair cells," appear to significantly amplify repair processes by activating endogenous cells to proliferate, differentiate, and effect the actual tissue repair.

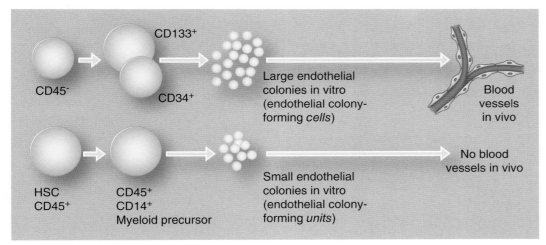

Figure 7-15. Endothelial cells. Endothelial cells of donor origin may be observed following allogeneic bone marrow transplantation [63]. Cells with an endothelial phenotype can originate by two different processes [10]. Endothelial cells with the ability to generate blood vessels in vivo or give rise to endothelial colonies in collagen gels arise from a stem/progenitor cell that is CD133+ and CD45−. Additionally, a macrophage lineage–derived cell, *ie*, CD14+ and CD45+, may give rise to cells in endothelial colonies that are CD45−, CD31+, von Willebrand factor, and Tie 2+ [36]. Colonies formed are generally smaller, and this cell is unable to give rise to blood vessels in vivo [10]. A schematic of these populations is presented here. There is a need for caution in the interpretation of clinical studies of endothelial precursors because of the potential diversity of effector cell populations. Endothelial and hematopoietic precursors circulate in the blood in myocardial infarction [64], and their frequency is associated with severity of coronary artery disease [65]. Their numbers are decreased, as are circulating side population stem cells, and the cells are dysfunctional in smokers [66]. The number recovers following smoking cessation [67]. HSC—hematopoietic stem cell.

Established and Potential Nonhematopoietic Stem/Progenitor Cell Populations in Bone Marrow and the Circulation

Cell Population	Study
Multipotential mesenchymal stromal cells	Dominici *et al.* [62]
Fibroblasts/myofibroblasts	Abe *et al.* [70]; McAnulty [71]
Endothelial cells	Yoder *et al.* [10]
Cytokeratin 5–positive epithelial cells	Gomperts *et al.* [69]
Smooth muscle or myofibroblasts/pericytes	Espinosa-Heidmann *et al.* [72]

Figure 7-16. Other potential stem cell populations in bone marrow. Bone marrow may harbor heterogeneous stem cell populations [68]. Gomperts *et al.* [69] reported a cytokeratin 5–positive stem cell population in bone marrow and circulation that can repair epithelial tissues. Limited evidence exists for a platelet-derived growth factor receptor (PDGFR+) cell from bone marrow that may be a myofibroblast/smooth muscle precursor that may become a periadventitial cell (pericyte). Bone marrow cells and circulating cells can give rise to subepithelial myofibroblasts in damaged lung, but the cell of origin remains undefined [70]. Clearly, additional studies are required to inventory the many potential stem cell populations in bone marrow. Are they separate or related cell populations? Is their relationship a function of the time of evaluation (eg, in development vs in the adult) or the methods employed to assess their presence? If multiple stem or progenitor cell types exist, this has implications for "plasticity," which implies that bone marrow cells can morph (transdifferentiate) into cells of other lineages. Cell fusion is an alternative explanation that likely applies, particularly to liver and Purkinje cells in the brain. If there are multiple stem cell populations in bone marrow, then claims of plasticity would require the demonstration that a purified hematopoietic stem cell, or other stem cell type, can give rise, at the single cell level, to progeny of different lineages. This has not been convincingly demonstrated.

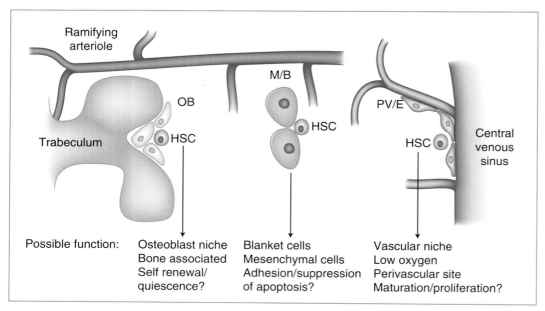

Figure 7-17. Hematopoietic microenvironment (HM). Shown is a schematic of the possible relationships between the HM and stem cell niche. The introduction outlined the controversies regarding the nature of the HM and stem cell niche. A possible unifying hypothesis might be that there are differing but closely associated microenvironments with differing roles. For example, mesenchymal blanket cells might promote hematopoietic stem cell (HSC) survival and suppress apoptosis (like feeder cells). Osteoblasts might promote HSC self-renewal, or quiescence and endothelial cells might activate HSCs for proliferation and migration. These different cell populations might provide different stimulatory and inhibitory ligands controlling cell proliferation and promotion or inhibition of differentiation in a manner similar to ectodermal control of limb bud mesenchymal cell differentiation or regeneration in newts and salamanders [73]. Substances with limited diffusion distances, such as Wnts or their ligands, could bind membrane receptors expressed by HSCs, thereby establishing a local topography of factors that regulate stem cell behaviors. Clinically, disturbance of any or all components of the HM, such as fibrosis, conversion of mesenchymal cells to adipocytes, or autoantibody depletion of endothelial cells, could lead to HSC loss (yellow marrow), dysplasias, and ultimately aplasias. As with HSCs, the HM is disturbed by chemotherapy agents and especially by radiation. Although recovery occurs, the effects of radiation on the HM may be long lasting [74]. M/B—mesenchymal/blanket cells; OB—osteoblasts; PV/E—perivascular/endothelial cells.

Potential Clinical Application of Nonhematopoietic Stem Cells From Bone Marrow*		
Cell Type	**Application**	**Trial Status/Company**
Mesenchymal cells	Ischemic heart disease	In trials (several centers)
	Repair of nonhealing fractures	In trials (Aastrom, Ann Arbor, MI)
	Peripheral vascular ischemia	In trials
	Spinal cord injury repair	Anecdotal reports
Chondrocytes (from MMSCs not cartilage biopsies)	Repair of cartilage	In trials (Osiris, Baltimore, MD)

*Note: these are examples, not an exhaustive list. More up-to-date information may be obtained by searching the National Institutes of Health Clinical Trials or company websites [77].

Figure 7-18. Clinical applications of mesenchymal (nonhemato-poietic) bone marrow cells. Based on their purported lineage relationships (*see* Figure 7-14), a primary application of multipotential mesenchymal stromal cells (MMSCs) has been in the repair of damaged connective tissues, primarily cartilage, bone, and tendons. Addition of bone marrow cells to bone fracture nonunions accelerates healing. However, bone marrow cells do not easily generate large amounts of bone [75], so the application to large defects still requires additional allogeneic bone or matrix materials. The application of various cytokines to accelerate the bone-forming process, primarily the bone morphogenic protein family [76], and potentially vascular endothelial growth factor to accelerate angiogenesis, is in progress. Clinical trials are being conducted in these areas [77]. Early in 2007, there were positive reports on the initial results of bioreactor-generated MMSCs for nonhealing fracture repair and a bone marrow MMSC–derived chondrocyte product for cartilage repair. There is a growing, largely anecdotal, literature showing that MMSCs can promote the repair of spinal cord injuries and improve ischemic vascular disease. All these additional potential applications need to be subjected to rigorous clinical trial evaluation using cells prepared according to current regulations, preferably by accredited (FACT-JACIE [Foundation for the Accreditation of Cellular Therapy-Joint Accreditation Committee] approved) cellular therapy facilities [78].

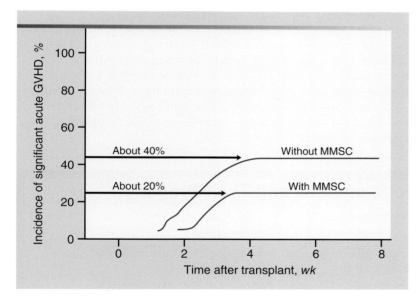

Figure 7-19. Application of mesenchymal (nonhematopoietic) bone marrow cells in the treatment of graft-versus-host disease (GVHD). A relatively new and developing clinical application of multipotential mesenchymal stromal cells (MMSCs) is to ameliorate GVHD. As noted earlier, GVHD arises as a consequence of the infusion of immunocompetent cells into an immunocompromised host. MMSCs were shown to suppress allogeneic responses in vitro—for example, mixed lymphocyte reactivity [79]—and have begun to be evaluated for immunomodulatory effects in vivo [80]. Initial trial results that build on anecdotal reports are encouraging in that MMSCs appear to reduce the incidence and or extent of GVHD. Anecdotal reports further indicate that MMSCs mitigate the symptoms of established severe GVHD. There remain a number of unanswered questions, including whether the use of MMSC therapy for GVHD will exacerbate the risks of tumor relapse and whether this cellular therapy might have broader applications, such as treatment of autoimmune diseases.

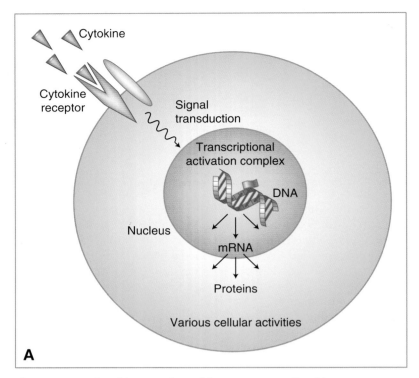

	Diseases Associated with
B	**Abnormal Cytokine Activities**
Erythropoietin is deficient in anemia of renal failure, with excess production in many polycythemic disorders	
Thrombopoietin receptor is abnormal in congenital amegakaryocytic thrombocytopenia	
G-CSFR (CSF3R) exhibits mutations in a portion of cases of severe congenital neutropenia	
IL-5 is abnormal in some eosinophilic states	
IL-6 levels are abnormal in Castleman disease, atrial myxoma, multiple myeloma, and a variety of inflammatory conditions	
FLT3 tandem duplications and mutations occur in myelodysplasias and acute myeloid leukemias	

Figure 7-20. Cytokines and cytokine receptors. Cytokines are soluble factors, mostly glycoproteins, produced by a wide variety of cells in the body. **A**, Cytokines interact with cells via specific membrane receptors. Following the interaction of the cytokine with the receptor, different signaling pathways and secondary messengers are activated. These in turn signal the up-regulation of transcriptional complexes and the initiation of gene expression, leading to altered cellular functions. Cytokines can be grouped into "families" based on structure, primary cellular targets, and receptor specifications/activation. In this section, the various classifications are employed to provide examples and familiarize readers with these options. Cytokines or their receptors can be therapeutic targets, and the receptors can be activated by agonists and inhibited by antagonists. Drugs acting according to these principles, such as inhibitors of tumor necrosis factor (TNF) or TNF receptors and inhibitors of vascular endothelial growth factor, are in clinical use and many more are under development and evaluation, including agents intended, for example, to counter radiation effects on hematopoiesis as a result of nuclear terrorism [81]. **B**, Abnormalities of cytokine production, mutations [82], or abnormalities in cytokine receptor functions [83] are associated with disease. Several of these defects have been recognized and defined only recently, and it is likely additional abnormalities will be defined. G-CSFR—granulocyte colony-stimulating factor receptor; IL—interleukin.

Cytokines Acting on Hematopoietic Stem Cells and Their Progeny

Cytokine	Abbreviation	Primary Function(s)
Granulocyte colony-stimulating factor	G-CSF	Induction/amplification of neutrophil differentiation
Granulocyte-macrophage colony-stimulating factor	GM-CSF	Induction/amplification of granulocyte and monocyte differentiation; enhances dendritic cell functions
Macrophage colony-stimulating factor	M-CSF	Induction/amplification of monocyte and macrophage differentiation, bone remodeling
Erythropoietin	EPO	Produced by kidney peritubular cells in response to hypoxia; primary regulator of red cell production
Thrombopoietin	TPO	Primary regulation of platelet production
Stem cell (Steel) factor	SCF	Acts on stem cells; synergizes with G-CSF in neutrophil production; promotes mast cell generation

Figure 7-21. Colony-stimulating factors (CSFs) and direct activators of hematopoiesis. CSFs, erythropoietin and thrombopoietin, are multifunctional stimulators of hematopoietic stem and progenitor cells. These cytokines also act on differentiating hematopoietic cells. In some instances, they regulate the functional status of mature hematopoietic cells, such as granulocyte CSF (G-CSF) and granulocyte-macrophage CSF (GM-CSF). Their functions include promotion of survival and proliferation of stem/progenitor cells, induction of differentiation or commitment of progenitor cells, amplification of progenitor cell proliferation and differentiation, and stimulation of differentiated cell functions. Cytokines often act cooperatively (synergistically) to amplify cell production and cellular functions [37]. These glycoproteins also may have effects, perhaps indirectly, on systems outside hematopoietic tissues. Erythropoietin appears to be neuroprotective. M-CSF is critical to bone development and remodeling. G-CSF plays a role in T-cell differentiation, and GM-CSF is involved in dendritic cell development and function.

Interleukins

Interleukin	Source	Activity
IL-1α and IL-1β	Macrophages, dendritic cells, epithelial cells	Endogenous pyrogen, stimulates IL-2 release from T cells
IL-2	T cells	Stimulates T cells, B cells, NK cells
IL-3	T cells, mast cells	**Stimulates multilineage hematopoietic progenitor cells**
IL-4	Th2 cells, mast cells	Stimulates B cells and dendritic cells, important in production of IgE and IgG1, activity on hematopoietic progenitors as a cofactor with other cytokines
IL-5	Th2 cells, mast cells	Stimulates eosinophil progenitors, B cells
IL-6	T cells, fibroblasts, monocytes, endothelial cells	**Stimulates hematopoietic progenitors and megakaryocyte progenitors, induces acute-phase proteins, B-cell differentiation, and plasmacyte growth**
IL-7	Stromal cells	Acts on pre-B cells, thymocytes, T cells
IL-8	Monocytes, endothelial cells	**Chemotaxis; mobilizes hematopoietic stem cells**
IL-9	Th2 cells	Stimulates mast cell proliferation, erythroid progenitor cells
IL-10	Monocytes, macrophages, T cells, B cells	Suppresses cytokine production, stimulates proliferation of mast cells as a cofactor
IL-11	Stromal cells, endothelial cells, epithelial cells	**Synergy with other hematopoietic cytokines to stimulate hematopoietic progenitors, stimulates megakaryocytopoiesis, inhibits osteogenesis and adipogenesis, induces acute-phase proteins**
IL-12	Dendritic cells, macrophages	**Synergy with other colony-stimulating factors to stimulate hematopoietic progenitors, stimulates NK cells, CD8+ cells, CD4+ Th1 cells, induces IFN-γ production**
IL-13	Th2 cells, mast cells	**Synergy with other cytokines to stimulate hematopoietic progenitors, IgE production; stimulates B-cell proliferation**
IL-14	T cells	Enhances B-cell proliferation
IL-15	Epithelial cells, bone marrow stromal cells, monocytes, macrophages	Stimulates NK and T cells
IL-16	T cells	Chemotaxis for T cells, monocytes, and eosinophils; induces IL-2 receptor expression
IL-17	Th17 cells, CD8+ cells, NK cells	Autoimmune inflammatory responses, neutrophil mobilization
IL-18	Monocytes, macrophages	Induces IFN-γ, GM-CSF production; suppresses IL-10 production
IL-19	Monocytes	Induces Th2 responses, keratinocyte effects
IL-20	Monocytes	**Stimulates keratinocytes; activity on multipotential hematopoietic progenitors as a cofactor**
IL-21	CD4+ T cells	Stimulates B, T, and NK cells
IL-22	Activated T cells	Stimulates keratinocytes, enhances keratinocyte migration
IL-23	Dendritic cells	Induces production of IL-6, IL-17, and TNF; expands (amplifies) Th17 cells
IL-24	Th2 cells, monocytes	Induces tumor cell apoptosis, keratinocyte effects
IL-25	Th2 cells, macrophages, mast cells	Suppresses IL-17–induced autoimmune inflammatory responses; induces Th2 responses
IL-26	Activated T cells	Biological activity has not been defined
IL-27	Dendritic cells	Inhibits production of Th17 cells
IL-28	Epithelial cells, endothelial cells, macrophages, dendritic cells	Antiviral responses
IL-29	Epithelial cells, endothelial cells, macrophages, dendritic cells	Antiviral responses
IL-30		Originally defined as p28 of the heterodimeric cytokine IL-27 (p28 and EBI3)
IL-31	Th2 cells	Involved in skin inflammatory responses
IL-32	T cells, monocytes, NK cells, epithelial cells	Induces TNF-α, IL-1, IL-6, and IL-8 production
IL-33	Endothelial cells	Induces Th2 responses

IL-1 family: IL-1α, IL-1β, IL-18, IL-33.
IL-10 family: IL-10, IL-19, IL-20, IL-22, IL-24, IL-26.
IL-12 family: IL-12, IL-23, IL-27.
IL-12 (p70) and IL-10 are activated via Toll receptors (TRs) 1, 2, and 6. IL-12 (p70) is also activated by TRs 3, 4, 5, 8, and 11.

Figure 7-22. Interleukins (ILs). This group of cytokines was named based on the original observations that these factors were produced by and acted upon "leukocytes" and played an important role in communication between these cells. This family of glycoproteins has grown dramatically and continues to grow. Some of the activities assigned to earlier interleukins have been defined more specifically,

Continued on the next page

Figure 7-22. *(Continued)* leading to new interleukins. Also, as the family of interleukins has increased in number, the diversity of actions has grown. The actions of the interleukins that target hematopoietic cells are shown in *bold*. The subfamilies that are related on a structural basis are listed. Clinically, interleukins are primarily employed in immunotherapeutic protocols, many of which are still under development or evaluation. Although several interleukins target hematopoietic progenitor cells, clinically they have proved either minimally useful, *eg*, IL-3, or too toxic, *eg*, IL-6. As noted, several interleukins are generated when Toll receptors, which underlie innate immune responses, are activated by bacterial products or double- or single-stranded RNAs. GM-CSF—granulocyte-macrophage colony-stimulating factor; IFN—interferon; NK—natural killer; Th—T helper; TNF—tumor necrosis factor.

Chemokines with Significant Hematopoietic Activities

Chemokine	Actions	Relevance
CXCR4	Receptor for CXCL12 (SDF1)	This receptor targets cells to move along a concentration gradient of SDF1 involved in mobilization
		Antagonized by AMD3100
SDF1	Ligand for CXCR4	Chemoattractant for stem cells
		Involved in migration
		Produced by irradiated (damaged) bone marrow endothelial cells

Figure 7-23. Chemokines. Chemokines are a large family of molecules, with more than 70 members. As their name implies, they are involved in stimulating cellular activities, especially motion and migration. Only those chemokines that have major involvement in hematopoiesis are listed. Chemokines play an important role in stem cell homing. A successful outcome of stem cell transplantation depends on homing, engraftment, and repopulation by hematopoietic stem cells (HSCs), and these are complex processes [84]. Human stem cell engraftment in nonobese diabetic severe combined immunodeficient (NODSCID) mice is critically dependent on CXCR4 expression by CD34+ stem cells [85]. Such cells migrate in response to the expression of stromal-derived factor-1 (SDF1; CXCL12), the receptor for CXCR4 [86]. AMD3100 is an antagonist of CXCR4 and is useful in increasing the mobilization of CXCR4-expressing stem cells in individuals who are often heavily pretreated with chemotherapy and who exhibit poor mobilization of HSCs to cytokines alone [87].

A. Other Factors with Roles in Hematopoiesis

Factor	Actions
Interferons	Generally suppress stem cell activities
	Used clinically in treatment of chronic myelogenous leukemia
	Interferon-α is activated by TRs 3, 4, 7, 8, and 9
PGE	Amplifies stem cells in zebra fish and mice
	Promotes hematopoiesis following chemotherapy or radiation
	Interacts with the Wnt pathway
TGF-β	Biphasic action
	Stimulates hematopoiesis at some (generally low) concentrations
	Inhibits at higher concentrations
VEGF	Survival factor
	Modulation of differentiation
	Involved in angiogenesis of malignancies

B. Negative Regulators of Hematopoiesis

Factor	Source(s)	Function
AcSDKP	Undefined	Inhibits hematopoietic stem cell entry into cell cycle
Inhibin	Sertoli cells, granulosa cells	Inhibits proliferation of hematopoietic progenitors
MCP-1	Endothelial cells, smooth muscles cells	Inhibits cycling of hematopoietic progenitor cells
MIP-1α	Macrophages, fibroblasts, T cells, B cells, mast cells	Inhibits hematopoietic stem cell entry into cell cycle
SOCS	Induced by cytokines	Negative regulator of Jak/Stat pathway
TGF-β	Macrophages, fibroblasts, osteoblasts, osteoclasts	Inhibits hematopoietic stem/progenitor cell proliferation
TNF-α	T cells, mast cells, macrophages, fibroblasts	Inhibits hematopoietic stem/progenitor cell proliferation
		May also stimulate proliferation of other cell types

Figure 7-24. Other factors influencing hematopoiesis. **A**, A number of diverse factors influence hematopoietic activities but do not readily fit into cytokine families. Some of these are described in the table, which is not an exhaustive list of all factors that can have effects. However, if patients are identified with abnormal levels of these factors, hematopoietic consequences may ensue. For example, endothelial cells respond to vascular endothelial growth factor (VEGF). There are three primary isoforms: VEGF 121, which lacks a heparin-binding domain, and VEGFs 165 and 189, which have heparin-binding domains and associate with extracellular matrix. There are two VEGF receptors: Dlk-1 and KDR. VEGF acts to stimulate endothelial cell proliferation and migration and angiogenesis. VEGF is involved in several hematologic malignancies [88]. Some cytokines, such as interferons, are employed clinically. **B**, There are also inhibitors of hematopoiesis [89]. Some of these have been employed during chemotherapy to protect stem cells. AcSDKP—*N*-acetyl-seryl-aspartyl-lysyl-proline; MCP—monocyte chemotactic protein; MIP—macrophage inflammatory protein; PGE—prostaglandin E; SOCS—suppressor of cytokine signaling; TGF—transforming growth factor; TNF—tumor necrosis factor; TRs—Toll receptors.

A — Examples of Clinical Applications of Cytokines

Application	Cytokines Employed
Stimulation/amplification of cell production	G-CSF–neutrophils
	GM-CSF–neutrophils/dendritic cells
	EPO–red cells
	TPO–platelets
Mobilization of stem cells for collection by apheresis	G-CSF primarily
	GM-CSF secondarily
In vitro amplification of stem cells, *eg*, with cord blood	Multiple, usually as mixtures including SCF, IL-6, FLT3, TPO
Kostmann's neutropenia	G-CSF

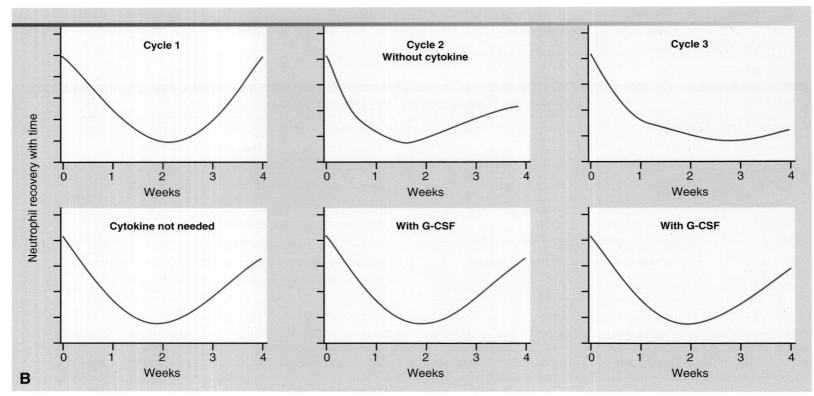

Figure 7-25. Clinical applications of cytokines: stimulation of cell production. **A**, Cytokines are employed to increase production of critical cell populations—for example, stimulation of red cell production in anemic patients by erythropoietin (EPO) or granulocytes in chemotherapy patients by granulocyte colony-stimulating factor (G-CSF). **B**, Because the production of progeny from hematopoietic stem cells (HSCs) involves extensive proliferation and because most chemotherapeutic agents target cycling cells, the HSC system is a primary target for damage by chemotherapy. The administration of cytokines can accelerate recovery following chemotherapy but only if an adequate pool of HSCs remains. Consequently, cytokines do not permit a significant escalation of chemotherapy doses. However, they do permit shortening of the interval between chemotherapy treatments, which in turn, increases effective dose intensity. EPO improves anemia, but more slowly than do blood cell transfusions. There is evidence that increasing red cell mass improves the outcomes of radiation therapy, probably by decreasing tissue hypoxia, and there is increased interest in the use of EPO in anemic elderly populations. To reduce the frequency of administration, longer-acting versions of EPO have been developed. Recently, the effectiveness of some of these preparations has been questioned and an increased risk of deaths has been reported to the Food and Drug Administration [18]. Clearly, cytokines are powerful drugs that need to be used with caution. GM-CSF—granulocyte-macrophage colony-stimulating factor; IL-6—interleukin 6; SCF—stem cell factor; TPO—thrombopoietin.

Stem Cell Source	Time to 500 Neutrophils, *d*	Time to 20,000 Platelets, *d*
Bone marrow	17–21	20–30+*
Bone marrow and daily G-CSF	10–12	20+
Nonmobilized blood stem cells	20–25	20+*
G-CSF (or GM-CSF*) mobilized blood stem cells	9–15	10–15

*A small proportion of patients, especially those receiving total-body irradiation, have delayed platelet recovery. Ranges of median values are listed because mean values are influenced by outliers. Presentation of the cumulative percentage of subjects achieving the target cellularity versus days provides a more comprehensive picture of cell recoveries.

Figure 7-26. Cytokine acceleration of hematopoietic cell regeneration following transplantation. When bone marrow is employed as a transplant product, neutrophil and platelet recovery is relatively slow following high-dose therapy and transplantation. Recovery to 500 neutrophils/μL requires about 19 days and to 20,000 platelets/μL, about 21 days. Consequently, there is an emphasis on the use of granulocyte colony-stimulating factor (G-CSF) or granulocyte-macrophage CSF (GM-CSF) administration to accelerate neutrophil recovery and thrombopoietin (TPO) to accelerate platelet recovery. Interleukin-6 was also evaluated for acceleration of platelet recovery, but this agent has toxicities. Neutrophil and platelet recovery is similarly slow following blood stem cell transplantation, when the cells are collected by apheresis in "steady state," that is, without mobilization. In contrast, transplantation of adequate numbers of G-CSF– or GM-CSF–mobilized blood stem cells results in initial neutrophil and platelet reconstitution in 9 to 15 days and 10 to 15 days, respectively [90]. However, platelet recoveries to 100,000/μL were faster using G-CSF. Clinical outcomes did not differ significantly. The additional administration of G-CSF or TPO following transplantation does not further accelerate reconstitution and adds significant costs. In addition to accelerating cellular reconstitution, cytokines such as G-CSF reduced the incidence of infections as well as transfusion requirements. Also, longer-acting versions of these cytokines, such as pegylated G-CSF, have been introduced into clinical practice.

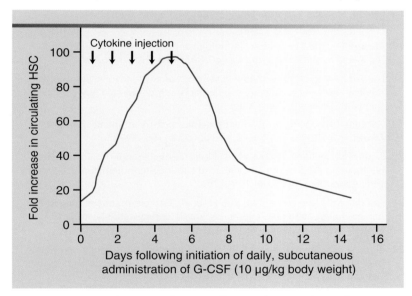

Figure 7-27. Mobilization of stem cells into the circulation by cytokines for collection. Cytokines make it much easier and faster to collect a sufficient number of hematopoietic stem cells (HSCs) for transplantation, and significantly accelerate the kinetics of granulocyte and platelet engraftment. These agents are injected subcutaneously daily for 5 days, and the mobilized stem/progenitor cells are then harvested by apheresis and employed for transplantation following high-dose therapy. In normal donors, a sufficient stem cell dose is 2×10^6 CD34+ cells/kg, but for optimal immunologic recovery, 10×10^6 CD34+ cells/kg is preferred [91]. Such cell numbers can usually be collected in one or two aphereses in normal donors. In heavily pretreated autologous donors, three or more aphereses may be required to collect an adequate cell dose. Granulocyte-macrophage colony-stimulating factor (GM-CSF) mobilizes a slightly different population of stem cells than does granulocyte CSF (G-CSF), including dendritic cell precursors; however, in clinical use there is generally no difference in outcomes [90,92]. However, GM-CSF has a slightly higher incidence of side effects and is less frequently used. Although the addition of erythropoietin to G-CSF improves mobilization in mice, there is no advantage in humans. Addition of stem cell factor to G-CSF enhances mobilization somewhat, but because of its activities on mast cells, anaphylactic-related reactions may occur and this disadvantage generally outweighs its advantages; therefore, it is rarely employed clinically.

Potential New Agents for Amplification of HSCs in vitro	
Agent	**Action**
Stromal cells	Provide putative niches
Polycomb genes	Promote HSC self-renewal
Wnt	Amplifies adult stem cells

Figure 7-28. Cytokine amplification of hematopoietic stem cell (HSC) numbers in vitro. In some situations, such as the use of cord blood cells for transplanting to an adult, the number of HSCs might be lower than desired on a CD34+ cells per kilogram basis. To overcome this problem, a portion of the harvest (with the remainder frozen for direct application) may be subjected to culture in vitro to expand the available pool of stem cells. A variant on this theme has been to direct the stem cells to differentiate toward a desirable precursor, such as megakaryocytes to improve platelet recovery in the recipient. Although such approaches have had modest success, there are ongoing attempts to improve this process using newer agents or modified culture procedures using stromal cells or bio-reactors. One problem may be that currently approved cytokines are primarily differentiation-inducing rather than stem cell–amplifying agents. Consequently, a danger of culturing stem cells in vitro with such cytokines is that although cell numbers are increased dramatically and progenitor cells are increased moderately, stem cell numbers may be minimally increased and, with time, extensively self-renewing stem cells may be lost by differentiation to progenitor cells. Stromal cells [93] and newer agents such as polycomb gene products; HoxB4 [94]; and modifiers of Wnt [95], hedgehog, and notch ligands that act in stem cell self-renewal and the earliest stages of differentiation might find a role in manipulation of stem cell production and differentiation in vitro [13,96].

References

1. Weissman IL, Anderson DJ, Gage F: Stem and progenitor cells: origins, phenotypes, lineage commitments, and transdifferentiations. *Annu Rev Cell Dev Biol* 2001, 17:387–403.

2. Taichman RS, Emerson SG: The role of osteoblasts in the hematopoietic microenvironment. *Stem Cells* 1998, 16:7–15.

3. Yin T, Li L: The stem cell niches in bone. *J Clin Invest* 2006, 116:1195–1201.

4. Calvi LM, Adams GB, Weibrecht KW, et al.: Osteoblastic cells regulate the haemopoietic stem cell niche. *Nature* 2003, 425:841–846.

5. Ahmed N, Khokher MA, Hassan HT: Cytokine-induced expansion of human CD34+ stem/progenitor and CD34+CD41+ early megakaryocytic marrow cells cultured on normal osteoblasts. *Stem Cells* 1999, 17:92–99.

6. Arai F, Hirao A, Suda T: Regulation of hematopoietic stem cells by the niche. *Trends Cardiovasc Med* 2005, 15:75–79.

7. Visnjic D, Kalajzic Z, Rowe DW, et al.: Hematopoiesis is severely altered in mice with an induced osteoblast deficiency. *Blood* 2004, 103:3258–3264.

8. Nilsson SK, Johnston HM, Whitty GA, et al.: Osteopontin, a key component of the hematopoietic stem cell niche and regulator of primitive hematopoietic progenitor cells. *Blood* 2005, 106:1232–1239.

9. Kiel MJ, Yilmaz OH, Iwashita T, et al.: SLAM family receptors distinguish hematopoietic stem and progenitor cells and reveal endothelial niches for stem cells. *Cell* 2005, 121:1109–1121.

10. Yoder MC, Mead LE, Prater D, et al.: Redefining endothelial progenitor cells via clonal analysis and hematopoietic stem/progenitor cell principals. *Blood* 2007, 109:1801–1809.

11. Allen TD, Dexter TM: The essential cells of the hemopoietic microenvironment. *Exp Hematol* 1984, 12:517–521.

12. Crouse DA, Mann SL, Sharp JG: Segregation and characterization of lymphohematopoietic stromal elements. *Kroc Found Ser* 1984, 18:211–231.

13. Park IK, Qian D, Kiel M, et al.: Bmi-1 is required for maintenance of adult self-renewing haematopoietic stem cells. *Nature* 2003, 423:231–233.

14. Beausejour CM, Campisi J: Ageing: balancing regeneration and cancer. *Nature* 2006, 443:404–405.

15. Vieyra DS, Jackson KA, Goodell MA: Plasticity and tissue regenerative potential of bone marrow-derived cells. *Stem Cell Rev* 2005, 1:65–69.

16. Herzog EL, Chai L, Krause DS: Plasticity of marrow-derived stem cells. *Blood* 2003, 102:3483–3493.

17. Alverez-Dolado M: Cell fusion: biological perspectives and potential for regenerative medicine. *Front Biosci* 2007, 12:1–12.

18. Food and Drug Administration: FDA 2007 safety alerts for drugs, biologics, medical devices, and dietary supplements. http://www.fda.gov/medwathc/safety/2007/safety07.htm#Aranesp.

19. Verfaillie CM: Multipotent adult progenitor cells: and update. *Novartis Found Symp* 2005, 265:55–61; discussion 61–65, 92–97.

20. Serafini M, Dylla SJ, Oki M, et al.: Hematopoietic reconstitution by multipotent adult progenitor cells: precursors to long-term hematopoietic stem cells. *J Exp Med* 2007, 204:129–139.

21. Goodell MA, Rosenzweig M, Kim H, et al.: Dye efflux studies suggest that hematopoietic stem cells expressing low or undetectable levels of CD34 antigen exist in multiple species. *Nat Med* 1997, 3:1337–1345.

22. Bitan M, Shapira MY, Resnick IB, et al.: Successful transplantation of haploidentical mismatched peripheral blood stem cells using CD133+-purified stem cells. *Exp Hematol* 2005, 33:713–718.

23. Storms RW, Green PD, Safford KM, et al.: Distinct hematopoietic progenitor compartments are delineated by the expression of aldehyde dehydrogenase and CD34. *Blood* 2005, 106:95–102.

24. Robinson SN, Seina SM, Gohr JC, et al.: Evidence for a qualitative hierarchy within the Hoechst-33342 'side population' (SP) of murine bone marrow cells. *Bone Marrow Transplant* 2005, 35:807–818.

25. Uchida N, Fujisaki T, Eaves AC, et al.: Transplantable hematopoietic stem cells in human fetal liver have a CD34(+) side population (SP) phenotype. *J Clin Invest* 2001, 108:1071–1077.

26. Abe S, Lauby G, Boyer C, et al.: Transplanted BM and BM side population cells contribute progeny to the lung and liver in irradiated mice. *Cytotherapy* 2003, 5:523–533.

27. Hogan CJ, Shpall EJ, McNiece I, et al.: Multilineage engraftment in NOD/LtSz-scid/scid mice from mobilized human CD34+ peripheral blood progenitor cells. *Biol Blood Marrow Transplant* 1997, 3:236–246.

28. Ueda T, Yoshida M, Yoshino H, et al.: Hematopoietic capability of CD34+ cord blood cells: a comparison with CD34+ adult bone marrow cells. *Int J Hematol* 2001, 73:457–462.

29. Lang P, Schumm M, Greil J, et al.: A comparison between three graft manipulation methods for haploidentical stem cell transplantation in pediatric patients: preliminary results of a pilot study. *Klin Padiatr* 2005, 217:334–338.

30. Hess DA, Wirthlin L, Craft TP, et al.: Selection based on CD133 and high aldehyde dehydrogenase activity isolates long-term reconstituting human hematopoietic stem cells. *Blood* 2006, 107:2162–2169.

31. Gorantla S, Sneller H, Walter L, et al.: Human immunodeficiency virus type 1 pathobiology studied in humanized balb/c-rag2-/-{gamma}c-/- mice. *J Virol* 2007, 81:2700–2712.

32. Petriz J: Flow cytometry of the side population (SP). In *Current Protocols in Cytometry.* New York: John Wiley & Sons; 2007:S(39), unit 12.8.

33. Witt CM, Robey EA: Thymopoiesis in 4 dimensions. *Semin Immunol* 2005, 17:95–102.

34. Pelayo R, Miyazaki K, Huang J, et al.: Cell cycle quiescence of early lymphoid progenitors in adult bone marrow. *Stem Cells* 2006, 24:2703–2713.

35. Moretta L, Ferlazzo G, Bottino C, et al.: Effector and regulatory events during natural killer-dendritic cell interactions. *Immunol Rev* 2006, 214:219–228.

36. Bailey AS, Willenbring H, Jiang S, et al.: Myeloid lineage progenitors give rise to vascular endothelium. *Proc Natl Acad Sci U S A* 2006, 103:13156–13161.

37. Munugalavadla V, Kapur R: Role of c-Kit and erythropoietin receptor in erythropoiesis. *Crit Rev Oncol Hematol* 2005, 54:63–75.

38. Deutsch VR, Tomer A: Megakaryocyte development and platelet production. *Br J Haematol* 2006, 134:453–466.

39. Lensch MW, Daley GQ: Origins of mammalian hematopoiesis: in vivo paradigms and in vitro models. *Curr Top Dev Biol* 2004, 60:127–196.

40. Cheshier SH, Morrison SJ, Liao X, et al.: In vivo proliferation and cell cycle kinetics of long-term self-renewing hematopoietic stem cells. *Proc Natl Acad Sci U S A* 1999, 96:3120–3125.

41. Abkowitz JL, Linenberger ML, Persik M, et al.: Behavior of feline hematopoietic stem cells years after busulfan exposure. *Blood* 1993, 82:2096–2103.

42. Kessinger A: Collection of autologous peripheral blood stem cells in steady state. *Baillieres Best Pract Res Clin Haematol* 1999, 12:19–26.

43. Kessinger A, Sharp JG: Circulating hematopoietic stem cell transplantation. In *Handbook of Stem Cells, vol 2, Adult and Fetal Stem Cells.* Boston: Elsevier Academic Press; 2004:685–694.

44. Wang L, Cerdan C, Menendez P, et al.: Derivation and characterization of hematopoietic cells from human embryonic stem cells. *Methods Mol Biol* 2006, 331:179–200.

45. Pearson S: Embryonic stem cells: not just from humans. *Genetic Engineering & Biotechnology News* February 15, 2007:1.

46. Balducci L: Anemia, cancer and aging. *Cancer Control* 2003, 10:478–486.

47. Guralnik J, Ershler W, Schrier S, et al.: Anemia in the elderly: a public health crisis in hematology. *Hematology Am Soc Educ Program* 2005, 528–532.

48. Liang Y, Van Zant G, Szilvassy SJ: Effects of aging on the homing and engraftment of murine hematopoietic stem and progenitor cells. *Blood* 2005, 106:1479–1487.

49. Rossi DF, Bryder D, Zahn JM, et al.: Cell intrinsic alterations underlie hematopoietic stem cell aging. *Proc Natl Acad Sci U S A* 2005, 102:9194–9199.

50. Rothstein G: Disordered hematopoiesis and myelodysplasia in the elderly. *J Am Geriatr Soc* 2003, 51(3 Suppl):S22–S26.

51. Vescio R, Schiller G, Stewart AK, et al.: Multicenter phase III trial to evaluate CD34(+) selected versus unselected autologous peripheral blood progenitor cell transplantation in multiple myeloma. *Blood* 1999, 93:1858–1868.

52. Gazitt Y, Reading CC, Hoffman R, et al.: Purified CD34⁺ Lin⁻ Thy⁺ stem cells do not contain clonal myeloma cells. *Blood* 1995, 86:381–389.

53. Vose JM, Bierman PJ, Lynch JC, et al.: Transplantation of highly purified CD34⁺ Thy⁻1⁺ hematopoietic stem cells in patients with recurrent indolent non-Hodgkin's lymphoma. *Biol Blood Marrow* 2001, 7:680–687.

54. Stewart AK, Vescio R, Schiller G, et al.: Purging of autologous peripheral-blood stem cells using CD34 selection does not improve overall or progression-free survival after high-dose chemotherapy for multiple myeloma: results of a multicenter randomized controlled trial. *J Clin Oncol* 2001, 19:3771–3779.

55. Diehn M, Clarke MF: Cancer stem cells and radiotherapy: new insights into tumor radioresistance. *J Natl Cancer Inst* 2006, 98:1755–1757.

56. Barrett J: Improving outcome of allogeneic stem cell transplantation by immunomodulation of the early post-transplant environment. *Curr Opin Immunol* 2006, 18:592–598.

57. Wollert KC, Meyer GP, Lotz J, et al.: Intracoronary autologous bone-marrow cell transfer after myocardial infarction: the BOOST randomized controlled clinical trial. *Lancet* 2004, 364:141–148.

58. Rosenzweig A: Cardiac cell therapy—mixed results from mixed cells. *N Engl J Med* 2006, 355:1274–1277.

59. Engelmann MG, Theiss HD, Henniing-Theiss C, et al.: Autologous bone marrow stem cell mobilization induced by granulocyte colony-stimulating factor after subacute ST-segment elevation myocardial infarction undergoing late revascularization: final results from the G-CSF-STEMI (granulocyte colony-stimulating factor ST-segment elevation myocardial infarction) trial. *J Am Coll Cardiol* 2006, 48:1712–1721.

60. Koide Y, Morikawa S, Mabuchi Y, et al.: Two distinct stem cell lineages in murine bone marrow. *Stem Cells* 2007, 25:1213–1221.

61. Wilson A, Trumpp A: Bone-marrow haematopoietic-stem-cell-niches. *Nat Rev Immunol* 2006, 6:93–106.

62. Dominici M, Le Blanc K, Mueller I, et al.: Minimal criteria for defining multipotent mesenchymal stromal cells. The International Society for Cellular Therapy position statement. *Cytotherapy* 2006, 8:315–317.

63. Ikpeazu C, Davidson MK, Halteman D, et al.: Donor origin of circulating endothelial progenitors after allogeneic bone marrow transplantation. *Biol Blood Marrow Transplant* 2000, 6:301–308.

64. Massa M, Rosti V, Ferrario M, et al.: Increased circulating hematopoietic and endothelial progenitor cells in the early phase of acute myocardial infarction. *Blood* 2005, 105:199–206.

65. Kunz GA, Liang G, Cuculi F, et al.: Circulating endothelial progenitor cells predict coronary artery disease severity. *Am Heart J* 2006, 152:190–195.

66. Michaud SE, Dussault S, Haddad P, et al.: Circulating endothelial progenitor cells from healthy smokers exhibit impaired functional activities. *Atherosclerosis* 2006, 187:423–432.

67. Kondo T, Hayashi M, Takeshita K, et al.: Smoking cessation rapidly increases circulating progenitor cells in peripheral blood in chronic smokers. *Arterioscler Thromb Vasc Biol* 2004, 24:1442–1447.

68. Kucia M, Reca R, Jala VR, et al.: Bone marrow as a home of heterogeneous populations of nonhematopoietic stem cells. *Leukemia* 2005, 19:1118–1127.

69. Gomperts BN, Belperio JA, Burdick MD, et al.: Mobilization of circulating progenitor epithelial cells with keratinocyte growth factor aids in airway repair [abstract]. *Blood* 2006, 108:281.

70. Abe S, Boyer C, Liu X, et al.: Cells derived from the circulation contribute to the repair of lung injury. *Am J Respir Crit Care Med* 2004, 170:1158–1163.

71. McAnulty RJ: Fibroblasts and myofibroblasts: their source, function and role in disease. *Int J Biochem Cell Biol* 2007, 39:666–671.

72. Espinosa-Heidmann DG, Reinoso MA, Pina Y, et al.: Quantitative enumeration of vascular smooth muscle cells and endothelial cells derived from bone marrow precursors in experimental choroidal neovascularization. *Exp Eye Res* 2005, 80:369–378.

73. Odelberg SJ: Cellular plasticity in vertebrate regeneration. *Anat Rec B New Anat* 2005, 287:25–35.

74. Schmidt CM, Doran GA, Crouse DA, et al.: Stem and stromal cell reconstitution of lethally irradiated mice following transplantation of hematopoietic tissue from donors of various ages. *Radiat Res* 1987, 112:74–85.

75. Sharp JG, Murphy BO, Gohr JC, *et al.*: Promises and pitfalls of stem cell therapy for promotion of bone healing. *Clin Orthop Relat Res* 2005, 435:52–61.

76. Huang Y, Kaigler D, Rice K, *et al.*: Combined angiogenic and osteogenic factor delivery enhances bone marrow stromal cell-driven bone regeneration. *J Bone Miner Res* 2005, 20:848–857.

77. Wilan KH, Scott CT, Herrera S: Chasing a cellular fountain of youth. *Nat Biotechnol* 2005, 23:807–815.

78. Preti RA: Bringing safe and effective cell therapies to the bedside. *Nat Biotechnol* 2005, 23:801–804.

79. Aggarwal S, Pittenger MF: Human mesenchymal stem cells modulate allogeneic immune cells responses. *Blood* 2005, 105:1815–1822.

80. Le Blanc K, Ringden O: Mesenchymal stem cells: properties and role in clinical bone marrow transplantation. *Curr Opin Immunol* 2006, 18:586–591.

81. Pellmar TC, Rockwell S, Radiological/Nuclear Threat Countermeasures Working Group: Priority list of research areas for radiological nuclear threat countermeasures. *Radiat Res* 2005, 163:115–123.

82. Kiyoi H, Naoe T: FLT3 mutations in acute myeloid leukemia. *Methods Mol Med* 2006, 125:189–197.

83. Germeshausen M, Ballmaier M, Welte K: Incidence of CSF3R mutations in severe congenital neutropenia and relevance for leukemogenesis: results of a long-term survey. *Blood* 2007, 109:93–99.

84. Chute JP: Stem cell homing. *Curr Opin Hematol* 2006, 13:399–406.

85. Peled A, Petit I, Kollet O, *et al.*: Dependence of human stem cell engraftment and repopulation of NOD/SCID mice on CXCR4. *Science* 1999, 283:845–848.

86. Lapidot T, Kollet O: The essential roles of the chemokine SDF-1 and its receptor CXCR4 in human stem cell homing and repopulation of transplanted immune-deficient NOD/SCID/B2m(null) mice. *Leukemia* 2002, 16:1992–2003.

87. Broxmeyer HE, Hangoc G, Cooper S, *et al.*: Interference of the SDF-1/CXCR4 axis in mice with AMD3100 induces rapid high level mobilization of hematopoietic progenitor cells and AMD3100 acts synergistically with G-CSF and MIP-1 alpha to mobilize progenitors. *Blood* 2001, 96:3371a.

88. Podar K, Anderson KC: The pathophysiologic role of VEGF in hematologic malignancies: therapeutic implications. *Blood* 2005, 105:1383–1395.

89. Larsen L, Ropke C: Suppressors of cytokine signaling: SOCS. *APMIS* 2002, 110:833–844.

90. Arora M, Burns LJ, Barker JN, *et al.*: Randomized comparison of granulocyte colony-stimulating factor versus granulocyte-macrophage colony-stimulating factor plus intensive chemotherapy for peripheral blood stem cell mobilization and autologous transplantation in multiple myeloma. *Biol Blood Marrow* 2004, 10:395–404.

91. Sharp JG, Kessinger A, Lynch JC, *et al.*: Blood stem cell transplantation: factors influencing cellular immunological reconstitution. *J Hematother Stem Cell Res* 2000, 9:971–981.

92. Hohaus S, Martin H, Wassmann B, *et al.*: Recombinant human granulocyte and granulocyte-macrophage colony-stimulating factor (G-CSF and GM-CSF) administered following cytotoxic chemotherapy have a similar ability to mobilize peripheral blood stem cells. *Bone Marrow Transplant* 1998, 22:625–630.

93. Kusadasi N, Koevoet JL, van Soest PL, *et al.*: Stromal support augments extended long-term ex vivo expansion of hemopoietic progenitor cells. *Leukemia* 2001, 15:1347–1358.

94. Friel J, Schiedlmeier B, Geldmacher M, *et al.*: Stromal cells selectively reduce the growth advantage of human committed CD34+ hematopoietic cells ectopically expressing HOXB4. *Growth Factors* 2006, 24:97–105.

95. Willert K, Brown JD, Danenberg E, *et al.*: Wnt proteins are lipid-modified and can act as stem cell growth factors. *Nature* 2003, 423:448–452.

96. Akala OO, Clark MF: Hematopoietic stem cell self-renewal. *Curr Opin Genet Dev* 2006, 16:496–501.

ACKNOWLEDGMENTS

We thank Kaity Fucinaro and Susan Brusnahan for excellent assistance in typing this chapter and Sydney Clausen for preparation of the figures. The author's research that provided some of the background for this chapter was supported by the National Institute of Aging, the National Heart, Lung and Blood Institute of the National Institutes of Health, State of Nebraska LB506, and Nebraska Research Initiative Funds. This support is gratefully acknowledged. We thank our colleagues Marcel Devetten, MD, Ann Kessinger, MD, and David Crouse, PhD, for their helpful comments and advice.

INDEX

A

Acanthocytes, 179
Acrocyanosis, 171
Acute biphenotypic leukemia, 100
Acute erythroid leukemia, 99
Acute lymphoblastic leukemia, 86
Acute megakaryoblastic leukemia, 99
Acute myeloid leukemia
  age and incidence of, 86
  chemical exposure and, 85, 87
  classification of, 88
  diagnosis of, 85
  histology of, 90–91, 93, 95, 97–98
  overview of, 85
  poor risk factors in, 103
  progression from myelodysplastic
    syndrome to, 114, 116
  signs and symptoms of, 86
  subtypes of, 94–100
  treatment of, 101–108
Acute myelomonocytic leukemia, 98
Acute panmyelosis with myelofibrosis, 100
Acute promyelocytic leukemia, 94, 108
Adult T-cell leukemia/lymphoma, 2, 21, 39
Age
  in amyloidosis, 81
  lymphoma and, 25, 41–42
  in myelodysplastic syndrome, 109
  in plasma cell disorders, 63, 67
AIDS-associated lymphoma, 21, 43
Alkylating agents
  myeloid leukemia from, 96
Allogeneic bone marrow transplantation
  in acute myeloid leukemia, 106–107
  in multiple myeloma, 72
Allogeneic stem cell transplantation
  in multiple myeloma, 63, 72
Alloimmune hemolytic anemia, 193
Amyloidosis, 80–82
Anaplastic large B-cell lymphoma, 16
Anaplastic large cell lymphoma, 20, 38
Anemia, 175–200.
See also specific disorders
  alloimmune hemolytic, 193
  autoimmune hemolytic, 192
  of chronic disease, 185
  congenital dyserythropoietic, 188
  iron deficiency, 180–182
  macrocytic, 195–200
  microangiopathic hemolytic, 194
  microcytic, 176, 180–185
  in multiple myeloma, 68–69
  in myelodysplastic syndrome, 110–113
  normocytic, 176, 185–194
  overview of, 175
  pernicious, 199
  practical classification of, 176
Ann Arbor staging system
  Cotswolds modification of, 58
Anticoagulants
  bleeding induced by, 160
  natural, 147

Antiplatelet therapy
  targets of, 145
Atheroemboli, 171
Autoimmune hemolytic anemia, 192
Autologous bone marrow transplantation
  in acute myeloid leukemia, 106–107
Autologous stem cell transplantation
  in amyloidosis, 82
  in lymphoma, 31, 37, 47
  in multiple myeloma, 63, 70–71

B

Basophilia, 99
Basophilic stippling, 180
B-cell lymphoma, 7–17
  anaplastic large, 16
  classification of, 4
  diffuse large, 16–17, 46
  lymphoblastic, 17
  T-cell rich, 16
BCR/ABL gene
  in chronic myelogenous leukemia, 120
Bernard-Soulier syndrome, 157
Bisphosphonates
  in multiple myeloma, 74–75
Bite cells, 179
Blasts
  in leukemia, 90–91, 93, 95, 97–99
Bleeding disorders, 148–160.
See also specific disorders
Bone
  lymphoma of, 47
  in multiple myeloma, 68–69, 74–75
  plasmacytoma of, 78
Bone marrow failure
  anemia in, 188
Bone marrow involvement
  in amyloidosis, 80
  in lymphoma, 10, 22
Bone marrow transplantation
  in acute myeloid leukemia, 104, 106–107
  in chronic myelogenous leukemia,
    123–124
  endothelial cells after, 211
Buerger disease, 172
Burkitt lymphoma, 17, 40
Burkitt-like lymphoma, 16

C

Calciphylaxis, 170
Cancer. See also specific disorders
  anemia in, 187
  hypercoagulability in, 76, 162
Central nervous system involvement
  in lymphoma, 23, 46
Chemotherapy.
See also specific agents and regimens
  in acute myeloid leukemia, 101–106, 108
  in amyloidosis, 81–82
  in chronic myelogenous leukemia, 122
  in lymphoma, 28–50

  in macroglobulinemia, 80
  in multiple myeloma, 70, 72–73
  toxicity and oncogenicity of, 50, 85,
    96, 110
Childhood
  leukemia in, 86, 138
  warfarin-induced skin necrosis in, 167
Chromosomal abnormalities
  in acute myeloid leukemia, 92–94
  in acute promyelocytic leukemia, 94
  in chronic myelogenous leukemia, 119
  in diffuse large B–cell lymphoma, 17
  in marginal zone lymphoma, 14
  in multiple myeloma, 70
Chronic disease
  anemia of, 185
Chronic eosinophilic leukemia, 127
Chronic idiopathic myelofibrosis, 131–132
Chronic lymphocytic leukemia, 7
Chronic myelogenous leukemia, 118–125
  clinical and laboratory features of, 118–121
  cytogenetics of, 119–120
  diagnosis of, 137
  histology of, 121
  treatment of, 122–125
Chronic myeloid leukemia, 85, 137
Chronic myelomonocytic leukemia, 85,
  136–137
Chronic neutrophilic leukemia, 126
Coagulation
  disseminated intravascular, 154
  in normal hemostasis, 141–143, 146–147
Cold agglutinin test, 192
Colony-stimulating factors, 214
Compartment syndrome
  in hemophilia, 159
Congenital disorders
  predisposition to myeloid disorders and, 87
Congenital dyserythropoietic anemia, 188
Coombs' test, 191
Cryoglobulinemia, 170
Cutaneous involvement
  in hemostatic and thrombotic disorders,
    149, 151–154, 156, 158–160, 163–172
  in lymphoma, 18, 36, 46
Cutaneous T-cell lymphoma, 18, 46
Cytokines, 214–220
  clinical applications of, 218–220
  diseases in abnormalities of, 214
  hematopoiesis and, 216–217
  in malignant plasma cells, 74

D

Dacryocytes, 179
Dasatinib, 122, 124
Deep venous thrombosis, 76, 163–165
Diffuse large B-cell lymphoma, 16–17, 46
Dimorphic red blood cells, 178
Disseminated intravascular coagulation, 154
Drug-induced thrombocytopenia, 151–153
Durie-Salmon staging criteria
  in multiple myeloma, 69

E

Ecchymosis, 149, 151
Embolism
  pulmonary, 165–166
Endocarditis
  melanoma-induced emboli in, 166
Endothelial cells
  after bone marrow transplantation, 211
Epstein-Barr virus
  lymphoma associated with, 21, 43
Essential thrombocythemia, 133–134
Extramedullary myeloid tumor, 109

F

FAB subtypes
  in acute myeloid leukemia, 92
Factor V Leiden, 162
Fibrinolysis
  physiologic, 147
Fibronecrosis
  in mediastinal lymphoma, 47
Folate
  deficiency of, 198–199
  digestion and absorption of, 197
Follicular lymphoma, 8–11
  cytogenetics of, 10
  grades of, 9
  histologic progression in, 11
  treatment of, 29–32
Follicular Lymphoma International
  Prognostic Index, 26
French-American-British classification
  of myelodysplastic syndromes, 111

G

Gangrene
  in heparin-induced thrombocytopenia, 153
Gastrointestinal involvement
  in lymphoma, 12, 23, 45
Gemtuzumab
  in acute myeloid leukemia, 105
Granulomatosis
  lymphomatoid, 16

H

Hemarthrosis
  in hemophilia, 158
Hematopoietic stem cells, 201–220
  aging and, 208
  characteristics of, 204, 206
  diseases in abnormal function of, 206
  generation of, 204
  overview of, 201–203
  potential clinical uses for, 207, 209
  progenitor cells and, 205
  self-renewal and differentiation of, 203
  sources of, 207
  in transplantation, 208.
    See also Stem cell transplantation
Hemolytic anemia
  alloimmune, 193
  autoimmune, 192
  diagnosis of, 189–190
  microangiopathic, 194

  spherocytic, 191
Hemophilia, 157–158
  acquired, 159
  other bleeding disorders versus, 160
Hemorrhage
  in hemophilia, 158
Hemostasis
  disorders of, 148–160.
    See also specific disorders
  normal, 141–147
Henoch-Schönlein purpura, 169
Heparin-induced thrombocytopenia,
  152–153
Hereditary hemorrhagic telangiectasia, 168
Hereditary spherocytosis, 70, 72–73,
  82, 191
Hodgkin lymphoma, 53–61
  classification of, 5, 53
  diagnosis and staging of, 58
  pathologic features of, 53–57
  prognostic factors in, 59
  treatment and follow-up of, 60–61
Howell-Jolly bodies, 180
Human immunodeficiency virus
  lymphoma associated with, 21, 43
Human T-cell leukemia and lymphoma
  virus-1, 2, 21
Hypercalcemia
  in multiple myeloma, 68–69
Hypercoagulable states, 161
  cancer-associated, 76, 162
  deep venous thrombosis as, 163–165
Hypereosinophilic syndrome, 127–128
Hypocellular myelodysplastic syndrome, 114

I

Imatinib
  in chronic myelogenous leukemia,
  122, 124–125
Immune-mediated thrombocytopenia, 151
Immunodeficiency
  lymphoproliferative disorders
  associated with, 5, 21–22, 43
Immunoglobulin D myeloma, 77
Immunophenotyping
  of acute myeloid leukemia, 92
  of lymphoma, 8, 10
Infections
  in lymphoma pathogenesis, 2, 21
  purpura in, 170
Interferon
  in chronic myelogenous leukemia, 125
  in cutaneous lymphoma, 36
Interleukins
  overview of, 215–216
International Prognostic Index
  in lymphoma, 26
International Staging System
  in multiple myeloma, 69
Intravascular lymphoma, 16
Iron deficiency anemia, 180–182

J

Jaw osteonecrosis
  in multiple myeloma, 75

Juvenile myelomonocytic leukemia, 85, 138

K

Klippel-Trenaunay-Weber syndrome, 172

L

Leukemia
  acute biphenotypic, 100
  acute erythroid, 99
  acute lymphoblastic, 86
  acute megakaryoblastic, 99
  acute myeloid, 86–109.
    See also Acute myeloid leukemia
  acute myelomonocytic, 98
  acute promyelocytic, 94, 108
  adult T-cell, 2, 21
  chronic eosinophilic, 127
  chronic lymphocytic, 7
  chronic myelogenous, 118–125
  chronic myeloid, 85, 137
  chronic myelomonocytic, 85, 136–137
  chronic neutrophilic, 126
  classification of lymphoproliferative, 4–5
  juvenile myelomonocytic, 85, 138
  plasma cell, 63, 65, 77
Leukemia cutis, 171
Lipedema, 172
Lung cancer
  digital ischemia in, 166
Lymphedema, 172
Lymphocyte-predominant Hodgkin
  lymphoma, 53, 56–57
Lymphoma
  adult T-cell, 2, 21
  anaplastic large cell, 20, 38
  anemia in, 187
  B-cell, 7–17.
    See also B-cell lymphoma
  Burkitt, 17, 40
  Burkitt-like, 16
  classification of, 4–6
  diffuse large B-cell, 16–17
  follicular, 8–11, 29–32
  histologic transformation in, 6
  Hodgkin, 53–61.
    See also Hodgkin lymphoma
  immunodeficiency-associated, 21–22, 43
  intravascular, 16
  MALT, 14–15, 23, 33–34
  mantle cell, 11–12, 32–33
  marginal zone, 13–15, 34–35
  natural killer cell, 19
  non-Hodgkin, 1–50.
    See also Non-Hodgkin lymphoma
  plasmablastic, 16
  postrelapse survival in, 48–49
  prognostic factors in, 22–27
    ability to tolerate treatment as, 24
    age and disease site and, 25, 41
    Follicular Lymphoma International
      Prognostic Index in, 26
    International Prognostic Index in, 26
    recently defined, 27
  small lymphocytic, 7–8, 29
  survival by type in, 28

T-cell, 18–21.
See also T-cell lymphoma
treatment of, 28–50
  ability to tolerate, 24
  approach to, 28
  bone, 48
  central nervous system, 46
  cutaneous, 47
  in elderly patients, 41–42
  follow-up after, 50
  gastrointestinal, 45
  in immunodeficiency, 43
  initial response and, 47–49
  palliation in, 49
  in pregnancy, 44
  regimens in, 28–46
Lymphomatoid granulomatosis, 16
Lymphoproliferative syndromes.
See also specific disorders
  classification of, 4–5
  immunodeficiency-associated, 21–22

M

M protein
  in MGUS, 66–68
Macrocytic anemia, 176, 195–200
Macroglobulinemia, 79–80
MALT lymphoma, 14–15, 23, 33–34
Mantle cell lymphoma, 11–12
  gastrointestinal involvement in, 12, 23
  treatment of, 32–33
Marginal zone lymphoma, 13–15, 34–35
Mean corpuscular volume
  in anemia classification, 195
Mesenchymal cells, 213
Microangiopathic hemolytic anemia, 194
Microcytic anemia, 176, 180–185
Monoclonal antibodies.
See also specific agents
  in lymphoma, 32
Monoclonal gammopathy of unknown
  significance, 63–66
Mucosa-associated lymphoid tissue
  lymphoma, 14–15, 23, 33–34
Multiple myeloma, 67–77
  anemia in, 187
  complications of, 74–76
  cytogenetics of, 70
  diagnosis of, 68
  epidemiology of, 67
  laboratory and clinical features of, 67–68
  staging of, 69
  treatment of, 70–74
  variant forms of, 77
Multipotential mesenchymal stromal cells, 211
Mycosis fungoides, 18, 36
Myelodysplastic disorders, 109–117.
See also specific disorders
  classification of, 95, 111–112
  overview of, 85
Myelodysplastic syndrome, 109–110
  anemia in, 186
  histology of, 113–114
  International Prognostic Scoring System
    in, 115–116
  treatment of, 117

Myelodysplastic/myeloproliferative disorders, 85, 136–138
Myelofibrosis
  acute panmyelosis with, 100
  chronic idiopathic, 131–132
Myeloid disorders, 85–138.
See also specific disorders
  acute myeloid leukemia as, 86–109
  classification of, 88, 111–112, 118
  conditions predisposing to, 87
  myelodysplastic, 109–117
  myelodysplastic/myeloproliferative, 136–138
  myeloproliferative, 118–135
  overview of, 85
Myeloid sarcoma, 109
Myeloma. *See* Multiple myeloma
Myeloproliferative disorders, 118–135.
See also specific disorders
  classification of, 118
  clinical features of, 118–119
  overview of, 85
  platelet disorders and splenomegaly in, 155

N

Natural killer cell lymphoma, 19
Necrosis
  warfarin-induced skin, 167
Neuropathy
  in multiple myeloma, 76
Nodular sclerosis Hodgkin lymphoma, 53–55
Non-Hodgkin lymphoma, 1–50.
See also specific disorders
  B-cell, 7–17
  causes of, 1
  classification of, 4–6
  diagnosis of, 1–4
  overview of, 1
  pretreatment workup in, 4
  T-cell, 18–21
Nonsecretory multiple myeloma, 77
Normocytic anemia, 176, 185–194
  diagnosis of, 189–192
  differential diagnosis of, 185

O

Osteonecrosis of jaw
  in multiple myeloma, 75

P

Parasites
  intra-erythrocyte, 180
Perfusion scintigraphy
  in pulmonary embolism, 165
Peripheral neuropathy
  in multiple myeloma, 76
Peripheral T-cell lymphoma, 19, 39
Pernicious anemia, 199
Petechiae, 149, 151
Philadelphia chromosome
  in chronic myelogenous leukemia, 119
Plasma cell disorders, 63–82.
See also specific disorders
  amyloidosis as, 80–82
  classification of, 5, 65
  epidemiology of, 65

leukemia as, 63, 65, 77
  macroglobulinemia as, 79–80
  monoclonal gammopathy of unknown
    significance as, 63–66
  multiple myeloma as, 67–77
  overview of, 63
  plasmacytoma as, 78–79
  POEMS syndrome as, 78
Plasmablastic lymphoma, 16
Plasmacytoma, 78–79
Platelets
  disorders of, 150–157.
    See also specific disorders
    in myeloproliferative syndromes, 155
  normal function of, 141–145
POEMS syndrome, 65, 78
Polychromasia
  in hemolytic anemia, 200
Polycythemia vera, 129–131
Post-thrombotic syndrome, 164
Pregnancy
  lymphoma in, 44
Primary myelodysplastic syndrome, 109–110
Progenitor cells, 205
Psoralen photochemotherapy
  in cutaneous lymphoma, 36
Pulmonary embolism, 165–166
Purpura
  in hemostatic and thrombotic disorders,
    149, 151, 153
  thrombotic thrombocytopenic, 153
  in vascular disorders, 168–171

Q

5q- syndrome, 115

R

Race
  in plasma cell disorders, 63
Radiotherapy
  acute myeloid leukemia from, 85
  in Hodgkin lymphoma, 60–61
  in non-Hodgkin lymphoma, 35–36
Red blood cells
  abnormal, 178–180
  normal, 177
Renal disease
  anemia in, 186
  in multiple myeloma, 68–69
Rituximab, 29–30, 32, 38, 80

S

Sarcoma
  myeloid, 109
Schilling test, 197
Schistocytosis, 194
Senile purpura, 169
Sézary syndrome, 18, 36
Sickle cells, 178
Sideroblasts, 111–113
Small lymphocytic lymphoma, 7–8, 29
Spherocytes, 179
Spherocytic hemolytic anemia, 191
Spherocytosis
  hereditary, 191

Splenomegaly, 34, 155
Stem cell transplantation
  allogeneic, 63, 72
  autologous.
    See Autologous stem cell transplantation
  cell selection in, 208
  in lymphoma, 31, 37, 47
  in multiple myeloma, 63, 70–72
Stem cells
  hematopoietic.
    See Hematopoietic stem cells;
    Stem cell transplantation
  nonhematopoietic, 210, 212–213
Storage pool disease, 157
Systemic amyloidosis, 80–82

T

Target cells, 178
T-cell lymphoma, 18–21
  adult leukemia and, 2, 21, 39
  classification of, 5
  cutaneous, 18, 46
  lymphoblastic, 22, 40
  peripheral, 19, 39
T-cell rich B-cell lymphoma, 16

Telangiectasia, 149, 168
Thalassemia, 183–184
Thalassemia major, 190
Thrombin
  role of, 147
Thromboangiitis obliterans, 172
Thrombocythemia
  essential, 133–134, 155–156
  in polycythemia vera, 155
Thrombocytopenia, 150–151
  schistocytosis and, 194
Thrombocytosis, 135, 155
Thrombosis
  deep venous, 76, 163–165
  disorders of, 161–172.
    See also specific disorders
    clinical features of, 148–149
  in heparin-induced thrombocytopenia, 152
  risk factors for, 161
Thrombotic thrombocytopenic purpura, 153
Topoisomerase II inhibitors
  myeloid leukemia from, 96
Tumor
  extramedullary myeloid, 109
Tyrosine kinase inhibitors
  in chronic myelogenous leukemia, 124

V

Vascular disorders
  purpura in, 168
Vascular endothelium
  normal function of, 141–143, 145
Vascular malformations
  cutaneous, 171
Viral infection
  leukemia/lymphoma associated with, 2, 21
Vitamin B$_{12}$
  absorption and transport of, 196, 198–199
  deficiency of, 198–199
Von Willebrand disease, 159–160

W

Warfarin
  disorders induced by, 153, 1667
World Health Organization classification
  of acute myeloid leukemia, 89
  of myelodysplastic syndromes, 111–112
  of myeloid neoplasms, 88
  of myeloproliferative diseases, 118
  of polycythemia vera, 130

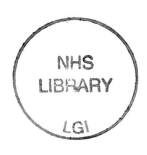